Dakshesh Parikh • Pala B. Rajesh
Editors

Tips and Tricks in Thoracic Surgery

Springer

Editors
Dakshesh Parikh
Department of Pediatric Surgery
Birmingham Women's and
Children's Hospital
NHS Foundation Trust
Birmingham
United Kingdom

Pala B. Rajesh
Regional Department of Thoracic Surgery
Birmingham Heartlands Hospital
Birmingham
United Kingdom

ISBN 978-1-4471-7353-3 ISBN 978-1-4471-7355-7 (eBook)
https://doi.org/10.1007/978-1-4471-7355-7

Library of Congress Control Number: 2017964009

Printed on acid-free paper

This Springer imprint is published by the registered company Springer-Verlag London Ltd. part of Springer Nature.
The registered company address is: The Campus, 4 Crinan Street, London, N1 9XW, United Kingdom

Our respective families for their dedication, love, patience and support throughout our career.

Our patients, colleagues and staff for their support and trust to allow us to perform to our best in the specialty.

Foreword

Every thoracic surgeon needs "Tips and Tricks"! You never have enough of them and any or all may come in handy someday.

The authors have run a very successful course for thoracic surgeons in Birmingham, England, for many years. This textbook in many respects is an extension of that course. That course is predominantly for trainees, but this book is for practitioners of every level. This book will become a resource for the everyday problems and the occasional unusual one. The authors have selected an outstanding group of "expert" contributors from around the world. This international group of surgeons offers unique perspectives on a variety of problems facing thoracic surgeons.

Lung failure is a challenging problem facing physicians and surgeons. There is still an important role for lung volume reduction surgery (LVRS) in carefully selected patients. LVRS is an important stand-alone procedure or as a "bridge" to transplant. Both areas are ably covered by Drs. Wood and Mulligan who have extensive experience with both.

In many parts of the world, lung infections and the management of complications pose major challenges for thoracic surgeons. In some countries, these problems are infrequent, but in other countries quite common. Drawing on the experience of surgeons who regularly deal with empyema, tuberculosis, and hydatid disease will be invaluable to all. This is true of trauma management as well.

Mediastinal tumors are uncommon for most surgeons. However, they do occur on a regular basis. Understanding the principles of management of tumors and associated conditions is valuable.

Esophageal surgery is the most challenging area of commonly practiced thoracic surgery. This book deals with benign and malignant disease. The authors are acclaimed experts. Their chapters deal with technical aspects and important management issues.

I hope the thoracic surgery community looks forward to this important text as much as I do. There is something in it for everyone: trainee or practicing surgeon. ENJOY!

Boston, MA, USA — Douglas J. Mathisen

Preface

A number of textbooks and atlases of adult and Pediatric thoracic surgery have been published. These are either textbooks for reference or descriptive atlases of operative techniques. Information relating to surgical results and outcomes is scattered in the literature. Outcomes and complications in thoracic surgery are dependent on the competence of the surgeon and the team. Surgical practice and operative technique are transferred by competence-based training to the new generation of surgeons. These surgeons require mentoring and support in their initial years of independent practice. This is especially true for those carrying out occasional procedures or as a sub-specialty interest in Pediatrics. The experts have acquired these skills by experience over the years, the knowledge gained is key to the outcome and reduction in the complications associated with the surgery. We believe that this book will be a useful resource to the trainee and the newly appointed thoracic surgeon.

This book includes 37 chapters that are aimed at the higher surgical trainees and serve as a useful adjunct to all newly appointed adult and Pediatric thoracic surgeons. We believe the expert contributors have discussed pathology in their chapters that may be useful to senior consultants undertaking surgery outside their comfort zone. Thoracic surgery is a high-risk specialty and requires attention to detail. Tips and tricks from experienced surgeons will contribute to improving outcomes and reduce complications.

In spite of our objective to allow contributors freedom to share their experience, tips and tricks of their surgical practice, we made every effort to achieve a uniform style. The authors were carefully chosen for their recognized expertise from around the world. The effort involved in making this textbook a reality has been exhausting and exhilarating. We sincerely hope the final result does justice to the original aim.

We would like to express our gratitude for the time and expertise provided by all the contributing authors. We express our sincere thanks to Melissa Morton, Senior Editor, at Springer and her editorial assistants and project managers especially Andre Tournois, Suganya Selvaraj and Georgette who have encouraged and helped us throughout this project.

Birmingham, UK Dakshesh Parikh
Birmingham, UK Pala B. Rajesh

Contents

Part I

Lung

Congenital Lung Malformations

1

Jörg Fuchs

Abstract

Congenital lung lesions are mostly diagnosed by a routine antenatal ultrasound scanning. Many remain asymptomatic immediately after birth but are likely to present later in life with symptoms of pneumonic infection or a persistent lesion in adults can be confused with malignancy. Controversy amongst the surgeons is to resect these asymptomatic lesions electively or to resect only if presented with infection on follow-up. With the advent of thoracoscopic resections and reduced morbidity with minimally invasive resections, elective resection has become more attractive. There is definitely increased morbidity once the lesion becomes infected with need for blood transfusion, wider resection, post-operative air leaks and risk of conversion to open thoracotomy. The subspecialization in Pediatric thoracic surgery may improve overall outcome of this and many other Pediatric thoracic surgical conditions.

Keywords

Antenatal diagnosis · Congenital cystic lung lesions · Congenital pulmonary airway malformations · Congenital cystic adenomatoid malformations · Pulmonary sequestrations · Lung agenesis · Bronchopulmonary foregut cysts · Congenital lobar emphysema · Hydrops fetalis · VATS · Lobectomy · Segmental resection Partial lobectomy

J. Fuchs
Department of Pediatric Surgery and Pediatric Urology, University of Tuebingen, Tuebingen, Germany
e-mail: Joerg.fuchs@med.uni-tuebingen.de

D. Parikh, P.B. Rajesh (eds.), *Tips and Tricks in Thoracic Surgery*,
https://doi.org/10.1007/978-1-4471-7355-7_1

1.1 Introduction

This chapter describes congenital malformations of the lung such as lung agenesis and hypoplasia, congenital pulmonary adenomatoid malformation, lung sequestration, bronchopulmonary cysts and congenital lobar emphysema. All these entities are rare and their incidences difficult to determine. Despite different hypotheses, the aetiology of congenital lung malformations is not yet finally clear. Many of these malformations can be detected antenatally. Clinical symptoms are vary from asymptomatic course to life-threatening conditions [1].

Surgical treatment plays a key role for the successful treatment of all these entities with relatively low mortality and morbidity rates [2–4].

1.2 Lung Agenesis/Aplasia

Lung agenesis is very rare and includes absence of the bronchus, lung parenchyma and pulmonary vessels. There are approximately 200 cases described in the literature. More than 50% of the patients may die within the first years of life. However, some children with unilateral disease survived with a normal expectation of life (Fig. 1.1). Relevant prognostic factors for survival are associated anomalies of the heart, intestinal and urinary tract. Leading symptoms are dyspnoea, thoracic asymmetry and a secondary scoliosis [5]. Clinical symptoms depend on the existence of a uni- or bilateral affection. A respiratory distress syndrome is frequent; survival is minimal in bilateral constellations. Pulmonary hypertension is the leading criterion for the severity of the disease.

Lung hypoplasia implies a reduced number of alveoli and a hypoplasia of the pulmonary artery. Lung hypoplasia is associated with several syndromes or

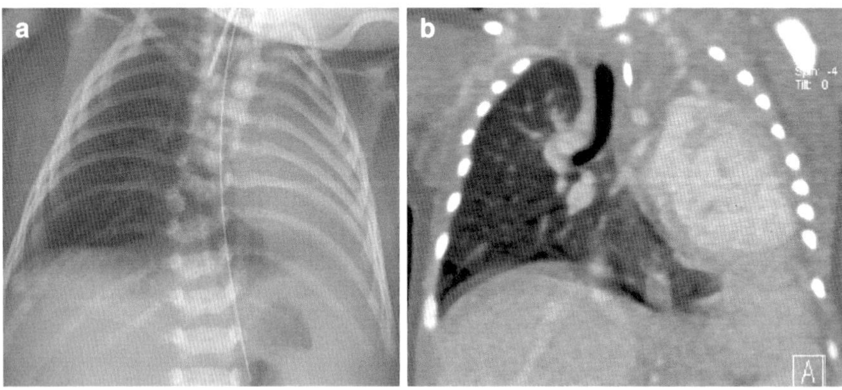

Fig. 1.1 Newborn with congenital unilateral lung agenenis on the left side. X-ray with complete shifting of the mediastinum to the right side (**a**). Corresponding CT scan with complete absence of the left lung (**b**)

associations such as Potter syndrome, bilateral renal dysplasia, congenital diaphragmatic hernia, Scimitar syndrome, trisomy 13/15/18 or a severe scoliosis [6].

The diagnosis is established through chest X-ray, CT scan, echocardiography and bronchoscopy. The initial treatment includes a wide spectrum of measures ranging from supportive care such as a simple oxygen application to ECMO therapy. The further therapeutic approach depends on the underlying disease and has to take the surgical correction of associated congenital malformations into account [7, 8].

1.3 Cystic Lung Lesion

Isolated lung cysts are malformations of the terminal respiratory tract and histologically include cartilage, smooth muscles and glandular structures. They occur as singular or multiple cysts (Fig. 1.2). Incidence rates are notably higher in patients with Down syndrome in combination with congenital heart disease.

Clinical symptoms during the newborn period are varying depending on the size of the lesions and ranging from nearly asymptomatic clinical conditions to a severe respiratory distress syndrome. A pneumothorax with mediastinal shift caused by a cyst rupture can occur as emergency situation in every age group. Later, infections (pneumonia or lung abscess) are the leading symptom.

The treatment depends on the clinical symptoms and the size of the cyst. Spontaneous regression is possible. However, in symptomatic cases, the treatment of choice is the surgical resection. Whenever possible a lung sparing surgery should be performed (enucleation or wedge resection) [9]. Multiple cysts localized in one lobe can be managed by lobectomy. The best surgical approach is VATS. However, conventional thoracotomy should be preferred in cases of severe respiratory compromise or infection because of intolerance of the intrathoracic pressure during thoracoscopy or adhesions after an inflammation with difficulties to identify the anatomical structures [10, 11].

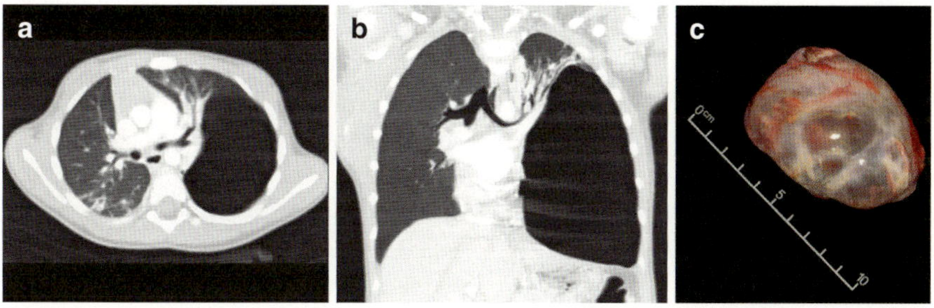

Fig. 1.2 Congenital lung cyst in a 2-year-old girl, diagnosed after a simple respiratory infection. Extension of the isolated cyst on CT scan (**a**, **b**). Completely excised specimen after thoracoscopic resection (**c**)

1.4 Congenital Pulmonary Airway Malformation CPAM

The term "congenital pulmonary airway malformation" (CPAM) has been recently introduced in the nomenclature for the historical description of the former congenital cystic adenomatoid malformation (CCAM). The incidence is approximately 1:25,000–35,000. This malformation accounts for 25% of all congenital lung malformations and is mainly located on the left side (60%). Bilateral involvement is rare and occurs in approximately 6% of all cases. In up to 25%, a hybrid lesion (CCAM + lung sequestration) can be identified. There exist different clinical and histopathological classifications of CPAM (Table 1.1) [2].

Histologically, the CPAM has mainly four different appearances, which include polypoid changes of the mucosa, presence of mucous-secreting cells, absence of cartilage and inflammation.

The routine ultrasound examination in the second pregnancy trimester is reliable. The accuracy of the antenatal diagnostic workup in congenital lung lesions can be improved through MRI. Regarding the clinical risk stratification, prenatal ultrasound is able to distinguish between the macrocystic (single or multiple cysts with a diameter larger than 5 mm, good prognosis) and microcystic (solid mass with cysts smaller than 5 mm, poor prognosis) subtype. Meanwhile the CPAM volume-to-head circumference ratio (CVR) plays an additional key role for the risk stratification. CVR > 1.6 is predictive for a high risk of hydrops with poor prognosis. This parameter represents an indication for a possible prenatal intervention (laser ablation, thoraco-amniotic shunting) including lung resection as an EXIT (ex utero intrapartum therapy) procedure. However, the first step is the maternal steroid administration with a response in up to 90% of all cases. Therefore the maternal steroid administration can significantly improve the foetal survival [2, 3, 12].

Postnatal clinical symptoms include acute respiratory distress syndrome (approximately 60–80% of all cases), later recurrent pulmonary infections in the CPAM area, failure to thrive and reactive airway disease. Previously it has been postulated

Table 1.1 Classification of CPAM [37, 38]

	Anatomical classification (prenatal ultrasound)	Stocker classification (classical)
Size of the cysts	Macrocystic: >5 mm Microcystic: <5 mm	I: >2 cm II: <2 cm III: solid
Associated malformation	Microcystic	II
Prognosis		
• Favourable	Macrocystic	I
• Unfavourable	Microcystic	III
Echogenicity in ultrasound		
• Solid	Microcystic	III
• Cystic	Macrocystic	I, II

that the mesenchymal tissue of CPAM possesses a neoplastic potential. Malignant transformations (bronchoalveolar carcinoma, pulmoblastoma, rhabdomyosarcoma and myxosarcoma) have been described in 2–14% [13–15].

Most authors recommend contrast CT scan or MRI in older children as postnatal imaging for an exact description of the malformation and identification of a hybrid lesion or an atypical blood supply.

Respiratory compromises in neonates are almost always indication for an emergency lobectomy via conventional muscle-sparing thoracotomy or thoracoscopy (Fig. 1.3). In rare cases of multilobular involvement, a pneumonectomy or parenchyma preserving surgery might be indicated. Pneumonectomy performed in young infant is highly morbid condition and may result in mortality.

There exists a controversial debate in the literature regarding the role of surgical treatment in asymptomatic cases. Arguments for observation are the unknown natural history with the chance of spontaneous regression [12]. Reasons for the surgical treatment are the high risk of infection, which may render surgery more difficult, the malignant transformation without typical signs in imaging, the risk of

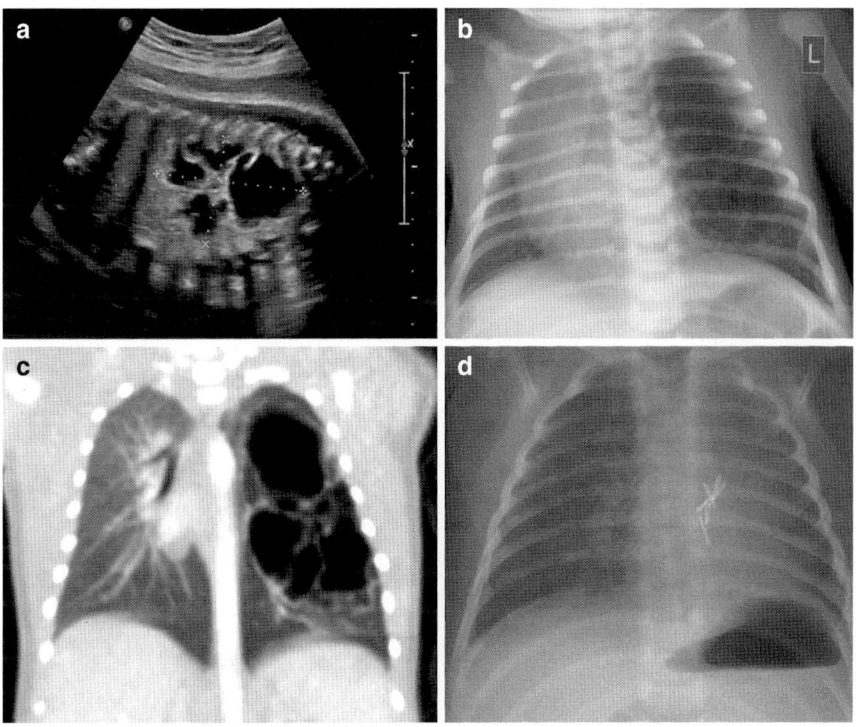

Fig. 1.3 CPAM in a newborn, antenatally diagnosed in the 22nd Gestational week. Ultrasound scan during pregnancy (**a**). Postpartal chest X-ray (**b**). Postpartal CT scan with a mediastinal shift to the right side (**c**). Postoperative chest X-ray after thoracoscopic lower lobe resection on day 8 after birth (**d**)

pneumothorax because of a rupture of the cyst and the fast post-operative recovery in young asymptomatic children [16]. The optimal time point for an elective surgical treatment in asymptomatic children is the third to sixth month of life because of the compensatory lung growth up to 5 years of age [15, 17].

1.5 Congenital Lobar Emphysema

Congenital lobar emphysema (CLE) is characterized by a lobar overexpansion based on a bronchial pathology. In this condition the passage of air takes place into the lobe during inspiration, whereas there is only a limited expulsion of air during expiration (air trapping). There exist several reasons for the bronchial pathology (endobronchial obstruction through inspissated mucus, dysplasia of the cartilages and extrinsic obstruction caused by an aberrant vessel) [18]. The left upper lobe is involved in up to 50% of cases followed by the right middle lobe and right upper lobe. The pathology in the lower lobes is extremely uncommon.

Clinical symptoms vary widely ranging from very mild symptoms with a sporadic diagnosis to acute respiratory distress syndrome including a foetal hydrops.

The prenatal diagnosis is established through the classical ultrasound scan or MRI. In these examinations CLE can be distinguished from other congenital lung malformations. In approximately 25–50% of all cases, postnatal diagnoses are made directly after birth. Here, the diagnostic tools are chest X-ray and CT scan. An echocardiography is necessary to exclude cardiac malformations; a preoperative bronchoscopy is essential for delineation of an intrinsic cause for CLE.

In the constellation of mild clinical symptoms, a conservative treatment can be successful. If the child presents with respiratory distresses, an emergency thoracotomy is indicated [19]. The anaesthesiological management during surgery might be a challenge because of the air trapping with a massive overextension of the affected lobe. A selective intubation can prevent this problem, but this depends on the clinical tolerance of the child. The thoracoscopic resection may be difficult because of the small working space resulting from the rigid overextended lobe; it may be possible only in selected cases (Fig. 1.4).

1.6 Lung Sequestration

Lung sequestration is represented by a microcystic mass of non-functioning pulmonary tissue without communication to the main tracheobronchial tree. Two different forms of lung sequestrations: extrapulmonary and intrapulmonary sequestrations are described. An extrapulmonary lung sequestration is completely separated from the normal lung tissue and incorporated by separate covering visceral pleura. It can appear above, within and below the level of the diaphragm and has a separate arterial blood supply from the aorta (Fig. 1.5). Associated occurrence of other congenital malformations (CDH, congenital heart disease, skeletal abnormalities) is frequent. Extralobar sequestrations predominantly occur in males (3:1) [2]. In some

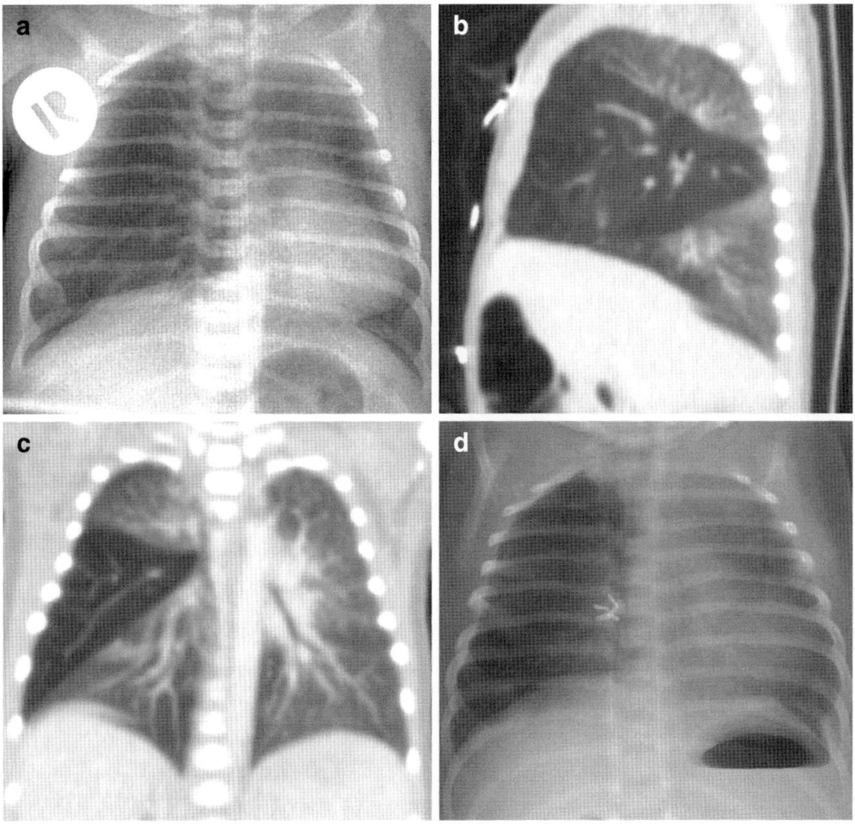

Fig. 1.4 Congenital lobar emphysema in a 4-week-old newborn. Conventional X-ray with an overexpansion of the right lung (**a**). Corresponding CT scan with the pathology in the middle lobe (**b**, **c**). Postoperative X-ray after thoracoscopic middle lobe resection (**d**)

cases the atypical blood supply can lead to a high cardiac output failure. Under these circumstances an emergency treatment might become necessary (surgery or coiling). The venous drainage is systemic or through the portal vein.

In contrast, an intrapulmonary sequestration is usually refined to one single lung lobe (predominance of the left side). Communications with the oesophagus or stomach are possible in 10% of all cases. Bilateral cases and so-called hybrid lesions (combination of CPAM and intrapulmonary lung sequestration) are uncommon.

The venous drainage of the lung sequestration is mainly into the pulmonary vein but can be variable and from the diagnostic point of view a challenging aspect (Fig. 1.5) [20].

Clinical symptoms range from asymptomatic situations over recurrent infections with haemoptysis to emergency situations in cases of high cardiac output failure. In analogy to the CPAM, a foetal hydrops can occur in some cases resulting from the compression of the inferior cava vein compromising the cardiac output.

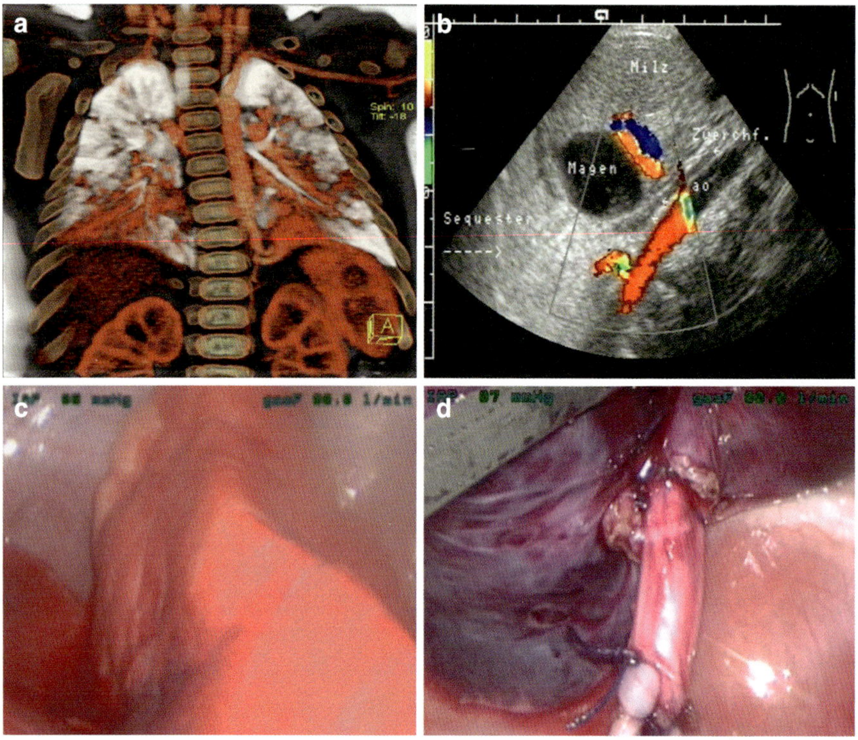

Fig. 1.5 Extrapulmonary lung sequestration in a 6-month-old baby, diagnosed antenatally. CT scan (reconstruction) (**a**) and Doppler ultrasound (**b**) with an atypical arterial blood supply from the abdominal aorta. Intraoperative aspect before (**c**) and after (**d**) ligation of the vessels within the inferior pulmonary ligament

The prenatal diagnosis has an important significance in lung sequestration. The classical appearance on prenatal ultrasound is an echodense and homogeneous structure with an atypical blood supply detected on Doppler ultrasound. However, differentiation from CPAM, hybrid lesions or neuroblastoma can be challenging. Adzick et al. reported that 75% of antenatally diagnosed bronchopulmonary sequestrations can resolve spontaneously [21].

The postnatal diagnostic workup includes chest X-ray, Doppler ultrasound with identification of the blood supply, thoracic CT scan and in selected cases an angiography [22].

Lobectomy is the treatment of choice in intrapulmonary sequestrations, whereas simple resection (enucleation) is preferred in isolated extrapulmonary sequestrations. The thoracoscopic approach should be chosen in all cases of extrapulmonary sequestration. It is a safe and fast surgical procedure, which often makes a chest tube unnecessary. The feeding systemic arterial vessels are mostly located in the inferior pulmonary ligament and arise from the abdominal aorta. Therefore a careful dissection of the ligament is necessary through which a severe bleeding is prevented.

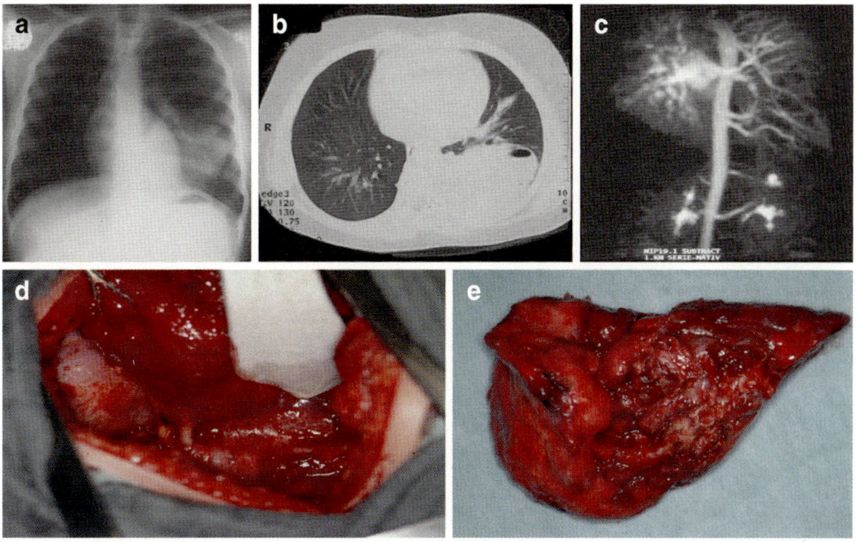

Fig. 1.6 Intrapulmonary lung sequestration within the left lower lobe in a 5-year-old boy. Conventional chest X-ray (**a**). CT scan with compression of the healthy upper lobe (**b**). Vascular reconstruction showing an atypical blood supply with two arteries from the aorta (**c**). Intraoperative view on the two arteries within the inferior pulmonary ligament (**d**). Completely resected lower lobe (**e**)

Lobectomies can be performed as an open or thoracoscopic procedure. They are mainly depending on the expertise of the surgeon. In the literature there is a controversial discussion between promotion of lungs sparing procedures (wedge resection) and lobectomies (Fig. 1.6). Atypical or nonanatomic lung resections often lead to recurrent infections and should be avoided. The optimal time point for surgery is within the first 3–6 months of life [2, 17].

1.7 Bronchogenic Cyst

A bronchogenic cyst develops from an abnormal budding from the tracheobronchial tree. It is usually located along the trachea and bronchial structures. However, so-called ectopic location has been described within the lung parenchyma or in the tongue, the neck or below the diaphragm [23].

Histologically, the wall of the cysts is lined by ciliated columnar epithelium. Some cysts may contain cartilage, and they can have a communication with the tracheobronchial tree.

The clinical spectrum is wide and ranges from asymptomatic children over respiratory symptoms in the newborn period to complications such as infections including lung abscess, atelectasis or haemorrhage.

The diagnosis can be made antenatally using ultrasonography. In older children the pathology is possibly detected as an incidental finding during investigation for

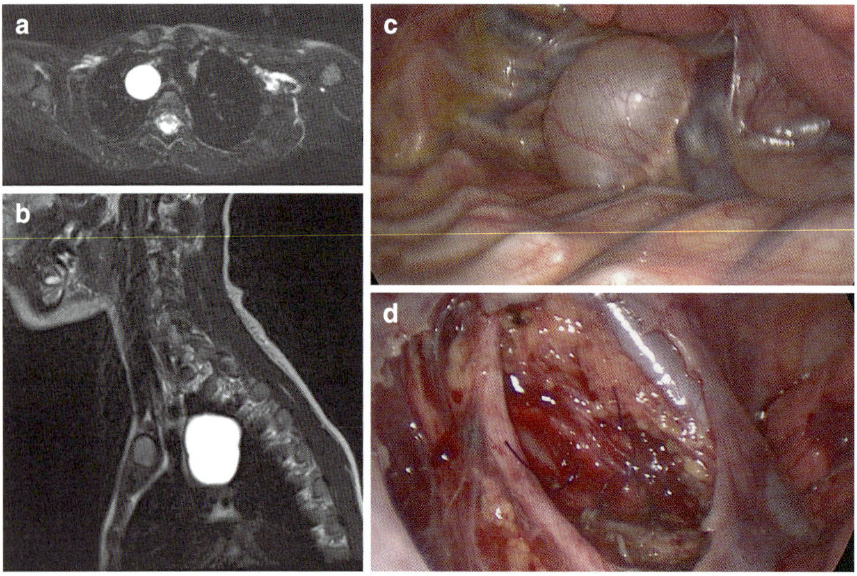

Fig. 1.7 Bronchogenic cyst in a boy with recurrent pulmonary infection. MRI showing a cyst filled with fluid (**a**, **b**). Intraoperative aspect during thoracoscopy before (**c**) and after (**d**) resection. The main bronchus has been sutured because of a connection from the cyst to the bronchial tree

infections or on a chest X-ray. CT scan or MRI can confirm the diagnosis displaying a homogeneous mass with smooth margins.

Complete excision of the cysts is the treatment of choice (Fig. 1.7). Malignant transformations have been described. A lobectomy is necessary in cases of intrapulmonal cysts. The majority of affected patients can be managed using a thoracoscopic approach [2, 24].

1.8 Technical Tips and Tricks for Thoracic Surgery in Congenital Lung Malformation

1.8.1 Thoracoscopic Resection

One of the important aspects for a successful thoracoscopic lung resection is a good selection of the patients. Candidates for MI lung surgery should be in clinically stable conditions without additional major congenital malformations such as heart diseases. Previous pneumonia is a risk factor for conversion to open surgery [25, 26]. In small children MIS for thoracic pathologies is possibly limited because of the distension of the affected lobe or the rigidity of pulmonary structures (e.g. lobar emphysema). This results in a small working space within the chest. Also, mechanical ventilation during surgery can be relevantly hampered because of lung compression and increased intrathoracic pressure. Finally, the intraoperative carbon dioxide uptake might represent an anaesthesiological issue that needs further evaluation [27].

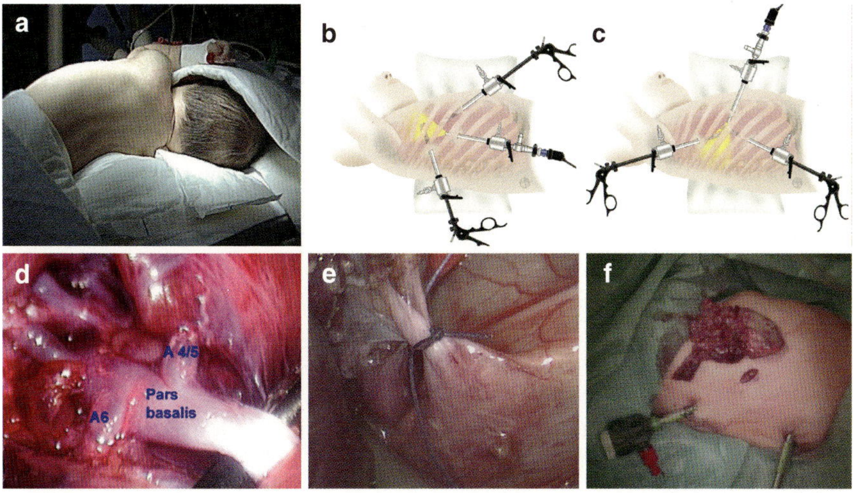

Fig. 1.8 Technical aspects of thoracoscopic lung resection with demonstration of the position of the child (**a**). Trocar positioning for an upper lobe resection (**b**), and for a middle/lower lobe resection (**c**). Exploration of the pulmonary arteries within the fissura (**d**). Dissection and ligation of the pulmonary vein (**e**). Retrieval of a CPAM through a 2 cm trocar incision (**f**)

The procedures should be performed in a lateral decubitus position and if possible using single lung ventilation. Single-lung ventilation leads to a larger working space and can be realized in infants and children below 6 years of age by a main stem intubation or by blocking the ipsilateral bronchus using a Fogarty® catheter. In older children (above 25 kg), the anaesthesiologist can use a commercial double-lumen endotracheal tube [28]. In noninflammatory congenital lung malformations, destruction of the affected lobe with bipolar forceps or LigaSure® can improve the working space. This is nearly necessary in all cases of CPAM or CLE [29, 30].

For the surgical procedures 3 or 4 ports are necessary. Positioning of the trocars depends on the procedure and is different for the lower/middle and upper lobe resections (Fig. 1.8). However, different options for the trocar positions have been suggested. Finally, trocar positions depend on the personal experience of the surgeon and the access to the anatomical structure within the lobar fissure from anterior or posterior. Initially, the chest should be insufflated only with a low pressure in order to induce a collapse of the lung and to allow adaptation of the child. The initial pressure should not exceed 3 mmHg (flow 1.5 L/min) and should then slowly be raised to 5–6 mmHg. Dissection of the anatomical structures should be performed with the monopolar hook. This device gives a comparatively good tactile feedback to the surgeon. It allows an accurate visualization of the border between the different anatomical structures and sufficiently seals the vessels located around the bronchus wall or feeding the lymph nodes. However, other surgeons strictly promote LigaSure® for dissection.

In contrast to the open approach, the chronological order of dissection of anatomical structures is management of the lung arteries, then bronchus and finally pulmonary veins.

For the *upper lobe resections*, a 5 mm camera port should preferably be placed in the mid-axillary line. The two working trocars should be inserted in the posterior and anterior axillary line cranially to the camera port. After identification of the interlobar fissure, the segmental artery A2 has to be clipped or sealed. In the next step, A1 and A3 have to be identified. This can be difficult because of the overlying pulmonary veins V1–3, which must be divided beforehand. The preservation of V4 and V5 is mandatory to protect the venous drainage from the middle lobe or lingula. After this step the main bronchus and the segmental bronchus B1–3 are identified. The transection of the bronchus can be realized in infants with clips or suturing in older children with a meanwhile available 5 mm stapler or 10 mm stapler device. The separation of the lobes is facilitated using the LigaSure® [31].

For the *lower/middle lobe resections*, the camera port should be positioned in the anterior axillary line. The working ports are then located cranially and caudally from the camera trocar in the mid-axillary line. The first step is the dissection of the oblique fissure with identification of the pars basalis including the arteries A6, A4/5 and A2. After clipping or sealing the feeding arteries, identification of the lower bronchus with the branches B6, B4/5 and B7–10 is possible. The bronchus management should be realized in the same fashion as described above. An intraoperative bronchoscopy can be helpful to identify all these structures, especially in cases of anatomical variations. There exist several classical variations in the segmental arteries A4 and A5 [32]. However, the key for a successful thoracoscopic lung resection is the consequent dissection and identification of all anatomical structures, which allows the unambiguous assignment of vessels and bronchi to the specific lobes [33]. The final step is the dissection of the inferior pulmonary ligament with dissection of the lower branches of the pulmonary vein from V4/5. A transthoracic traction suture through the lower lobe allows an excellent exploration of the inferior pulmonary vein, and a safe ligation of this vein is possible (Fig. 1.8).

The removal of the resected lung specimen is usually possible through the extension of a port incision (2–3 cm). Certainly, a destruction of the resected lobe helps retrieving the specimen. This procedure has no negative impact for the histological investigation.

Minimally invasive lung segmentectomies have been described by several authors being applicable for segment 6, lingula segments and upper lobe segments. The thoracoscopic segmentectomy is a challenging procedure with higher complication rates compared to lobectomies [34]. The border between affected segments and healthy lung tissue is identifiable after dissection of the segmental bronchus following the ventilation of the lower lobe [25].

1.9 Muscle-Sparing Thoracotomy

Whenever possible a thoracotomy should be performed as muscle-sparing posterolateral procedure. Historically, the classical posterolateral approach has been the gold standard as access to the thoracic cavity. However, this is one of the most painful surgical incisions. The muscle-sparing thoracotomy (MST) means less acute and chronic pain, a better function of lung and shoulder, faster recovery and superior cosmetic results [35]. MST is realized performing a skin incision of 5–10 cm length in line with the fourth or fifth intercostal space. The latissimus dorsi muscle and the trapezius muscle are exposed, and the triangle fascia is incised along the posterior border of the latissimus; the serratus fascia is incised in the same way. A small retractor is used to spread the ribs, while a second retractor is placed at a right angle to retract the latissimus anteriorly and the paraspinal muscles posteriorly. Generally, the incision through the fifth intercostal space is the optimal approach for an excellent visualization of nearly all congenital anomalies. In cases of intrapulmonary lung sequestration on the left lower lobe, the sixth intercostal space may permit a better overview and handling of the anomalous vessels. Management of the malformation starts with the dissection of lung arteries, followed by ligation of the pulmonary vein. Now the lung lobe is sufficiently mobile and the bronchial tree can easily be managed. Generally, surgeons should carefully close the bronchus without narrowing the neighbouring airways. This can be realized with a separate surgical supply of the subsegment bronchus (e.g. B6 and B7–10 on the lower lobe resection to prevent a stenosis on the remnant B4/5) [36].

References

1. Adzick NS. Management of fetal lung lesions. Clin Perinatol. 2003;30(3):481–92.
2. Azizkhan RG, Crombleholme TM. Congenital cystic lung disease: contemporary antenatal and postnatal management. Pediatr Surg Int. 2008;24(6):643–57.
3. Baird R, Puligandla PS, Laberge JM. Congenital lung malformations: informing best practice. Semin Pediatr Surg. 2014;23(5):270–7.
4. Aspirot A, Puligandla PS, Bouchard S, Su W, Flageole H, Laberge JM. A contemporary evaluation of surgical outcome in neonates and infants undergoing lung resection. J Pediatr Surg. 2008;43(3):508–12.
5. Nazir Z, Qazi SH, Ahmed N, Atiq M, Billoo AG. Pulmonary agenesis—vascular airway compression and gastroesophageal reflux influence outcome. J Pediatr Surg. 2006;41(6):1165–9.
6. Page DV, Stocker JT. Anomalies associated with pulmonary hypoplasia. Am Rev Respir Dis. 1982;125(2):216–21.
7. Backer CL, Kelle AM, Mavroudis C, Rigsby CK, Kaushal S, Holinger LD. Tracheal reconstruction in children with unilateral lung agenesis or severe hypoplasia. Ann Thorac Surg. 2009;88(2):624–30.
8. Berrocal T, Madrid C, Novo S, Gutierrez J, Arjonilla A, Gomez-Leon N. Congenital anomalies of the tracheobronchial tree, lung, and mediastinum: embryology, radiology, and pathology. Radiographics. 2004;24(1):e17.
9. Lal R, Lama TK, Bhatnagar V. Congenital lung cyst. Eur J Pediatr Surg. 1999;9(5):334–6.
10. Mattioli G, Buffa P, Granata C, et al. Lung resection in pediatric patients. Pediatr Surg Int. 1998;13(1):10–3.
11. Rothenberg SS. Thoracoscopic lung resection in children. J Pediatr Surg. 2000;35(2):271–4.
12. Tsao K, Hawgood S, Vu L, et al. Resolution of hydrops fetalis in congenital cystic adenomatoid malformation after prenatal steroid therapy. J Pediatr Surg. 2003;38(3):508–10.
13. Libretti L, Ciriaco P, Casiraghi M, Arrigoni G, Zannini P. Pleuropulmonary blastoma in the area of a diagnosed congenital lung cyst. Ann Thorac Surg. 2008;85(2):658–60.
14. Priest JR, Williams GM, Hill DA, Dehner LP, Jaffe A. Pulmonary cysts in early childhood and the risk of malignancy. Pediatr Pulmonol. 2009;44(1):14–30.

15. Puligandla PS, Laberge JM. Congenital lung lesions. Clin Perinatol. 2012;39(2):331–47.
16. Laberge JM, Puligandla P, Flageole H. Asymptomatic congenital lung malformations. Semin Pediatr Surg. 2005;14(1):16–33.
17. Beres A, Aspirot A, Paris C, et al. A contemporary evaluation of pulmonary function in children undergoing lung resection in infancy. J Pediatr Surg. 2011;46(5):829–32.
18. Azizkhan RG, Grimmer DL, Askin FB, Lacey SR, Merten DF, Wood RE. Acquired lobar emphysema (overinflation): clinical and pathological evaluation of infants requiring lobectomy. J Pediatr Surg. 1992;27(8):1145–51.
19. Cataneo DC, Rodrigues OR, Hasimoto EN, Schmidt AF Jr, Cataneo AJ. Congenital lobar emphysema: 30-year case series in two university hospitals. J Bras Pneumol. 2013;39(4):418–26.
20. Alivizatos P, Cheatle T, de Leval M, Stark J. Pulmonary sequestration complicated by anomalies of pulmonary venous return. J Pediatr Surg. 1985;20(1):76–9.
21. Adzick NS, Harrison MR, Crombleholme TM, Flake AW, Howell LJ. Fetal lung lesions: management and outcome. Am J Obstet Gynecol. 1998;179(4):884–9.
22. Saeed A, Kazmierski M, Khan A, McShane D, Gomez A, Aslam A. Congenital lung lesions: preoperative three-dimensional reconstructed CT scan as the definitive investigation and surgical management. Eur J Pediatr Surg. 2013;23(1):53–6.
23. Vaos G, Zavras N, Antypas G. Bronchogenic cyst of the lung mimicking a pulmonary hydatid cyst in a child. Pediatr Surg Int. 2005;21(5):383–5.
24. Rothenberg SS. Thoracoscopic pulmonary surgery. Semin Pediatr Surg. 2007;16(4):231–7.
25. Rothenberg SS, Shipman K, Kay S, et al. Thoracoscopic segmentectomy for congenital and acquired pulmonary disease: a case for lung-sparing surgery. J Laparoendosc Adv Surg Tech A. 2014;24(1):50–4.
26. Vu LT, Farmer DL, Nobuhara KK, Miniati D, Lee H. Thoracoscopic versus open resection for congenital cystic adenomatoid malformations of the lung. J Pediatr Surg. 2008;43(1):35–9.
27. Bishay M, Giacomello L, Retrosi G, et al. Hypercapnia and acidosis during open and thoracoscopic repair of congenital diaphragmatic hernia and esophageal atresia: results of a pilot randomized controlled trial. Ann Surg. 2013;258(6):895–900.
28. Dingemann C, Zoeller C, Bataineh Z, Osthaus A, Suempelmann R, Ure B. Single- and double-lung ventilation in infants and children undergoing thoracoscopic lung resection. Eur J Pediatr Surg. 2013;23(1):48–52.
29. Rothenberg SS. First decade's experience with thoracoscopic lobectomy in infants and children. J Pediatr Surg. 2008;43(1):40–4.
30. Rothenberg SS, Middlesworth W, Kadennhe-Chiweshe A, et al. Two decades of experience with thoracoscopic lobectomy in infants and children: standardizing techniques for advanced thoracoscopic surgery. J Laparoendosc Adv Surg Tech A. 2015;25(5):423–8.
31. Albanese CT, Sydorak RM, Tsao K, Lee H. Thoracoscopic lobectomy for prenatally diagnosed lung lesions. J Pediatr Surg. 2003;38(4):553–5.
32. Seitz G, Warmann SW, Szavay PO, et al. Thoracoscopic lobectomy as a treatment option for persistent middle lobe syndrome in children. Pediatr Int. 2010;52(2):e79–81.
33. Fuchs J, Kirschner HJ, Warmann SW, Schellinger K, Baden W, Szavay P. Thoracoscopic anatomical lung resection in children. Zentralbl Chir. 2007;132(3):247–50.
34. Johnson SM, Grace N, Edwards MJ, Woo R, Puapong D. Thoracoscopic segmentectomy for treatment of congenital lung malformations. J Pediatr Surg. 2011;46(12):2265–9.
35. Kunisaki SM, Powelson IA, Haydar B, et al. Thoracoscopic vs open lobectomy in infants and young children with congenital lung malformations. J Am Coll Surg. 2014;218(2):261–70.
36. Mattioli G, Asquasciati C, Castagnetti M, Bellodi S, Rossi G, Jasonni V. Muscle-sparing thoracotomy combined with mechanically stapled lung resection for benign lung disorders: functional results and quality of life. Pediatr Surg Int. 2006;22(6):491–5.
37. Adzick NS, Harrison MR, Glick PL, et al. Fetal cystic adenomatoid malformation: prenatal diagnosis and natural history. J Pediatr Surg. 1985;20(5):483–8.
38. Stocker JT, Madewell JE, Drake RM. Congenital cystic adenomatoid malformation of the lung. Classification and morphologic spectrum. Hum Pathol. 1977;8(2):155–71.

Lung Volume Reduction Surgery for Severe Emphysema

2

Douglas E. Wood

Abstract
Lung volume reduction surgery (LVRS) was reincarnated in the early 1990s as a promising therapy to palliate symptoms and improve quality of life in patients disabled by severe emphysema. Controversy regarding the reliability and risks of the surgery as well as long-term durability stifled the initial proliferation of LVRS and led to the historic National Emphysema Treatment Trial (NETT). There are now strong data from large case-controlled series, from several small randomized trials, and from the large randomized multi-institutional NETT that confirm improvement in pulmonary function, exercise capacity, and quality of life in select patients with severe emphysema.

Keywords
Emphysema · Lung reduction · LVRS

2.1 Introduction

Over the last century, a number of surgical interventions have been proposed to improve the symptoms and quality of life in patients with severe emphysema. Costochondrectomy and thoracoplasty were performed in an attempt to alter the configuration of the chest cavity, and phrenic nerve ablation or induced pneumoperitoneum were attempted to restore the curvature of the diaphragm. Numerous efforts were made to treat the airway component of chronic obstructive pulmonary disease—using airway de-enervation procedures or prosthetic devices to support

D.E. Wood, M.D., F.A.C.S., F.R.C.S.Ed.
Department of Surgery, University of Washington, Seattle, WA, USA
e-mail: dewood@u.washington.edu

D. Parikh, P.B. Rajesh (eds.), *Tips and Tricks in Thoracic Surgery*,
https://doi.org/10.1007/978-1-4471-7355-7_2

the membranous trachea. Improvement of pulmonary blood flow was the intent of pleurodesis. Each of these procedures enjoyed a period of popularity, but each were ultimately found to be ill-advised resulting in severe life-threatening complications with negligible clinical benefit [1].

Dr. Otto Brantigan and his colleagues at the University of Maryland approached patients in a different fashion by attempting to reduce the hyperinflation of emphysematous lungs. They hypothesized that surgical removal of lung volume could restore radial traction on terminal bronchioles, improving respiratory airflow obstruction and diaphragmatic excursion. In 1959, Dr. Brantigan reported his experience with 33 patients [2]. Although symptomatic improvement was reported in most patients, the operative mortality was high, and the procedure was never widely adopted.

The modern era of lung volume reduction surgery (LVRS) was first described by Dr. Joel Cooper and his colleagues at Washington University in 1994 [3]. Using a median sternotomy to perform bilateral stapled wedge resections on patients with heterogeneous emphysema and plethysmographic evidence of hyperinflation resulted in an objective improvement in forced expiratory volume in 1 s (FEV_1) of 82% [3]. These exciting results led to a rapid dissemination of LVRS throughout the United States in both academic and community centers. Although early results were encouraging, there were a number of criticisms of the published reports relating to small patient numbers, variable selection criteria, lack of patient randomization, incomplete follow-up, and lack of long-term results. Concern regarding potential excessive morbidity and mortality of LVRS as well as the reliability and durability of clinical benefit led to a moratorium of Medicare coverage for LVRS in December, 1995, ultimately resulting in the large randomized National Emphysema Treatment Trial (NETT), published in 2003.

2.2 The National Emphysema Treatment Trial

Although many physicians felt that the case for LVRS was compelling without a randomized trial, this was balanced by criticism of the adequacy of LVRS evaluation. First of all, it was felt that the majority of reports involved small numbers of patients with vague or variable patient selection criteria. Secondly, since each of these series were case controlled without randomized assessments, it was not possible to confirm that the outcomes were truly attributable to the surgical procedure rather than other aspects of patient selection and medical care of the highly select patient subgroup. Thirdly, all authors reported mean results with most not providing standard deviation data in the objective outcomes. When standard deviation was provided, they were often greater than the mean improvement, representing patients with negative outcomes or minimal improvement. Careful review of these data revealed that 20–50% of patients actually had negligible objective improvement in FEV_1 in the initial series [4, 5]. Fourthly, most series were weakened by incomplete follow-up allowing follow-up selection bias to cloud the interpretation of the results. Short-term follow-up possibly obscured the potential long-term deleterious effects of LVRS with some authors showing an accelerated annual decline in FEV_1 in patients who had LVRS [5]. Incomplete follow-up certainly could have failed to include patients with poor outcomes who either suffered late mortality or refused to return the follow-up assessments. Finally, it was clear that there may also be an unintentional but systematic selection bias in the reporting of data. Although major academics centers reported positive outcomes and low operative morbidity and mortality, unreported outcomes were largely unknown.

As preliminary experience with LVRS accumulated, the NIH convened a conference to evaluate LVRS and concluded that there was "…a need for systemic study of LVRS selection criteria and long-term efficacy" [6]. The Agency for Health Care Policy and Research (AHCPR) also concluded that there was inadequate scientific data regarding efficacy and risk of LVRS and that "…a prospective trial of LVRS…. is both ethically supportable and scientifically essential" [7].

It was in this setting that the Health Care Finance Administration (HCFA), now known as the Center for Medicare and Medicaid Services (CMS), discontinued reimbursement for LVRS procedures. Because of an immediate and vociferous outcry from patients and their physicians, Medicare bowed to public and legislative pressure and agreed to fund the historic National Emphysema Treatment Trial (NETT) as a pioneering collaboration between the National Institutes of Health (NIH) and Medicare (CMS) in evaluating a new surgical procedure. The NETT developed as a multi-institutional prospective randomized clinical trial comparing medical therapy to LVRS in patients with severe emphysema. Seventeen clinical centers throughout the United States were involved in the trial, and the trial design has been well described and previously published [8]. Two unique aspects of the NETT deserve special mention. First of all, the collaboration between CMS and NIH was unique, with the cost of patient care within the trial reimbursed by Medicare, while the NIH supported the cost of the associated research questions. Secondly, this was the first time that a new surgical procedure was subjected to a rigorous multi-institutional trial so early in its development. Until LVRS, new procedures and interventions had primarily been evaluated by an evolutionary process of procedure refinement, observational studies, and occasional randomized controlled trials. Randomized trials had generally been performed late within the process of procedure development, well after the majority of indications and outcomes were believed to be well-known.

The Medicare decision to withhold reimbursement for LVRS outside of the NETT was highly controversial, with some believing that this decision moved uncomfortably close to policy makers determining appropriate medical therapy. Others suggested that Medicare policy was driven by an effort to control medical expenditures at the expense of a promising new therapy for emphysema patients. Editorials in medical and surgical journals were equally dogmatic in their support for or their disparagement of the NETT [9–11].

The primary outcome measures in the NETT were survival and maximum exercise capacity 2 years after randomization. Secondary outcome measures were quality of life, disease-specific symptoms, cost-effectiveness, pulmonary function, gas exchange, oxygen utilization, radiologic assessment, and psychomotor function.

Eligible patients were those with radiographic evidence of emphysema, severe airflow obstruction and hyperinflation, and those who could participate in pulmonary rehabilitation with the attainment of preset performance goals.

During the National Emphysema Treatment Trial, the Data Safety Monitoring Board (DSMB) carefully evaluated early outcomes, to detect both possible patient subgroups with marked benefit from LVRS who should no longer be subjected to randomization and patients who had excessive risks of LVRS and should no longer be included as candidates within the trial. In April, 2001, analysis by the DSMB identified a subgroup of patients with an increased risk of mortality after LVRS. These analyses suggested that a low FEV_1 (<20% predicted) combined with either a homogenous pattern of emphysema or a DLCO <20% predicted were associated with a 30-day mortality after surgery of 16%. Likewise, these patients were found to have only a small improvement in maximum exercise capacity at 6-month follow-up with a negligible improvement of functional outcomes for the surgical patients [12].

The NETT protocol was immediately changed to prevent further enrollment of patients identified as high risk for LVRS. This was quickly followed by a publication of the NETT high-risk results in the New England Journal of Medicine [12]. Unfortunately, these results were largely misinterpreted by the medical community and the lay press. Even leaders in national medical societies suggested that this denoted a poor outcome for LVRS overall rather than the appropriate identification of a small subset of patients with increased mortality risk with a negligible functional benefit.

In May 2003, the primary outcomes of the 5-year National Emphysema Treatment Trial were presented at the American Thoracic Society Annual Meeting in Seattle and simultaneously published in the New England Journal of Medicine [13, 14]. Overall, 1218 patients were randomized to undergo lung volume reduction surgery or continued medical therapy, and the overall mortality of 0.11 death per person year was identical in both treatment groups. A substantial improvement in exercise capacity at 24 months was defined as >10 W improvement in cycle ergometry. Using this definition, a 10 W or greater improvement was seen in 16% of surgical patients compared with 3% of medical patients ($p < 0.001$) [13]. In secondary outcome measures of FEV_1 and HRQOL as measured by the quality of well-being score (QWB), surgically treated patients showed significant improvement over medical patients at 6, 12, and 24 months.

Further analysis performed on the 1078 who were not at high risk demonstrated a 2.2% 30-day mortality and a 5.2% 90-day mortality after LVRS [15]. These excellent early outcomes matched the best of the single institution case-controlled series of LVRS previously published. However, the NETT demonstrated that, of patients undergoing LVRS, 14% remained hospitalized or living in a nursing rehabilitation facility 2 months after randomization compared to 3.3% of medically treated patients ($p < 0.001$). This discrepancy in independent living ultimately equalized between the two groups at 8 months post randomization. Changes in exercise capacity, 6-minute walk, FEV_1, quality of life, and dyspnea scale favored the surgery group at all time points. Just as importantly, a follow-up of both groups revealed a progressive decline from baseline in the medical therapy group, while the surgery group had improvements from baseline with a subsequent gradual decline over the 24-month follow-up [13].

One of the critical components of the NETT was to try to identify baseline characteristics and identify differential likelihood of benefit for patients considering LVRS. Although a large number of characteristics were examined, only upper lobe predominance of emphysema and baseline exercise capacity was associated with differences in predicting primary outcomes. These two characteristics allowed the NETT patients to be divided into four subgroups on the basis of combinations of upper lobe or non-upper lobe emphysema and low or high exercise capacity at baseline. Patients with upper lobe disease and low exercise capacity not only showed a favorable impact of surgery on exercise capacity and quality of life but also showed an improvement in survival in the surgically treated patients [13]. Patients with upper lobe disease and high exercise capacity demonstrated equal mortality, but surgically treated patients had a significant improvement in both exercise capacity and health related quality of life at 24 months. The patients with non-upper lobe disease and low exercise capacity had a similar risk of death regardless of the treatment group and did not show a significant difference in the maximum exercise capacity. However surgically treated patients did show an improvement in health-related quality of life. Finally, the patients with non-upper lobe disease and exercise capacity had both a higher risk of death and no significant benefit of surgery in improving exercise capacity or quality of life.

These clinical results provided reinforcement of many of the data provided in less rigorous case-controlled or randomized series, in spite of a very conservative statistical analysis. Although a randomized study, the NETT analysis compared patients to their baseline, similar to the case-controlled studies, in order to provide data regarding the changes to be anticipated after lung volume reduction surgery. However, when surgical treated patients are compared to the progressive decline in function of medically treated patients, these differences between groups appear even more profound. The NETT also revealed an unexpected and paradoxical relationship of outcomes to baseline exercise capacity, with those patients with low exercise capacity appearing to benefit the most from LVRS. This most likely relates to the very poor outcomes in the medically treated patients with this degree of disability and exercise limitation. Finally, the NETT provided evidence of an actual survival benefit in emphysema patients undergoing LVRS within the specific subgroup of upper lobe emphysema and low exercise capacity. Although this is just a subset of emphysema patients, this is the only time a treatment other than oxygen supplementation has been shown to provide a benefit on survival in patients with severe COPD.

A companion study of the cost-effectiveness of lung volume reduction was performed alongside the clinical NETT [14]. With the high-risk patients excluded, the cost-effectiveness ratio for lung volume reduction surgery compared to medical therapy was $190,000 per quality-adjusted life year at 3 years and $53,000 per quality-adjusted life year at 10 years. Subgroup analysis parallel to that described in the clinical paper revealed that the favorable subgroup with upper lobe emphysema and low exercise capacity had a cost-effectiveness ratio at 10 years of $21,000. This analysis certainly revealed that lung volume reduction surgery is costly relative to medical therapy, but with further analysis, this may show the procedure to be cost-effective if benefits can be maintained over time.

Complications in Brantigan's original work and in all of the modern reports of LVRS have been dominated by the complication of frequent and prolonged air leakage due to the friable nature of the underlying lung parenchyma. Simultaneous with the clinical development of LVRS, Dr. Cooper and his colleagues proposed the addition of a buttressing material along the surgical staple line in order to minimize postoperative air leaks [16]. Since then, a variety of buttressing materials have been used including bovine pericardium, PTFE, Teflon, and gel foam. Stammberger and colleagues confirmed the beneficial effect of buttressing material on surgical staple line in lung volume reduction surgery in a randomized study. This study showed a significantly shorter duration of postoperative air leaks in patients buttressed with bovine pericardium compared to surgical staples alone. These patients also had a significant decrease in the incidence of initial air leakage and a trend toward a shorter hospital stay [17].

Dr. Cooper's initial report of LVRS was a bilateral technique accomplished with a median sternotomy. Interest in applying the technique via video-assisted thoracic surgery (VATS) resulted in application of the procedure as a unilateral thoracoscopic approach. Experienced thoracoscopy centers reported unilateral lung volume reduction operations with mortality and hospital length of stays similar to that reported by Cooper [15, 18]. Unfortunately, nonrandomized comparisons suggested that unilateral LVRS produced a smaller improvement in FEV_1 compared to the bilateral procedure. Although no randomized comparisons have been performed, McKenna and his colleagues in Los Angeles reported a retrospective comparison of their unilateral versus bilateral LVRS procedures [19]. This study revealed a higher 1-year mortality after unilateral LVRS, presumed due to subsequent respiratory failure due to insufficient postoperative physiologic improvement. Since a number of additional studies have confirmed superior physiologic outcomes with no increase in preoperative morbidity or mortality after bilateral LVRS, the bilateral procedure has become the procedure of choice for the majority of LVRS candidates.

Centers preferring a thoracoscopic approach to LVRS adapted to the improved physiologic outcomes after bilateral LVRS and began performing bilateral VATS lung reduction procedures. Nonrandomized comparisons of outcomes after median sternotomy versus VATS demonstrated similar improvement in physiologic outcome. The National Emphysema Treatment Trial (NETT) randomized surgically treated patients between VATS and median sternotomy in 6 of the 17 clinical centers. Another eight centers formed LVRS by median sternotomy only and the remaining three centers performed only bilateral VATS procedures. In this large comparison of the two surgical techniques, patient characteristics and intraoperative outcomes were similar. There was no significant difference in operative mortality between techniques with a 90-day mortality of 5.9% for MS and 4.6% for VATS ($p = 0.67$) [20]. Patients in the sternotomy group required more ICU days postoperatively than patients in the VATS group but this difference was not statistically significant when the analysis was restricted to centers that randomized patients to both sternotomy and VATS. There was also no difference in the incidence of respiratory complications or other complications. However, the hospital length of stay tended to be longer for sternotomy patients who had a median length of stay of 9 days versus 8 days, respectively ($p = 0.05$) [20]. This also corresponded to a trend toward fewer patients living independently 30 days after surgery, 70.5% after sternotomy versus 80.9% after VATS ($p = 0.11$). Functional results and survival had a mean follow-up of 31.4 months with similar functional and physiological outcomes and no difference in overall mortality. These results appear to confirm that effective outcomes after can be achieved by either median sternotomy or VATS in experienced centers with the only benefit of VATS being a quicker functional recovery.

2.3 Patient Assessment

A wide variety of patients may be referred for consideration of lung volume reduction surgery, ranging from well-performing patients with subjective dyspnea during exercise to oxygen-dependent and wheelchair-bound respiratory cripples who are desperate to improve their quality of life. Preoperative medical management by a pulmonary physician is important to confirm the diagnosis of emphysema and the application of optimal medical management before consideration of surgical intervention. Initial screening studies should at least include pulmonary function tests including lung volumes and a chest CT scan. Important aspects to obtain from the history is smoking exposure, functional status, degree of disability, COPD exacerbations and hospitalizations, bronchospastic disease, and nature of secretions/sputum production along with recurrence of pulmonary infections.

2.3.1 Symptoms

Patients generally present with symptoms of exercise limitation, and dyspnea ranging from dyspnea on exertion to dyspnea at rest. Patients will commonly complain of shortness of breath with simple maneuvers that may produce diaphragmatic elevations such as bending over or postprandial gastric distention. They may also note substantial limitation in relatively simple activities like showering or performing similar activities of daily living. Some patients will note an ability to walk on the level for relatively long distances but become extremely dyspneic when walking up a slight incline or climbing a flight of stairs. More extreme patients report substantial dyspnea at rest that may be exacerbated when eating or talking; these patients concentrating the majority of their day on simple survival.

Tip: Patients with severe end-stage emphysema may present with a desperate level of symptoms and are willing to "try anything" to improve their quality of life. It is important to not allow the desperation of the severely symptomatic patient to influence the objective indications for lung volume reduction surgery.

Tip: It is very important to ascertain the patient's goals of therapy in order to both educate the patient and assure that the patient's goals are realistic and achievable.

2.3.2 Preoperative Work-Up

In general, eligible patients for LVRS will have a clinical and radiologic diagnosis of emphysema that is not confounded with concomitant pulmonary disease such as asthma, pulmonary fibrosis, or bronchiectasis. Patients will describe a moderately severe to very severe impairment in pulmonary function that is validated by spirometry showing an FEV1 less than 45% predicted. A requirement for eligibility for lung reduction surgery is objective evidence of hyperinflation on imaging (Fig. 2.1) and as measured by lung volumes, including a total lung capacity (TLC) of ≥100% predicted and a residual volume (RV) of ≥150% predicted.

Tip: Lung volumes can be measured by either helium dilution techniques or body plethysmography. Because of air trapping in some patients with severe emphysema, helium dilution techniques may significantly underestimate true lung volumes. Although helium dilution is more readily available, requires less extensive equipment, and is less expensive, it does not provide adequate accuracy for the assessment of patients for lung volume reduction surgery. Body plethysmography is necessary to attain accurate lung volumes for the assessment of surgical candidacy.

The pattern of emphysema is also a critical determinant in the potential eligibility for LVRS. Some have incorrectly assumed that eligible patients for LVRS will have giant bulla as targets for resection (Fig. 2.2a). However, indications for lung reduction are distinct from those of bullectomy; LVRS candidates have generalized

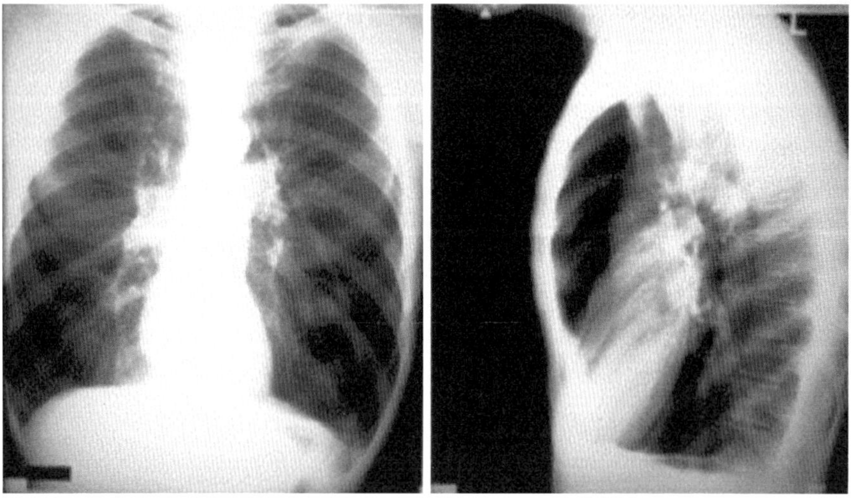

Fig. 2.1 Marked hyperinflation of emphysema as seen on PA and lateral chest x-ray. Note the flattened hemidiaphragms and increased AP diameter

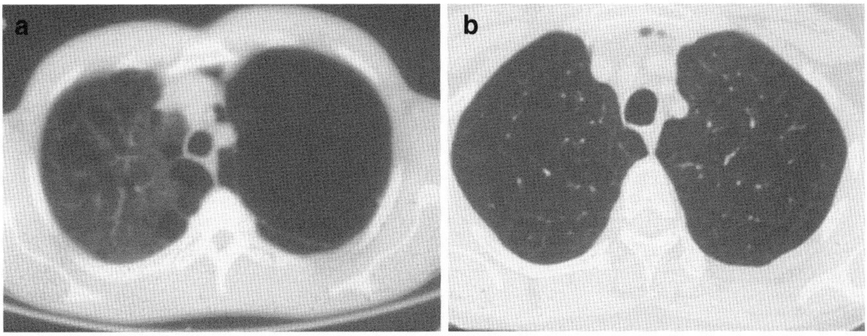

Fig. 2.2 (**a**) Chest CT of a patient with left upper lobe giant bulla. This may be appropriate for bullectomy, but bulla are not a requirement for LVRS. (**b**) Generalized upper lobe predominant emphysema with pattern of disease appropriate for LVRS

emphysema, with or without bullous changes (Fig. 2.2b). Marked heterogeneity with upper lobe predominance of emphysema (worse disease in the upper lung zones) is generally a requirement for most LVRS programs, and a reliable predictor of better postoperative outcomes.

Trick: Many programs prefer to use high-resolution CT scan to determine emphysema heterogeneity and the target zone for potential resection. We have long preferred perfusion imaging for providing a more accurate view of regional pulmonary blood flow which more directly correlates to functional pulmonary parenchyma. It is sometimes surprising that perfusion imaging does not directly match up to expected areas of poor pulmonary function on the basis of CT imaging alone. Most recently, we have adopted SPECT perfusion imaging to give highly accurate anatomic detail of pulmonary perfusion in order to refine eligibility for LVRS and allow for a personalized surgical approach based upon preoperative imaging.

Tip: Highly selected patients with lower lobe predominant emphysema may occasionally be candidates for lung reduction surgery if they have marked heterogeneity with relatively spared upper lobes combined with marked hyperinflation (generally an RV $\geq$ 250%) (Fig. 2.3).

Confirmed smoking cessation for at least 4 months is a requirement for lung volume reduction surgery.

Tip: Smoking abstinence can be confirmed with plasma cotinine level $\leq$ 13.7 ng/mL (or arterial carboxyhemoglobin $\leq$2.5% if using nicotine products).

Contraindications to LVRS include a history of recurrent bronchial infections with increased sputum production; cardiovascular comorbidities including significant coronary artery disease, recent MI, CHF, or uncontrolled hypertension or arrhythmias; pulmonary hypertension; and non-pulmonary comorbidities that cause significant functional limitation or could limit survival. Patients with significant pleural adhesions as demonstrated by preoperative imaging or a history of previous chest surgery or pleurodesis are not good candidates for lung reduction surgery.

Tip: Patients with an FEV1 < 20% combined with either homogeneous disease or DLCO < 20% are considered at "high risk" for LVRS, with a very high postoperative mortality and a low potential for functional benefit. These patients are

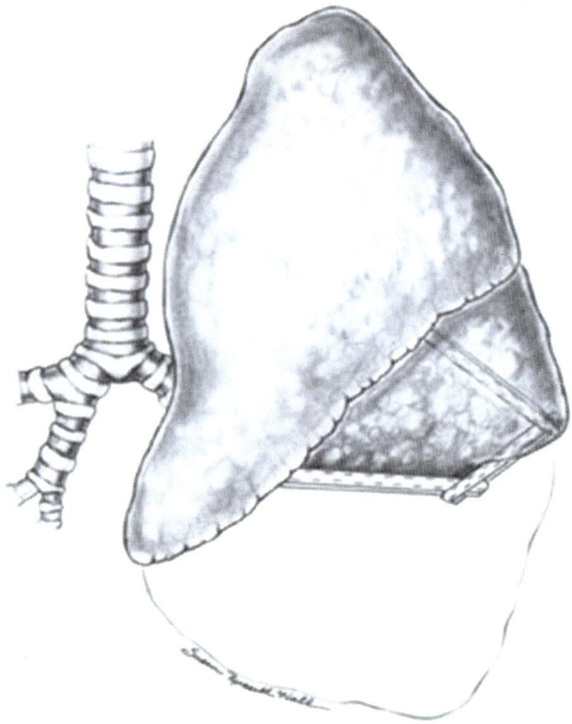

Fig. 2.3 Schematic drawing of left lower lobe LVRS, essentially performing a non-anatomic basilar segmentectomy using a buttressed stapler

contraindicated for lung reduction surgery and can be considered for lung transplantation.

Patients with lung cancer are not considered for lung volume reduction surgery and require a prioritization of their oncology management that generally precludes elective surgery for symptoms.

Tip: Some patients can have a very protracted natural history with lung cancer, particularly those with nonsolid lung nodules diagnosed as adenocarcinoma in situ. It may be appropriate to treat these patients for symptom management in spite of a presumed lung cancer diagnosis.

Trick: Some patients with suspected or diagnosed lung cancer may appear to not be operative candidates due to very poor pulmonary function. However, in patients who are candidates for LVRS and have the cancer in the area of planned lung reduction, curative intent resection can still be considered with the potential for a paradoxical improvement in postoperative pulmonary function.

2.4 Patient Preparation

A formalized pulmonary rehabilitation program has become a standard preoperative requirement for most patients being considered for lung volume reduction surgery. This is with the intent of both better clarifying candidacy for surgery as well as providing optimal preoperative preparation. Most programs require a post-rehabilitation assessment of the 6-minute walk test with a requirement that a patient be able to achieve at least a 140 m distance to be eligible for LVRS. Exercise capacity as determined by the maximum achieved cycle ergometry watts was an important part of the assessment during the National Emphysema Treatment Trial and has continued to be used by most centers as a part of the preoperative assessment. In this assessment a low exercise capacity is defined as a post-rehabilitation maximal workload at or below the sex-specific 40th percentile (25 W for women and 40 W for men).

Tip: Non-upper lobe distribution of emphysema combined with high exercise capacity (>25 W for women and >40 W for men) have higher mortality and lower benefit from lung volume reduction surgery and should not be considered for LVRS.

During the pulmonary rehabilitation program, all efforts should be made to maximize medical therapy. Systemic steroids should be weaned off or decreased to the lowest possible dose before surgery.

Tip: Systemic corticosteroid therapy is widely used in advanced COPD even though data only supports its role for short course therapy during exacerbations. Ideally, patients should be clinically stable on 20 mg prednisone or less prior to being considered for LVRS.

2.5 Operative Technique

Lung volume reduction surgery can be performed through a median sternotomy or with bilateral video-assisted thoracic surgery (VATS). As noted in the Introduction, while the original lung reduction procedure was done via a sternotomy, many surgeons have evolved to performing a bilateral VATS procedure. The advantages of a sternotomy are a single incision for a bilateral procedure, shorter operative time, ability to manually inspect and manipulate lung, and a more feasible evaluation of intraoperative staple line air leaks. A sternotomy is a stable and well tolerated surgical approach with relatively modest incisional impact on pulmonary function as compared to a lateral thoracotomy. In terms of incisional and operative pain, it is a trade-off between a single long midline incision and osteotomy and six bilateral intercostal incisions for VATS. The advantages of the VATS approach are the avoidance of a large sternotomy incision and the requirements for sternal precautions in the postoperative period. This also avoids potential sternotomy complications such as sternal wound infection or sternal nonunion. Other advantages of VATS include better cosmesis and easier postoperative mobilization. Most studies that have evaluated outcomes between sternotomy and VATS have shown an equivalent rate of complications and equal long-term functional outcomes. In comparisons between VATS and sternotomy in the National Emphysema Treatment Trial, there was a one day shorter hospitalization (8 days versus 9 days, $p < 0.05$) in patients having VATS LVRS but no difference in mortality, complications, or postoperative functional outcomes.

Tip: With essentially equivalent operative and functional outcomes between VATS and sternotomy, surgeons performing LVRS should choose the approach that they and their team are most comfortable with and that are tailored to the patient's anatomy and anticipated operative challenges.

2.5.1 Anesthetic Management

It is prudent to minimize or avoid premedication with sedatives to avoid respiratory depression in this group of severely ill patients. Most prefer to use a thoracic epidural catheter for both sternotomy and VATS approaches in order to minimize the need for postoperative systemic narcotics. Standard monitoring includes invasive arterial monitoring, pulse oximetry, and cardiac monitoring. Anesthesia induction and maintenance as well as the use of paralytics should allow for a planned extubation in the operating room at the completion of the procedure. A double lumen endotracheal tube is a necessity for both the open and VATS approaches. It is important to recognize that positive pressure ventilation can result in dynamic hyperinflation and/or pneumothorax, either of which can create hemodynamic instability.

Tip: Air trapping with auto-PEEP that produces hypotension is best managed by temporarily disconnecting the ventilator circuit from the endotracheal tube. Ventilating the patient with small tidal volumes and allowing longer expiratory times can avoid dynamic hyperinflation and its effects on venous return and systemic hypotension.

Tip: Pressure-controlled ventilation limits airway peak pressure, minimizing barotrauma and air leak.

2.5.2 Sternotomy Approach to LVRS

Patients undergoing open sternotomy are approached through a standard midline incision and full sternal osteotomy. Initially a unilateral longitudinal opening of the mediastinal pleura is made for exposure of the first half of the lung reduction procedure.

Trick: Keeping the contralateral mediastinal pleura intact during the first side of the procedure helps constrain the contralateral lung and avoid it being in the way or being inadvertently injured.

Tip: In symmetrical disease, there is no clear advantage of starting on either the right or left side. If one side is more severe or has anticipated technical challenges, like extensive pleural adhesions, it is generally better to do the less severe or simpler side first. If the more severe side is completed first, it may be more difficult to maintain a stable patient with single lung ventilation if it is compromised by air leak or minimal pulmonary reserve.

Tip: It is very important to be cautious during the cephalad portion of the pleural space opening to avoid inadvertent injury to the phrenic nerve which sometimes courses anteriorly enough to be threatened during the pleural opening. One should also identify and avoid injury to the cephalad extent of the internal mammary vein.

Tip: When opening the mediastinal pleura, it is helpful to make the opening close to the underside of the sternum in order to avoid a "curtain" of pleura that partially obscures the surgical field.

The lung is carefully manually inspected with all apical, mediastinal, and chest wall adhesions mobilized sharply to minimize the potential of underlying parenchymal injury and postoperative air leak. Complete mobilization of all lateral adhesions is necessary to allow the lung to reposition within the hemithorax after upper lobe lung reduction. Lack of adequate mobilization of adhesions may result in tearing of visceral pleura as the lung attempts to shift cephalad and may compromise the desired functional outcomes that benefit from smaller lung volumes and a repositioning of the diaphragm to a higher and more mechanically favorable position.

Trick: Basilar adhesions to the diaphragm do not need to be mobilized as these do not limit the ability of the post LVRS lung to reposition within the hemithorax.

Tip: Apical adhesions in the zone of planned resection can be taken down with relative impunity since minor underlying lung injury will be resected.

Tip: Apicomedial adhesions need to avoid injury to the phrenic nerves and the vagus nerve (on the left).

Trick: Hyperinflated emphysematous lung may be slow to deflate, even with contralateral single lung ventilation. Suction of secretions and placement of gentle ipsilateral suction through the endotracheal tube may facilitate deflation. This can be combined with gentle manual external pressure by the surgeon. Alternatively, a small incision may be made into the overinflated upper lobe in the area for planned resection in order to facilitate collapse and stapler application.

The target areas for planned resection are identified by chest CT and SPECT perfusion imaging. For most patients accepted for LVRS, this will be a fairly symmetrical pattern of upper lobe predominant disease, most severely impacting the apex and the upper portions of both the anterior and posterior segments. However, SPECT perfusion imaging provides important detail that may define important areas to be spared or opportunities for a tailored or deeper lung resection. Manual examination also helps refine the extent of the target area for resection. The most diseased portions of the lung remain inflated the longest and help the surgeon identify the best tissue margin for resection.

Tip: One advantage of sternotomy is the ability to manually manipulate and palpate the lung. This may decrease the potential of parenchymal air leaks from instrumentation of the lung and also provide manual feedback regarding the best demarcation of severely emphysematous lung to guide and refine the resection margins.

Trick: In an emphysema patient with a barrel chest, the deflated lung may lie very far posterior and be difficult to visualize. Since it is still partially filled with air, the simplest and least traumatic retractor is to float the lung with 1–2 L of warm irrigation in the chest.

A typical upper lobe LVRS will start with the anterior segment, the stapler being directed cephalad around the hilum with the cartridge and anvil along the medial

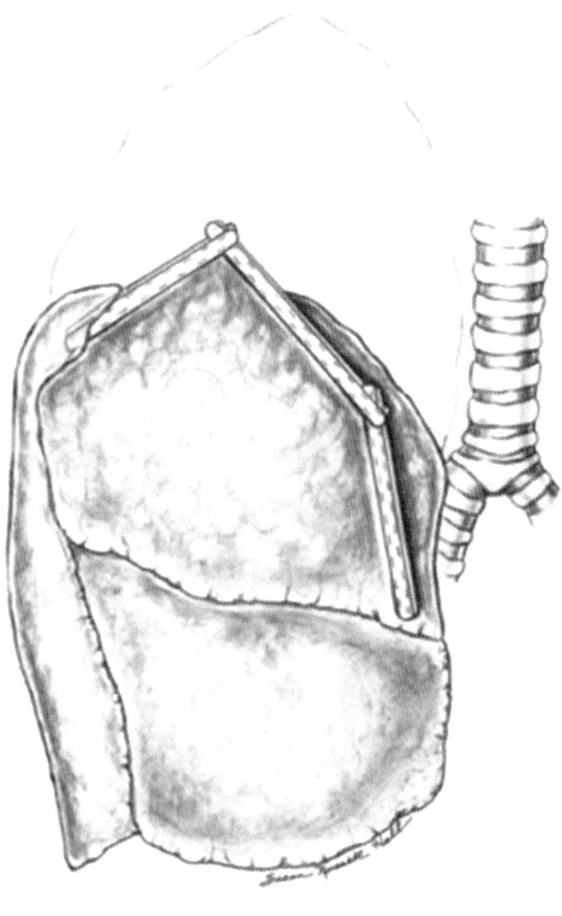

Fig. 2.4 Schematic drawing of right upper lobe LVRS, removing 60–80% of the RUL parenchyma using a buttressed stapler

and lateral surfaces of the upper lobe, respectively (Figs. 2.4 and 2.5a). An average lung reduction will target removing approximately 50–60% of the left upper lobe and 60–70% of the right upper lobe, but this can be modified depending on the extent of severe disease and the magnitude of hyperinflation. For example, in patients with severe upper lobe destruction and minimal residual function combined with marked hyperinflation (RV > 250% predicted), we will usually target removal of 80% or more of each upper lobe (excluding the lingula on the left). On the other hand, asymmetric presentation of disease may direct one to remove substantially less parenchyma on one side.

Tip: It is important to recognize that there is not one "standard" operation for lung volume reduction surgery, and the location and extent of resection should be carefully tailored based upon preoperative imaging, intraoperative findings, and the extent of hyperinflation on preoperative plethysmography.

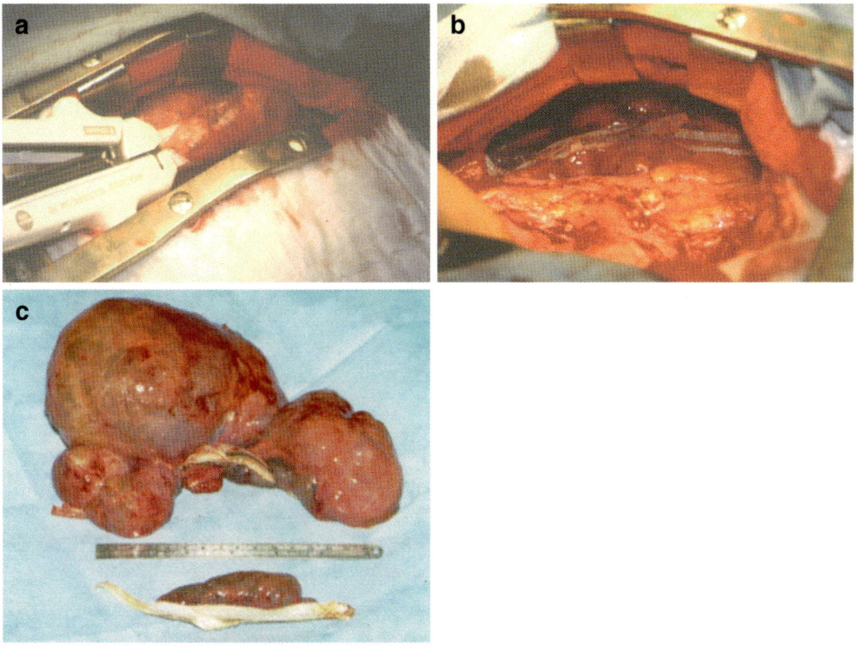

Fig. 2.5 (**a**) Buttressed surgical stapler starting a right upper lobe LVRS via a median sternotomy. The staple line begins along the anterior segment, progressively extending to the apical and posterior segments in repeated applications of the stapler. (**b**) A complete RUL lung reduction showing a buttressed staple line and smooth continuation of one staple firing to the next. (**c**) Resected specimen of RUL lung reduction, with approximately 60–70% of RUL excised

Tip: Buttressed staple lines are preferred by most surgeons performing lung reduction surgery due to their benefit in decreasing staple line air leaks. There are now a number of commercial products providing preloaded buttressing material for surgical staplers.

Progressive application of the stapler extends around the superior aspect of the hilum with gentle retraction of the lung anteriorly allowing the staple line to curve around the hilum and extend posteriorly to include a portion of the posterior segments (Fig. 2.5b, c). Some surgeons prefer to use the thickest possible staplers, especially due to the added thickness of the buttressing material. However, we have used a combination of medium and thick staplers depending on the underlying thickness of the parenchyma based on manual palpation.

Trick: Even with an open approach, the thoracoscopic staplers are easier to maneuver and provide more freedom of angulation for tailoring an optimal staple line with minimal trauma and with less need for a wider opening of the sternotomy.

Tip: The weakest link of the staple line is the junction of each progressive staple load. Therefore, the longest possible staple loads should be used when possible. One should also carefully line each subsequent firing of the stapler within the crotch of the previous staple firing to achieve a smooth resection line that has fewer areas of parenchymal tension that can result in possible tearing and air leak.

Trick: Using one hand to retract and spread the lung parenchyma while applying the stapler helps to avoid "wrinkles" of visceral pleura and parenchyma that are prone to tear on reinflation resulting in postoperative air leak.

When the first side resection is completed, it is valuable to control the reinflation of that lung while simultaneously evaluating for air leaks. The chest can be filled with warm irrigation and the unilateral lung gently reinflated. Once the lung is reinflated and there is no major air leak that needs to be addressed, a moist pack can be placed over the anterior aspect of the first lung to help keep it out of the field of the contralateral lung reduction, as well as to avoid injury to that lung during the second half of the procedure. The contralateral pleura is then opened to allow access for the second side of the procedure which is analogous to the procedure already described.

Tip: To provide the most control over lung reinflation, the anesthesiologist switches to ipsilateral single lung ventilation only, temporarily clamping the airway to the contralateral lung. With manual ventilation to a pressure of 15–20 mmHg, the lung is reinflated under direct vision. Steady handheld pressure provides the gentlest and most reliable inflation and parenchymal recruitment.

Trick: By holding a hand over the staple line as the lung inflates, one can manually protect the staple line from rapid inflation and overextension at the staple line. This provides tactile feedback of the degree of lung inflation; it also helps hold the staple line underwater for the air leak testing.

Tip: During the second half of the procedure, it is important to be very careful in avoiding over inflation of the first lung, particularly during the phase of single lung ventilation to that lung.

Trick: It is very easy for the anterior portion of each lung to be injured during the sternotomy closure. Covering the lung parenchyma with moist packs and/or coordinating ventilation during wire placement, along with temporary lung deflation during sternal approximation, can help avoid inadvertent injury.

We prefer to place both an anterior and posterior chest tube in each hemithorax at the completion of the procedure whether performing an open sternotomy approach or VATS (four tubes total).

2.5.3 VATS Approach to LVRS

The majority of the technical principles of lung reduction is identical between the open and the VATS approach. VATS provides better exposure for mobilization of posterior adhesions but does not benefit from the tactile feedback in determining staple resection margins or parenchymal thickness for choosing staple loads. VATS also requires more complete lung collapse for adequate visualization and stapler application and so may have additional benefit of making a purposeful venting hole in the part of the hyperinflated lung designated for resection. With the lateral approach and avoidance of mediastinal pleural opening, the phrenic nerve is readily visualized and readily protected during VATS LVRS. However, at the completion of the procedure, it can be substantially more challenging to identify areas of air leak on lung inflation with VATS.

Some surgeons use a supine position for bilateral sequential VATS lung reduction, both to avoid repositioning for sequential lateral approaches and to use gravity to assist in optimal enter apical exposure of both upper lobes. However, the supine position may make it more difficult to mobilize posterior adhesions. Many surgeons prefer a sequential lateral approach for VATS LVRS because of a preference for the extent of exposure and similarity to anatomical positioning to other VATS pulmonary procedures.

When the first side is completed, the operated lung is not aggressively recruited and is allowed to gradually reinflate with gentle ventilation from the anesthesiologist, analogous to the reinflation with the open technique but without manual support of the staple line.

Tip: It is critical that the chest drains from the first side are not kinked or obstructed during the second half of the procedure to avoid tension pneumothorax and intraoperative cardiovascular or respiratory collapse.

Trick: It may be difficult to apply the thoracoscopic stapler in areas of lung parenchyma that remained widened by air trapping. Placement of an atraumatic clamp to compress the underlying lung parenchyma may help create a crease in the lung to facilitate stapler application.

2.6 Postoperative Management

Lung volume reduction surgery carries a high morbidity with complications up to 60%. Anticipation and aggressive management of early postoperative complications, such as air leak, respiratory failure, and cardiac arrhythmias, are an important part of achieving successful long-term outcomes. Early extubation has the benefit of avoiding positive pressure ventilation and coughing or bucking that may produce barotrauma and air leaks in the underlying fragile emphysematous lung. With adequate epidural pain control and careful intraoperative anesthetic management, virtually all patients can be extubated in the operating room at the end of the procedure. These patients are typically managed in a specialized cardiothoracic ICU for the first 24 h postoperatively; stable patients are there and transitioned to a specialized thoracic surgery ward that has experience with chest tube management and the care of postoperative patients with severe emphysema.

Trick: Many patients undergoing LVRS have some component of CO_2 retention and subsequent hypoxic respiratory drive. It is common that caregivers in the postoperative care unit and cardiothoracic intensive care unit may attempt to achieve "normal" levels of oxygenation with O_2 saturation in the high 90s. However, this may result in a loss of hypoxic respiratory drive and progressive hypercarbia. Postoperative LVRS patients should be provided the minimal oxygen supplementation necessary to maintain oxygen saturation in the high 80s to low 90s, which may feel very uncomfortable to providers who care for other surgical patients and maintain a much higher oxygen saturation.

Tip: In the early postoperative period, it may be necessary to accept abnormally high levels of CO_2 as long as the patient is mentating appropriately and not in respiratory distress. This is particularly true in the first few hours after extubation when there may be a residual effect of the anesthetic on the patient's normal respiratory drive. It is worth being moderately tolerant of abnormal laboratory levels of CO_2 to avoid unnecessary re-intubation early after surgery.

The most common complication after lung volume reduction surgery is postoperative air leak, occurring in some degree with virtually every patient. Some surgeons prefer to avoid chest tube suction with a concern that it may create, exacerbate, or prolong an air leak. This may require accepting and tolerating a fairly large apical airspace as long as it does not result in any worsening of respiratory distress. Our center, along with many others, prefer early postoperative chest tube suction with the goal of minimizing the apical airspace, achieving optimal visceral to parietal pleural apposition, and achieving maximal cephalad excursion of the lung and diaphragm before adhesions fix the lung along the lateral chest wall.

Tip: After open lung reduction surgery, we treat both hemithoraces as a single connected space for the first 7–10 days postoperatively. In this early stage after surgery, we are cautious about removing any chest tubes until all air leaks have resolved. After 7–10 days, we assume a reestablishment of separate domains between the right and left hemithoraces and feel more confident about managing tubes independently.

Tip: It is important to not be impatient in the progression of chest tube management after LVRS. Aggressive efforts to prematurely clamp or remove chest tubes may result in a pneumothorax, loss of optimal lung expansion, and disruption of early formation of adhesions. Paradoxically, this may be a setback that actually prolongs the period of chest tube duration or, even worse, the potential functional benefit desired from lung reduction surgery.

Trick: Once generalized adhesions have formed, it is usually possible to remove all non-leaking chest tubes and discharge a patient with a solitary chest tube attached to a Heimlich valve for more prolonged air leak management.

As expected, pulmonary complications result in substantial postoperative morbidity. Maintenance of preoperative medications including inhalers and bronchodilators may be supplemented with short courses of corticosteroids to manage bronchospasm or COPD exacerbations. Aggressive pulmonary toilet with structured incentive spirometry, coughing, and deep breathing exercises combined with early mobilization can help minimize the challenges of retained secretions or postoperative pneumonia. Although prophylactic antibiotics are not indicated, postoperative care should include aggressive surveillance for pulmonary infection and a low threshold for initiation of antibiotics.

Tip: Early transfer of LVRS patients from the ICU to a standard thoracic surgery ward may facilitate early mobilization since this is a more routine part of the protocol and culture of surgical recovery outside of the intensive care unit.

Cardiovascular complications make up another part of common postoperative morbidity after LVRS. The most common of these are arrhythmias, occurring in up to 25% of patients. There is no indication for routine postoperative prophylaxis to prevent atrial arrhythmias, but if they occur they can be managed with calcium channel blockers, beta blockers, digoxin, and amiodarone as directed by cardiovascular treatment guidelines. Myocardial infarction and cardiac arrest are uncommon after LVRS, partly due to effective preoperative screening and management.

2.7 Alternative Interventions for Severe Emphysema

A majority of patients with severe emphysema will not be candidates for lung volume reduction surgery because of a lack of heterogeneous disease, inappropriate pattern of disease, mixed pulmonary pathology, very severe disease at high risk of early mortality, or other comorbidities. Even with fairly careful prescreening, only approximately one out of three patients referred for lung reduction surgery will ultimately be eligible for the procedure. Lung transplantation provides an alternative surgical intervention for patients with the most severe disease, particularly those with a very low FEV1 and DLCO or with homogeneous disease without targeted areas for resection. Some patients at the severe end of the spectrum of disease may simultaneously be candidates for LVRS or lung transplantation. In this case, consideration of the pros and cons of each procedure and integration of patient preferences can help direct the ultimate choice of therapy.

Tip: Coordinating a lung volume reduction program closely with a lung transplant program in the same center allows for the most streamlined and coordinated evaluation and optimal patient management.

Even with the initiation of the National Emphysema Treatment Trial, multiple investigators around the world began looking for less invasive endobronchial interventions that might achieve a similar physiologic benefit as identified in lung volume reduction surgery with a less invasive and less morbid approach. The most evolved approach has been the implantation of one way endobronchial valves in an attempt to produce focal areas of atelectasis and volume reduction analogous to that achieved by LVRS. Experience with endobronchial valves has demonstrated that the best results are obtained in heterogeneous emphysema where lobar ventilation can be isolated, and there is a little collateral ventilation. Randomized trials have been able to show statistically significant objective improvements in pulmonary function, yet small improvements that are marginally clinically significant [21, 22]. While endobronchial valves have been approved for clinical use in Europe, they have not yet been approved by the Food and Drug Administration (FDA) in the United States and are only available within ongoing clinical trials. Other endobronchial therapies have included coil implants to cause compression of adjacent lung tissue, biological LVRS and bronchial thermal vapor ablation to produce an inflammatory consolidated reaction, and airway bypass stents to create passages between the bronchi and emphysematous lobes to decrease hyperinflation. Each of these remains in clinical trials and awaits durable evidence of efficacy to obtain official approval and generalized access for patients and physicians seeking alternative interventions for the palliation of severe emphysema [23].

References

1. Deslauriers J. History of surgery for emphysema. Semin Thorac Cardiovasc Surg. 1996;8:43–51.
2. Brantigan O, Kress M, Mueller E. A surgical approach to pulmonary emphysema. Am Rev Respir Dis. 1959;39:194–202.
3. Cooper JD, Trulock EP, Triantafillou AN, et al. Bilateral pneumectomy (volume reduction) for chronic obstructive pulmonary disease. J Thorac Cardiovasc Surg. 1995;109:106–16.
4. Flaherty KR, Martinez FJ. Lung volume reduction surgery for emphysema. Clin Chest Med. 2000;21:819–48.
5. Fessler HE, Wise RE. Lung volume reduction surgery. Is less *really* more? Am J Respir Crit Care Med. 1999;159:1031–5.
6. Weinmann GG, Hyatt R, et al. Am J Respir Crit Care Med. 1996;154:1913–8.
7. Holohan FV, Handelsman H. Lung volume reduction surgery for end-stage chronic obstructive pulmonary disease. Washington, DC: Health Technology Assessment. US Department of Health and Human Services 1996, AHCPR, Publication #96-0062.
8. The National Emphysema Treatment Trial Research Group. Rationale and design of the National Emphysema Treatment Trial. A prospective randomized trial of lung volume reduction surgery. Chest. 1999;116:1750–61.
9. Wood DE, DeCamp MM. The national emphysema treatment trial: a paradigm for future surgical trials. Ann Thorac Surg. 2001;72:327–9.
10. Cooper JD. Paying the piper: the NETT strikes a sour note. Ann Thorac Surg. 2001;72:330–3.
11. Wood DE. Lung volume reduction surgery: tempest in a teapot. J Thorac Cardiovasc Surg. 2003;125:457–9.
12. National Emphysema Treatment Trial Research Group. Patients at high risk of death after lung-volume-reduction surgery. N Engl J Med. 2001;345:1075–83.
13. National Emphysema Treatment Trial Research Group. A randomized trial comparing lung volume reduction surgery with medical therapy for severe emphysema. N Engl J Med. 2003;348:2059–73.
14. National Emphysema Treatment Trial Research Group. Cost effectiveness of lung-volume-reduction surgery for patients with severe emphysema. N Engl J Med. 2003;348:2092–102.
15. Naunheim KS, Keller CA, Krucylak PE, et al. Unilateral video-assisted thoracic surgical lung reduction. Ann Thorac Surg. 1996;61:1092–8.
16. Cooper JD. Technique to reduce air leaks after resection of emphysematous lung. Ann Thorac Surg. 1994;57:1038–9.
17. Stammberger U, Klepetko W, Stamatis G, et al. Buttressing the staple line in lung volume reduction surgery: a randomized three-center study. Ann Thorac Surg. 2000;70:1820–5.
18. Keenan RJ, Landrenau RJ, Sciurba FC, et al. Unilateral thoracoscopic surgical approach for diffuse emphysema. J Thorac Cardiovasc Surg. 1996;111:308–16.
19. McKenna RJ Jr, Brenner M, Fischel RJ, et al. Should lung volume reduction for emphysema be unilateral or bilateral. J Thorac Cardiovasc Surg. 1996;112:1331–8.
20. National Emphysema Treatment Trial Research Group. The National Emphysema Treatment Trial: safety and efficacy of median sternotomy versus VATS for lung volume reduction surgery. J Thorac Cardiovasc Surg. 2004;127:1350–60.
21. Wood DE, Nader DA, Springmeyer SC, Elstad MR, Coxson HO, Chan A, Rai NS, Mularski RA, Cooper C, Wise RA, Jones PW, Mehta AC, Gonzalez X, Sterman DH. The IBV valve trial: a multicenter, randomized, double-blind trial of endobronchial therapy for severe emphysema. J Bronchology Interv Pulmonol. 2014;21:288–97.
22. Sciurba FC, Ernst A, Herth FJF, et al. A randomized study of endobronchial valves for advanced emphysema. N Engl J Med. 2010;363:1233–44.
23. Neder JA, O'Donnell DE. Update on nonsurgical lung volume reduction procedures. Can Respir J. 2016;2016:6462352. https://doi.org/10.1155/2016/6462352.

Primary Tumours

3

Lawrence Okiror, Maninder Singh Kalkat, and Pala B. Rajesh

Abstract

Lung cancer remains the leading cause of cancer deaths worldwide. A reduction in the smoking rates in the developed world has led to declining numbers of patients diagnosed with lung cancer. The role of surgery in the management of lung cancer patients encompasses the whole spectrum of the patient pathway including diagnosis, staging, resection with curative intent, palliation of advanced disease and multimodality treatment of selected patients. Advances in imaging and endoscopic staging techniques have led to better selection of patients likely to benefit from surgical resection. This has also reduced the need for invasive surgical staging. The advent of minimally invasive surgical techniques and a multidisciplinary approach to patient selection and optimization for surgery has led to falling perioperative mortality rates despite surgeons taking on increasingly older patients with multiple comorbidities. Large databases have led to validated risk-stratification models that guide patient selection for surgery. A number of randomised trials have helped clarify the role of surgery in multimodality treatment of lung cancer patients with locally advanced disease.

In spite of these advances, survival and cure rates from lung cancer remain dismally low. Newer strategies including screening of high-risk groups and early referral for imaging of patients with persisting chest symptoms are likely to result in more patients having early detection of their cancers with a potential for curative surgery. Advances in our understanding of tumour biology and the development of effective targeted treatments for patients with advanced disease may improve the prognosis of patients with advanced lung cancer with a potential role of surgery for palliative symptom control and multimodality treatment.

L. Okiror (✉) • M.S. Kalkat, MBBS, MCh, FRCS(CTh) • P.B. Rajesh
Regional Department of Thoracic Surgery, Birmingham Heartlands Hospital, Birmingham, UK
e-mail: Maninder.kalkat@heartofengland.nhs.uk

D. Parikh, P.B. Rajesh (eds.), *Tips and Tricks in Thoracic Surgery*,
https://doi.org/10.1007/978-1-4471-7355-7_3

Keywords
Surgery for lung cancer · Patient selection

3.1 Introduction

Lung cancer is the leading cause of cancer deaths worldwide accounting for more deaths than colon, breast and prostate cancers combined [1]. The majority of lung cancers are histologically of the non-small cell type (85%) with the rest being small cell lung cancer (SCLC). Surgical resection of non-small cell lung cancer (NSCLC) is only suitable in 25–30% of patients with early-stage disease [2]. A small number of patients with locally advanced and, exceptionally, metastatic NSCLC can be offered surgical resection as part of multimodality treatment [3]. The role of surgical resection for SCLC is controversial, and current guidelines recommend resection of early-stage disease only as part of clinical trials in a multimodality setting [4].

3.2 Assessment of Surgical Risk

Recent advances in thoracic anaesthesia, perioperative care and surgical techniques have led to improved outcomes with older patients and those with significant comorbidities now being offered surgical resection of lung cancer routinely. Careful preoperative evaluation with optimisation of comorbidities is, however, of paramount importance, particularly in patients with cardiovascular disease. The joint UK Society for Cardiothoracic Surgery and British Thoracic Society (SCTS/BTS) guidelines on risk assessment for surgical resection recommend a tripartite approach with screening for cardiovascular disease and risk estimation for perioperative death and for postoperative dyspnoea [4].

Estimation of risk of perioperative cardiac event starts with obtaining a careful clinical history. Any history of significant cardiac disease should prompt detailed cardiovascular evaluation including ECG, echocardiography and stress testing. If significant coronary artery disease is apparent following cardiac assessment, then early cardiology referral for percutaneous coronary intervention or surgical revascularisation as appropriate should be undertaken prior to lung resection.

Identification of cardiac risk factors should prompt cardiac investigations and referral for cardiac intervention prior to lung resection.

Estimation of perioperative and in-hospital death following lung resection is an important aspect of patient counselling prior to lung resection. In the UK, the in-hospital mortality after lobectomy for lung cancer was reported as 2.6% in 2003 [5]. More recently, this figure has been reported to be at 2.3% with the risk of death following pneumonectomy being 5.8%. Recent studies have showed that postoperative mortality after lung resections for lung cancer doubled between 30 and 90 days [6, 7]. As in-hospital mortality is low after lung resection, large databases from multiple institutions are required to develop a robust model that will provide a high degree of discrimination and be reproducible. Currently available models include the European Society of Thoracic Surgeons (ESTS) risk model derived from 3426 patients with 66 deaths and the Veterans Affairs risk model with 3516 patients and 184 deaths [8, 9]. The larger Thoracoscore derived from a database with over 15,000 patients and 338 deaths is currently recommended for use by the SCTS/BTS guidelines. However, it has limitations in its application to patients having lung cancer surgery [10]. More recently, a model to predict mortality at 30 and 90 days after lung cancer resection has been proposed which has the advantage of predicting risk beyond hospital admission and may be useful for counselling patients about the persisting risk of surgical morbidity and mortality up to 3 months after surgery [6].

Lung function testing enables estimation of the risk of perioperative respiratory complications and long-term postoperative breathlessness. Spirometry is cheap and easily accessible. FEV_1 was historically recommended with a cut-off figure of >40% predicted regarded as adequate pulmonary reserve for a lobectomy [11]. The value of FEV_1 in predicting postoperative complications is low even when the extent of resection is taken into account with calculated predicted postoperative FEV_1 ($ppoFEV_1$). Diffusion capacity of the lung for carbon monoxide (DL_{CO}) assesses properties of the alveolar-capillary interface including its integrity, thickness and surface area and the pulmonary capillary blood volume available for gas exchange. It has been shown to be an independent predictor of postoperative morbidity and mortality after lung resection at multivariate analysis [12]. A low DL_{CO} predicts not only postoperative complications but also long-term oxygen use and readmission for respiratory problems in the year after lung resection [13]. DL_{CO}, but not FEV_1, was shown to be independently prognostic for death after lung resection. In addition, patients with normal FEV_1 values can have very low values of DL_{CO} [14]. For these reasons, DL_{CO} and FEV_1 are recommended assessments for all patients prior to major lung resection for lung cancer by BTS and ERS/ESTS in their algorithms.

Cardiopulmonary exercise testing (CPET) is considered the gold standard test for assessing cardiopulmonary reserve preoperatively. The most commonly used and best validated parameter on the CPET is the maximal oxygen consumption (VO_2max). The VO_2max is a strong predictor of postoperative complications and accurately predicts postoperative exercise capacity [15]. The recommendations on when to perform CPET differ somewhat. The BTS and American College of Chest Physicians (ACCP) recommend performing CPET only on patients with moderate-to-high risk of postoperative dyspnoea [4] or low ppo values (<30%), respectively [16]. The ERS/ESTS, on the other hand, recommend CPET on all patients with reduced lung function (FEV_1 or DL_{CO} <80%) [17]. Generally, patients with a

VO_2max of >20 mL/kg/min of >75% predicted are considered low risk for postoperative complications, and it is expected that these patients would tolerate resection up to a pneumonectomy. Conversely a VO_2max of <10 mL/kg/min or <35% predicted are considered to be of high risk for postoperative complications, and it is recommended that these patients be counselled about minimally invasive surgery, sublobar resections or nonoperative treatment options for their lung cancer [4, 16].

Low technology tests such as shuttle-walk test (SWT), 6-minute walk test (6MWT) and stair-climbing test have been shown to correlate with CPET. Cut-off values such as a distance of <25 shuttles, <400 m and <22 m on the SWT, 6MWT and stair-climbing test, respectively, indicate high surgical risk, and it is recommended that these patients have a CPET [16].

3.3 Surgical Approaches and Extent of Lung Resection

Surgical access for lung resection has traditionally been performed through a thoracotomy. The most commonly used approach is a posterolateral thoracotomy although anterior and muscle-sparing thoracotomies are also performed. The intercostal space used may be varied in posterolateral thoracotomies to provide the best access for upper lobe versus lower lobe resections. Generally, upper lobectomies are better performed through a fourth or fifth space thoracotomy, while middle and lower lobectomy is best served by a fifth interspace thoracotomy.

Video-assisted thoracoscopic surgery (VATS) for lobectomy was first reported in the early 1990s. Uptake was initially slow due to concerns about safety, oncological equivalence and technical difficulties in learning the endoscopic skills to safely perform the operation. More recently VATS lobectomy has become more mainstream, and current evidence shows that for stage I NSCLC and patients with poor lung function, it may confer an advantage compared to open resection via thoracotomy [18–20].

3.4 Extent of Lung Resection

Every operation for lung cancer has three essential parts: establishing or confirming the diagnosis of cancer intraoperatively, complete resection of the tumour and systematic sampling or dissection of all ipsilateral lymph node stations potentially draining the site of the tumour. The goal of surgical management is complete resection. Incomplete resection where visible macroscopic tumour is left behind (R2) confers no therapeutic advantage. In contrast, despite appropriate preoperative assessment and intraoperative testing (frozen section analysis), R1 resections in which there is microscopic tumour found at bronchial resection margins or, more commonly, subclinical lymph node involvement with tumour is sometimes unavoidable.

If the diagnosis has not been established preoperatively, intraoperative diagnosis by frozen section analysis is mandatory. Intraoperative staging and assessment of resectability then ensue. The surgeon then proceeds to perform the appropriate lung resection and a systematic lymph node sampling or lymphadenectomy. The aim of surgery should be to perform an anatomical resection. For patients with adequate lung function, the standard resections include lobectomy, bronchoplastic lobectomy, bilobectomy, anatomic segmentectomy and pneumonectomy.

Lobectomy is the standard operation for lung cancer confined to the parenchyma of a single lobe. It is generally well tolerated with 30-day mortality rates reported as 2.5–3% in large modern series [6, 7].

Bilobectomy is performed for right-sided lung tumours in which there is crossing of the oblique or horizontal fissure or if there is involvement of bronchovascular structures of the middle lobe as well as either of the upper or lower lobes.

Sleeve lobectomy consists of lobectomy with resection of a circumferential segment of the adjacent main stem bronchus (Fig. 3.1). It is performed to spare the lung parenchyma as an alternative to pneumonectomy. The restoration of bronchial continuity is done by anastomosis of the proximal and distal bronchial resection edges. Several techniques have been described for this. We favour the use of absorbable sutures (4/0 polydioxanone or 4/0 polyglycolide) as a running continuous suture to the membranous bronchus and interrupted sutures to the anterior cartilaginous bronchus. Sleeve resections may involve a segment of the pulmonary artery as well as the bronchus (bronchovascular or "double sleeves"). The efficacy of sleeve resections as alternatives to pneumonectomy is now well established [21–23].

For bronchial sleeve resections, we favour the use of absorbable sutures (4/0 polydioxanone or 4/0 polyglycolide) as a running continuous suture to the membranous bronchus and interrupted sutures to the anterior cartilaginous bronchus.

A pneumonectomy is performed when lobectomy or its modifications are insufficient to remove all locoregional tumours. It is a radical procedure which can result in loss of more than half of a patient's lung function or pulmonary vascular bed. It is indicated for central tumours that involve the main stem bronchus, interlobar pulmonary arteries or tumour crossing the interlobar fissures. Mortality from pneumonectomy is variously reported as twice that of lobectomy, and right pneumonectomy carries a higher mortality than left mainly attributable to bronchopleural fistula [24, 25]. A significant number of patients requiring pneumonectomy to achieve complete resection particularly with lymph nodal involvement are now having induction treatment with chemotherapy and/or radiotherapy. This has helped bring down the rates of pneumonectomy by downstaging tumours leading to lesser resections. Pneumonectomy after induction treatment, particularly on the right side, carries a high mortality. Albain and associates in a randomised trial of 429 patients with T1-3, N2 and M0 NSCLC having chemoradiation alone or followed by surgery reported a pneumonectomy mortality rate of 26% [26]. Although lower mortality rates have been reported by Daly and associates with pneumonectomy after

Involvement of the diaphragm mandates en bloc resection of the involved diaphragm with a wide margin and reconstruction unless the defect is small in which case primary repair is performed.

3.7.2 T4 Disease

T4 tumours occur when there are satellite tumours in a separate lobe or when the primary tumour invades vital mediastinal structures. These tumours are generally deemed unresectable, but there are reports of good results from surgical resection in experienced hands [46].

3.7.3 T1–T3 N2 Disease

Involvement of ipsilateral mediastinal lymph node or subcarinal nodes forms the bulk of stage IIIA NSCLC. The prognosis from this is poor with surgery alone. The LACE Collaborative Group meta-analysis from 2008 showed a benefit of adjuvant chemotherapy in this group [49]. However, a third of patients did not complete adjuvant treatment, and two thirds had severe grade 3–4 adverse effects from it. More recent studies have showed better survival of up to 50% at 5 years especially if lobectomy is performed (as opposed to pneumonectomy) [27, 50]. The data from these trials emphasise the following principles in management of these patients: multimodality treatment is essential, patients with bulky mediastinal disease have a worse prognosis than those with disease limited to a single zone, and complete R0 resection is key.

Conclusion

The surgical management of NSCLC continues to evolve with widespread adoption of minimally invasive techniques. Better clinical staging has improved patient selection, and data from clinical trials has helped refine which patients with locally advanced disease are most likely to benefit from surgery. Multidisciplinary approaches to management are key, and although lung cancer remains the largest cancer killer, surgery remains the most effective modality at achieving a cure.

References

1. www.cancer.org. Accessed 22 Nov 2015.
2. Le Chevalier T. Adjuvant chemotherapy for resectable non-small cell lung cancer: where is it going? Ann Oncol. 2010;21(Suppl 7):vii196–8.
3. De Ruysscher D, Wanders R, van Baardwijk A, et al. Radical treatment of non-small cell lung cancer patients with synchronous oligometastases: long-term results of a prospective phase II trial (NCT 01282450). J Thorac Oncol. 2012;7:1547–55.

4. Lim E, Baldwin D, Beckles M, et al. Guidelines on the radical management of patients with lung cancer. Thorax. 2010;65(Suppl 3):iii1–27.
5. Treasure T, Utley M, Bailey A. Assessment of whether in-hospital mortality for lobectomy is a useful standard for the quality of lung cancer surgery: retrospective study. BMJ. 2003;327:73.
6. Powell HA, Tata LJ, Baldwin DR, Stanley RA, Khakwani A, Hubbard RB. Early mortality after surgical resection for lung cancer: an analysis of the English National Lung cancer audit. Thorax. 2013;68(9):826–34.
7. Pezzi CM, Mallin K, Mendez AS, Greer Gay E, Putnam JB Jr. Ninety-day mortality after resection for lung cancer is nearly double 30-day mortality. J Thorac Cardiovasc Surg. 2014;148(5):2269–77.
8. Berrisford R, Brunelli A, Rocco G, et al. The European Thoracic Surgery Database project: modelling the risk of in-hospital death following lung resection. Eur J Cardiothorac Surg. 2005;28:306–11.
9. Harpole DH Jr, MM DC Jr, Daley J, et al. Prognostic models of thirty-day mortality and morbidity after major pulmonary resection. J Thorac Cardiovasc Surg. 1999;117:969–79.
10. Bradley A, Marshall A, Abdelaziz M, et al. Thoracoscore fails to predict complications following elective lung resection. Eur Respir J. 2012;40:1496–501.
11. Armstrong P, Congleton J, Fountain SW, et al. BTS guidelines: guidelines on the selection of patients with lung cancer for surgery. Thorax. 2001;56:89–108.
12. Liptay MJ, Basu S, Hoaglin MC, et al. Diffusion lung capacity for carbon monoxide (DLCO) is an independent prognostic factor for long-term survival after curative lung resection for cancer. J Surg Oncol. 2009;100:703–7.
13. Bousamra M 2nd, Presberg KW, Chammas JH, Tweddell JS, Winton BL, Bielefeld MR, Haasler GB. Early and late morbidity in patients undergoing pulmonary resection with low diffusion capacity. Ann Thorac Surg. 1996;62(4):968–74.
14. Ferguson MK, Vigneswaran WT. Diffusing capacity predicts morbidity after lung resection in patients without obstructive lung disease. Ann Thorac Surg. 2008;85:1158–64.
15. Licker M, Schnyder JM, Frey JG, Diaper J, Cartier V, Inan C, Robert J, Bridevaux PO, Tschopp JM. Impact of aerobic exercise capacity and procedure-related factors in lung cancer surgery. Eur Respir J. 2011;37(5):1189–98.
16. Brunelli A, Kim AW, Berger KI, Addrizzo-Harris DJ. Physiologic evaluation of the patient with lung cancer being considered for resectional surgery: diagnosis and management of lung cancer, 3rd ed: American College of Chest Physicians evidence-based clinical practice guidelines. Chest. 2013;143(5 Suppl):e166S–90S.
17. Brunelli A, Charloux A, Bolliger CT, et al. ERS/ESTS clinical guidelines on fitness for radical therapy in lung cancer patients (surgery and chemo-radiotherapy). Eur Respir J. 2009;34:17–41.
18. Chen FF, Zhang D, Wang YL, Xiong B. Video-assisted thoracoscopic surgery lobectomy versus open lobectomy in patients with clinical stage I non-small cell lung cancer: a meta-analysis. Eur J Surg Oncol. 2013;39(9):957–63.
19. Zhang R, Ferguson MK. Video-assisted versus open lobectomy in patients with compromised lung function: a literature review and meta-analysis. PLoS One. 2015;10(7):e0124512.
20. Klapper J, D'Amico TA. VATS versus open surgery for lung cancer resection: moving toward a minimally invasive approach. J Natl Compr Canc Netw. 2015;13(2):162–4.
21. Schirren J, Bölükbas S, Bergmann T, et al. Prospective study on perioperative risks and functional results in bronchial and bronchovascular sleeve resections. Thorac Cardiovasc Surg. 2009;57:35–41.
22. Tronc F, Grégoire J, Rouleau J, et al. Long-term results of sleeve lobectomy for lung cancer. Eur J Cardiothorac Surg. 2000;17:550–6.
23. Yildizeli B, Fadel E, Mussot S, et al. Morbidity, mortality and long-term survival after sleeve lobectomy for nonsmall cell lung cancer. Eur J Cardiothorac Surg. 2007;31:95–102.
24. Shapiro M, Swanson SJ, Wright CD, et al. Predictors of major morbidity and mortality after pneumonectomy utilizing the Society for Thoracic Surgeons General Thoracic Surgery Database. Ann Thorac Surg. 2010;90:927–34.

25. Kozower BD, Sheng S, O'Brien SM, et al. STS database risk models: predictors of mortality and major morbidity for lung cancer resection. Ann Thorac Surg. 2010;90:875–81.
26. Darling GE, Abdurahman A, Yi QL, et al. Risk of a right pneumonectomy: role of bronchopleural fistula. Ann Thorac Surg. 2005;79:433–7.
27. Albain KS, Swann RS, Rusch VW, Turrisi AT 3rd, Shepherd FA, Smith C, Chen Y, Livingston RB, Feins RH, Gandara DR, Fry WA, Darling G, Johnson DH, Green MR, Miller RC, Ley J, Sause WT, Cox JD. Radiotherapy plus chemotherapy with or without surgical resection for stage III non-small-cell lung cancer: a phase III randomised controlled trial. Lancet. 2009;374(9687):379–86.
28. Daly BD, Fernando HC, Ketchedjian A, Dipetrillo TA, Kachnic LA, Morelli DM, Shemin RJ. Pneumonectomy after high-dose radiation and concurrent chemotherapy for nonsmall cell lung cancer. Ann Thorac Surg. 2006;82(1):227–31.
29. Ginsberg RJ, Rubinstein LV. Randomized trial of lobectomy versus limited resection for T1 N0 non-small cell lung cancer. Lung Cancer Study Group. Ann Thorac Surg. 1995;60(3):615–22.
30. Darling GE, Allen MS, Decker PA, Ballman K, Malthaner RA, Inculet RI, Jones DR, McKenna RJ, Landreneau RJ, Rusch VW, Putnam JB Jr. Randomized trial of mediastinal lymph node sampling versus complete lymphadenectomy during pulmonary resection in the patient with N0 or N1 (less than hilar) non-small cell carcinoma: results of the American College of Surgery Oncology Group Z0030 Trial. J Thorac Cardiovasc Surg. 2011;141(3):662–70.
31. Manser R, Wright G, Hart D, et al. Surgery for early stage non-small cell lung cancer. Cochrane Database Syst Rev. 2005;1:CD004699.
32. Allen MS, Darling GE, Pechet TT, Mitchell JD, Herndon JE 2nd, Landreneau RJ, Inculet RI, Jones DR, Meyers BF, Harpole DH, Putnam JB Jr, Rusch VW, ACOSOG Z0030 Study Group. Morbidity and mortality of major pulmonary resections in patients with early-stage lung cancer: initial results of the randomized, prospective ACOSOG Z0030 trial. Ann Thorac Surg. 2006;81(3):1013–9.
33. Lugg ST, Agostini PJ, Tikka T, Kerr A, Adams K, Bishay E, Kalkat MS, Steyn RS, Rajesh PB, Thickett DR, Naidu B. Long-term impact of developing a postoperative pulmonary complication after lung surgery. Thorax. 2016;71(2):171–6.
34. Hansen HJ, Petersen RH, Christensen M. Video-assisted thoracoscopic surgery (VATS) lobectomy using a standardized anterior approach. Surg Endosc. 2011;25(4):1263–9.
35. McKenna RJ Jr, Houck W, Fuller CB. Video-assisted thoracic surgery lobectomy: experience with 1,100 cases. Ann Thorac Surg. 2006;81(2):421–5; discussion 425–6.
36. Onaitis MW, Petersen RP, Balderson SS, et al. Thoracoscopic lobectomy is a safe and versatile procedure: experience with 500 consecutive patients. Ann Surg. 2006;244(3):420–5.
37. Shaw JP, Dembitzer FR, Wisnivesky JP, et al. Video-assisted thoracoscopic lobectomy: state of the art and future directions. Ann Thorac Surg. 2008;85(2):S705–9.
38. Swanson SJ, Herndon JE II, D'Amico TA, et al. Video-assisted thoracic surgery lobectomy: report of CALGB 39802—a prospective, multi-institution feasibility study. J Clin Oncol. 2007;25(31):4993–7.
39. Ali MK, Mountain CF, Ewer MS, Johnston D, Haynie TP. Predicting loss of pulmonary function after pulmonary resection for bronchogenic carcinoma. Chest. 1980;77(3):337–42.
40. Demmy TL, Curtis JJ. Minimally invasive lobectomy directed toward frail and high-risk patients: a case-control study. Ann Thorac Surg. 1999;68(1):194–200.
41. Sugiura H, Morikawa T, Kaji M, Sasamura Y, Kondo S, Katoh H. Long-term benefits for the quality of life after video-assisted thoracoscopic lobectomy in patients with lung cancer. Surg Laparosc Endosc Percutan Tech. 1999;9(6):403–8.
42. Petersen RP, Pham D, Burfeind WR, et al. Thoracoscopic lobectomy facilitates the delivery of chemotherapy after resection for lung cancer. Ann Thorac Surg. 2007;83(4):1245–9.
43. Billè A, Okiror L, Karenovics W, Choudhuri D, Routledge T. Thoracoscopic lobectomy: is a training program feasible with low postoperative morbidity? Gen Thorac Cardiovasc Surg. 2013;61(7):409–13.
44. Billè A, Okiror L, Harrison-Phipps K, Routledge T. Does previous surgical training impact the learning curve in video-assisted thoracic surgery lobectomy for trainees? Thorac Cardiovasc Surg. 2016;64(4):343–7.

45. Konge L, Petersen RH, Hansen HJ, Ringsted C. No extensive experience in open procedures is needed to learn lobectomy by video-assisted thoracic surgery. Interact Cardiovasc Thorac Surg. 2012;15(6):961–5.
46. Yildizeli B, Dartevelle PG, Fadel E, Mussot S, Chapelier A. Results of primary surgery with T4 non-small cell lung cancer during a 25-year period in a single center: the benefit is worth the risk. Ann Thorac Surg. 2008;86(4):1065–75.
47. Rusch VW, Giroux DJ, Kraut MJ, Crowley J, Hazuka M, Winton T, Johnson DH, Shulman L, Shepherd F, Deschamps C, et al. Induction chemoradiation and surgical resection for superior sulcus non-small-cell lung carcinomas: long-term results of Southwest Oncology Group Trial 9416 (Intergroup Trial 0160). J Clin Oncol. 2007;25(3):313–8.
48. Kunitoh H, Kato H, Tsuboi M, Shibata T, Asamura H, Ichinose Y, Katakami N, Nagai K, Mitsudomi T, Matsumura A, Nakagawa K, Tada H, Saijo N, Japan Clinical Oncology Group. Phase II trial of preoperative chemoradiotherapy followed by surgical resection in patients with superior sulcus non-small-cell lung cancers: report of Japan Clinical Oncology Group trial 9806. J Clin Oncol. 2008;26(4):644–9.
49. Pignon JP, Tribodet H, Scagliotti GV, Douillard JY, Shepherd FA, Stephens RJ, Dunant A, Torri V, Rosell R, Seymour L, Spiro SG, Rolland E, Fossati R, Aubert D, Ding K, Waller D, Le Chevalier T, LACE Collaborative Group. Lung adjuvant cisplatin evaluation: a pooled analysis by the LACE Collaborative Group. J Clin Oncol. 2008;26(21):3552–9.
50. Kim AW, Liptay MJ, Bonomi P, Warren WH, Basu S, Farlow EC, Faber LP. Neoadjuvant chemoradiation for clinically advanced non-small cell lung cancer: an analysis of 233 patients. Ann Thorac Surg. 2011;92(1):233–41.

Pulmonary Metastases

4

Cheng He, Cliff K.C. Choong, and Paul E. Van Schil

Abstract

Pulmonary metastasis is identified in patients managed with primary cancer elsewhere and is vigilantly followed up. Surveillance chest X-ray generally detects pulmonary nodule that may turn out to be a metastatic nodule. Preoperative investigations should include computed tomography of the chest with intravenous contrast and rule out the presence of other distant metastasis and nonrecurrence at primary site. Various approaches are available for thoracic surgeon to resect pulmonary metastasis. Video-assisted thoracoscopic approach has been popularised recently but has some limitations when the lesion is deeper, not visualised and centrally located metastasis. Bilateral and recurrent metastasis is also amenable to surgical resection.

Keywords

Pulmonary metastases · Metastasectomy · Soft tissue sarcoma · Video-assisted thoracoscopic surgery

C. He, M.B.B.S.
Department of Cardiothoracic Surgery, The Prince Charles Hospital, Chermside, QLD, Australia

C.K.C. Choong, M.B.B.S., F.R.C.S., F.R.A.C.S.
School of Rural Health, Monash University, Latrobe Regional Hospital, Traralgon, VIC, Australia

P.E. Van Schil, M.D., Ph.D. (✉)
Department of Thoracic and Vascular Surgery, Antwerp University Hospital, Edegem, Belgium
e-mail: paul.van.schil@uza.be

D. Parikh, P.B. Rajesh (eds.), *Tips and Tricks in Thoracic Surgery*,
https://doi.org/10.1007/978-1-4471-7355-7_4

4.1 Introduction

Surgical resection of lung metastases remains controversial, and its precise role has not been determined due to lack of prospective randomised studies [1]. Historically, Tudor Edwards [2] reported a sublobar resection for a soft tissue sarcoma of a metastasis from a previously amputated leg in 1927 from the Royal Brompton Hospital. The first long-term survival was reported by Barney and Churchill after pulmonary metastasectomy from a patient with metastatic renal cell cancer [3]. Early small series of pulmonary metastasectomy containing mixed cases of sarcomas and carcinoma suggested good outcome can be anticipated if patients could withstand the operation and no other metastasis is detected [4]. Mannix described, for the first time, resection of multiple pulmonary metastases from a patient with osteochondroma of the tibia [5]. In 1965, N. Thomford published a large series of 205 patients after pulmonary metastasectomy with 5-year survival rate of 30.3% [6].

Autopsy studies have demonstrated that about one-third of patients with cancer die with pulmonary metastases, but only a small percentage will have metastases confined solely to the lungs. Metastases from osteogenic and soft tissue sarcomas are often limited to the lung parenchyma (Fig. 4.1) [7]. Less commonly, patients with other solid organ neoplasms from the colon and breast or melanoma have isolated pulmonary metastases, but these may represent a subset of patients with favourable tumour biology. Synchronous liver and lung metastases may benefit from resection of all metastatic sites in selected patients whose primary tumour is completely irradicated. Resections of solitary and multiple pulmonary metastases from numerous primary neoplasms have been performed with long-term survival of

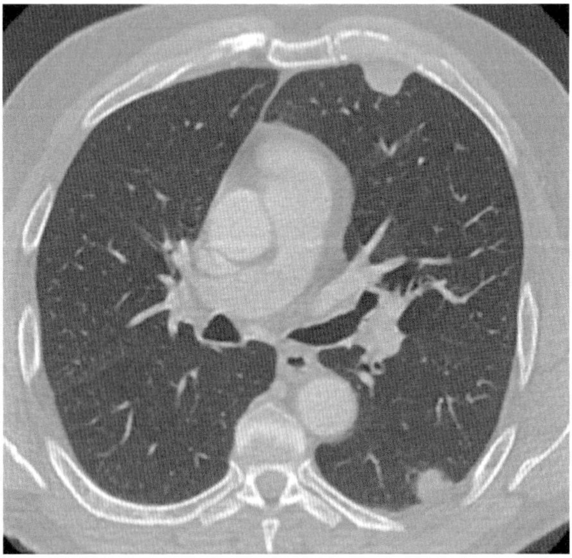

Fig. 4.1 Patient with myxofibrosarcoma of the left leg with lung metastases in close contact to the chest wall

20–40% in a retrospective study [8]. Long-term outcome with relatively good quality of life can only be maximised by patient selection and excluding other synchronous metastasis and control of primary disease, although some believe unresectability of pulmonary metastasis should only be the sole exclusion criteria [9]. It is mandatory to investigate all patients for the presence of extrapulmonary disease by positron emission tomography-computed tomography (PET-CT) prior to resection (Fig. 4.2). Preoperative workup must also ensure adequate cardiopulmonary reserve to undergo any resection. The goal of surgery is to identify all foci of parenchymal disease and ensure complete removal of malignancy whilst minimising the resection of normal lung tissue.

In general, most important prognostic factors related to long-term survival are complete resection, number of metastases, disease-free interval and specific histology [8]. Multidisciplinary evaluation is necessary to determine optimal diagnostic and therapeutic strategy. Effective systemic therapy may theoretically treat micrometastatic disease, thus increasing overall survival rate beyond that of immediate resection.

Repeat resection may be feasible and yield long-term survival. However, progression of metastatic involvement will reduce pulmonary reserve which may result in dyspnoea, respiratory insufficiency and severely diminished quality of life parameters.

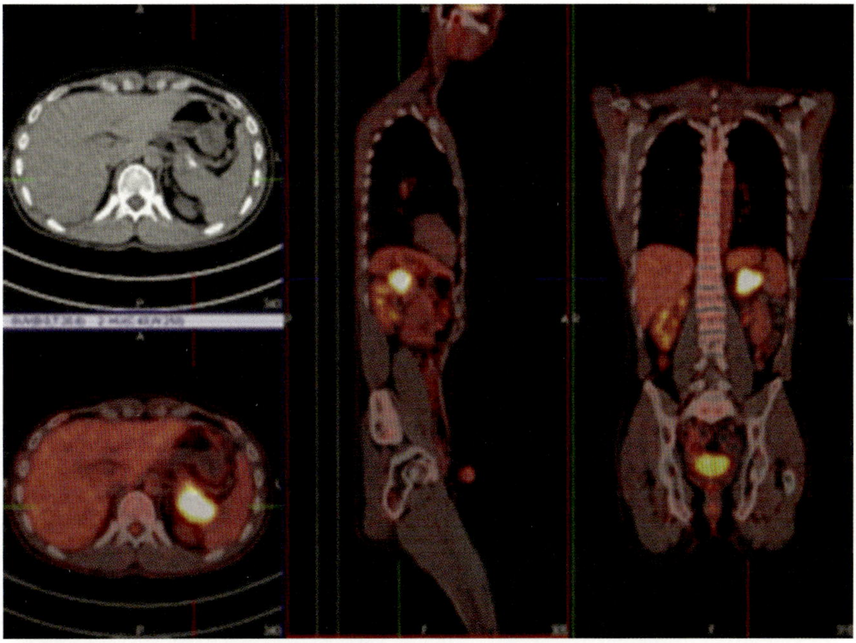

Fig. 4.2 Patient with osteosarcoma of the left tibia with bilateral lung metastases. Follow-up with PET-CT scanning also showed a large pancreatic metastasis that was removed by a bilateral subcostal incision

4.1.1 Not Every Lung Nodule Is a Metastasis

A new pulmonary lesion in patients with a known malignancy may represent metastatic disease, a new lung primary or a benign lesion. Chest CT remains the basic imaging tool of choice due to its high sensitivity (Fig. 4.3). There are no definitive imaging characteristics to discern metastases from other disease processes. However, metastatic pulmonary nodules are typically subpleural, located in the lung periphery, often being well-circumscribed with smooth margins. The presence of multiple nodules significantly increases the likelihood of metastatic disease.

Furthermore, the likelihood (i.e. the specificity) of a new solitary lung lesion being malignant is higher in patients previously treated for cancer. Among 1104 patients with solitary pulmonary nodules (SPNs) who underwent resection, SPNs were malignant in 63% of patients with no previous cancer compared to 82% and 79% of patients with a history of lung or extrapulmonary cancers, respectively [10]. The same study also correlated lesion size to likelihood of malignancy in patients with antecedent extrathoracic malignancy. Malignancy was found in 67% of nodules ≤1 cm in diameter and 91% for nodules >3 cm. Additionally, primary lung cancer was more likely if the nodule was >3 cm, whilst for lesions ≤3 cm, there was an equal likelihood of either primary lung cancer or metastasis.

4.1.2 Surgical Approach: Different Ways to Remove Lung Metastases

The choice of surgical approach depends on:

- Lesion characteristics: site, size, involvement of one or both lungs
- Imaging availability
- Patient performance status

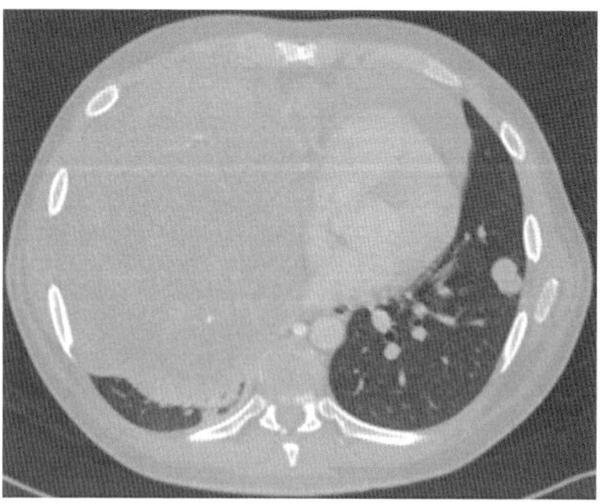

Fig. 4.3 A 21-year-old male patient with large extragonadal germ cell tumour with contralateral nodule which proved to be a lung metastasis

The surgical approach can be variable from median sternotomy, clamshell thoracotomy, lateral thoracotomy to video-assisted thoracoscopic surgery (VATS). Lateral thoracotomy offers excellent exposure of the hemithorax and enables detection of unknown lesions through bimanual palpation of the lung. Disadvantages of this approach are its postoperative musculoskeletal pain and respiratory compromise. Median sternotomy has been favoured by some owing to access to both lungs whilst reducing the degree of postoperative pain compared to thoracotomy. However, exposure of posterior aspects of both lungs and access to the lateral part of the left lower lobe may be challenging. Clamshell thoracotomy, similarly, allows broad access to both lungs by a single intervention but at the cost of postoperative pain. Whilst bimanual palpation of both hemithoraces may pick up occult disease otherwise missed by preoperative CT scan, this does not appear to offer any survival advantage compared to unilateral thoracotomy [11, 12].

As lymph node involvement implying further lymphatic spread in patients with known haematogenous metastases heralds a poor prognosis, a formal systematic lymph node dissection is recommended for correct staging [13–16].

4.1.2.1 Is VATS Indicated for Resection of Pulmonary Metastases?

Resection using VATS is attractive, given its minimally invasive nature, allowing improved postoperative recovery and decreased morbidity. Its use, however, is generally limited to lesions in the outer third of the lung and in cases without endobronchial involvement. Conversion to open thoracotomy may be required if the lesion cannot be confidently identified or for inaccessible deeper lesions. The primary criticism of VATS is the inability to fully inspect, with bimanual palpation, the deflated lung in its entirety. This deficiency results in a substantial number of nodules missed compared to thoracotomy. In a recent observer-blinded study from Denmark, 89 patients with 140 suspicious nodules on chest CT were evaluated. By VATS 87% of lesions could be localised. During thoracotomy 67 additional nodules were found of which 22 (33%) were metastases [17]. A survey from the European Society of Thoracic Surgeons (ESTS) reported 65% of surgeons believed palpation to be mandatory for adequate pulmonary metastasectomy [18]. Despite multiple studies demonstrating significant numbers of missed nodules with thoracoscopic surgery, removal of such occult nodules detected by bimanual palpation has not been shown to prolong survival. However, evidence from prospective comparative studies is not available.

It should be noted that VATS merely represents a specific approach to the thoracic cavity and that the thoracic surgeon should aim at complete removal of all identifiable lesions and at the same time perform a systematic lymph node dissection [19, 20]. Also, the Lung Metastasectomy Working Group recommends to perform a systematic lymph node dissection and indicates that video mediastinoscopy may play a role in more accurate staging of patients with lung metastases [21].

4.1.3 VATS Technique

- Generally, a three-port approach is used. Under single-lung ventilation, the camera port is inserted in the anterior axillary line at either the ninth or tenth intercostal space and can be used as a drain site later. The other two ports may be placed along the line of a thoracotomy incision, in case conversion is required. The principle of triangulating the lesion with the camera port at the apex still applies.
- Once pleural access is achieved, adhesions are freed with cautery to allow lung inspection. Pleural tenting may overly a subpleural lesion. A Duval retractor allows finger palpation once the pleural adhesions have been cleared. Under vision, the retractor may gently raise the lung area of concern towards the other port where the surgeon's finger lies waiting. Alternatively, gentle palpation of the lung with a long straight instrument may help localise the lesion. Once confirmed, the lesion is marked with either cautery or marking pen and stapler resection carried out.
- Resection specimens should be removed in containment devices to avoid port site recurrence of disease. A size 7 sterile glove often suffices and is an effective and economic alternative to commercially available options.

4.1.4 Finding Difficult Lesions

The likelihood of converting a VATS approach to thoracotomy due to inability to localise nodules was 63% in a study by Suzuki and colleagues, when lesion sizes were less than 10 mm or if located more than 5 mm from the pleural surface [22]. When lesions are difficult to localise with visual inspection or finger palpation, a number of alternative localisation techniques are available, to minimise the need for thoracotomy conversion.

Intraoperative imaging using a thoracoscopic ultrasound probe has allowed deep lesions to be accurately identified and resected. Sortini demonstrated localisation of all nodules seen on preoperative CT scan using this technique, allowing successful resection of lesions up to 5 cm deep from the pleural surface [23].

Percutaneous placement of hook wires and coils involves the risks of pneumothorax, pulmonary haemorrhage and significant pleural pain (Fig. 4.4a, b) [24, 25]. It is important to cut the wire at the skin surface before starting one lung ventilation to prevent dislodgement. Various percutaneously placed contrast/dyes, fiducial markers and radiotracers and bronchoscopically placed localisers have been reported, each with its own set of limitations [26–31]. Whilst useful as an adjunct to thoracoscopic resection, their use is institution and surgeon dependent.

4.1.4.1 Open Surgical Approach: Unilateral Disease

Classical open approach to unilateral consisted of a large posterolateral thoracotomy which is currently replaced in most centres by an anterolateral muscle-sparing

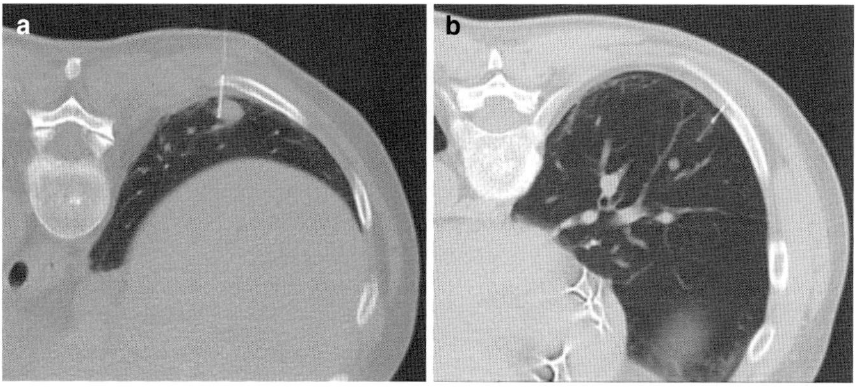

Fig. 4.4 Insertion of a harpoon wire in two lesions (**a**, **b**) in the right lower lobe which proved to be metastases of a malignant melanoma

thoracotomy whereby the latissimus dorsi muscle is pulled backwards and the thoracotomy opening allows manual palpation of the whole lung parenchyma.

4.1.5 Thoracotomy

- Double-lumen endotracheal tube is used.
- Patient is positioned in a lateral decubitus position.
- Standard anterolateral thoracotomy through the fifth intercostal space.
- Inferior pulmonary ligament is divided, as are any adhesions, to facilitate lung mobility.
- The lung is carefully held up by Duval retractors to allow careful bimanual palpation of the lung parenchyma.
- All palpable lesions should be accurately correlated to the preoperative imaging and marked by a suture.
- Since lung tissue will be distorted upon firing of the stapler, it is essential to precisely keep track of the boundaries of the lesion. This may be delineated with a tissue marking pen prior to resection, taking note especially of the boundary furthest away from the anticipated starting point of stapler resection.
- Aim for 1 cm resection margin, as a balance between resection completeness and lung preservation.
- Depending on the size of the thoracotomy, optimal positioning of the stapler to achieve the desired angle may necessitate bringing the endostapler through a planned chest tube site. The use of articulated endoscopic staplers may further assist in obtaining the ideal angle for resection.
- Smaller lesions may be removed by placing a clamp, removing the metastasis and oversewing the lung parenchyma with a continuous polypropylene suture underneath the clamp (Fig. 4.5a–c). Alternative methods include electrocoagulation and laser ablation, but these do not allow a complete pathological examination.

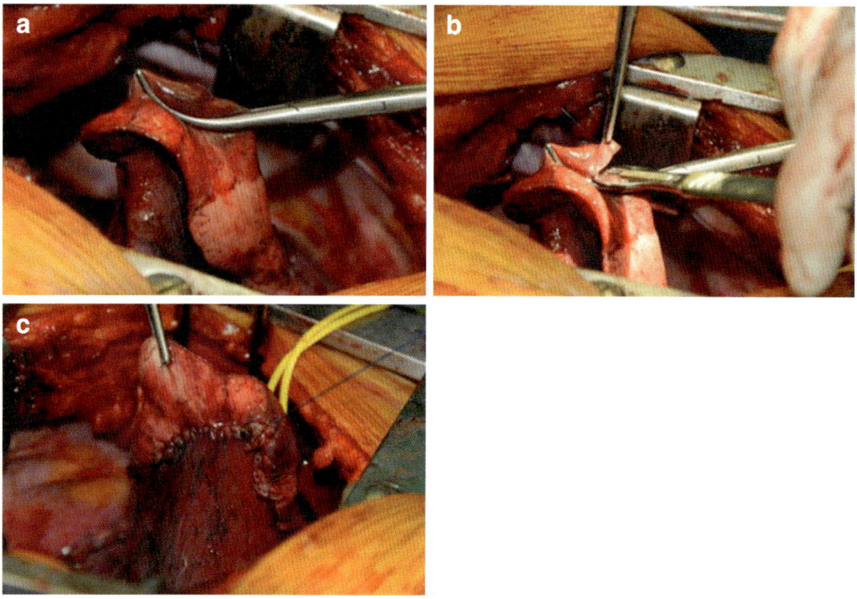

Fig. 4.5 Small wedge excision in a patient with presumed lung metastasis from colorectal cancer. This nodule was removed by placing a clamp underneath (**a**), sharp cutting with a knife (**b**), and oversewing of lung parenchyma with a continuous polypropylene suture (**c**). Pathology showed intrapulmonary lymph node

4.1.6 Central Lesions

- Careful examination of preoperative imaging will reveal the proximity of major hilar structures. The resection line should not compromise any major vascular structures. If there is any uncertainty, the fissure should be dissected to ascertain the exact location of the pulmonary artery branches, to enable safe stapler placement. Alternatively, anatomical resection may be required.

4.1.7 Open Surgical Approach: Bilateral Disease

Patients with known bilateral lesions can undergo sternotomy, bilateral anterior thoracotomy (clamshell incision) or bilateral sequential thoracotomy with a 4–6 weeks' interval.

4.1.8 Sternotomy

- A midline sternotomy is performed in the usual fashion as for cardiac surgery. The pleurae on both sides are widely opened. Lung mobility is improved by

division of the pulmonary ligaments on either side. Exposure of the left lung may be enhanced by instillation of warm water into the hemithorax or by putting large sterile gauzes behind the lung hilum.
- Lateral port sites for chest drains may be used for better angulation of staplers.

4.1.9 Bilateral Anterior Thoracotomies

- Patient is placed in the supine position, and both lungs may be accessed without the need for repositioning.
- Each hemithorax is entered via a sub-mammary incision through the fourth intercostal space, with single-lung ventilation. Further exposure, if required, may involve transection of the sternum, thereby converting to a clamshell incision.

4.2 Is Repeat Metastasectomy Feasible?

Retrospective evidence demonstrated recurrence of disease following metastasectomy in 53% of patients [8]. Five-year survival for patients who underwent repeat surgery for recurrent metastases was 44%. This is in stark contrast to a median survival of 8 months in patients who did not undergo further resection [32]. Repeat metastasectomy, it seems, may offer some degree of disease control in select patients. However, with each subsequent recurrence, the ability to achieve durable chest disease control, with additional resection, diminishes rapidly [32]. These retrospective reports lend support to the contention that pulmonary metastasectomy may be restricted only to radiologically visible lesions, obviating the need for bimanual palpation.

Conclusion

Pulmonary metastasectomy has an important role, in select patients, in offering the possibility of improved long-term survival, above what is possible with current systemic therapy alone. The goal of surgery in this setting is to remove all identifiable lung lesions whilst preserving as much normal lung parenchyma as feasible, to maintain pulmonary function and facilitate possible future resections as recurrences occur. Numerous surgical techniques are available, although focus in recent years has shifted towards a minimally invasive approach that minimises morbidity. The lack of comprehensive manual lung palpation with the thoracoscopic approach limits its potential to resect lesions not identified on preoperative imaging. However, current evidence does not show any survival advantage with thoracotomy compared to thoracoscopic metastasectomy, and no randomised studies are available. Certainly, careful surveillance imaging is critical to detect new disease as it appears, so that repeat resection may be considered.

References

1. Treasure T, Internullo E, Utley M. Resection of pulmonary metastases: a growth industry. Cancer Imaging. 2008;8:121–4. Epub 2008/04/30.
2. Pastorino U, Treasure T. A historical note on pulmonary metastasectomy. J Thorac Oncol. 2010;5(6 Suppl 2):S132–3. Epub 2010/06/05.
3. Barney JD, Churchill E. Adenocarcinoma of the kidney with metastasis to the lung cured by nephrectomy and lobectomy. J Urol. 1939;42:269–76.
4. Alexander J, Haight C. Pulmonary resection for solitary metastatic sarcomas and carcinomas. Surg Gynecol Obstet. 1947;85(2):129–46. Epub 1947/08/01.
5. Mannix EP Jr. Resection of multiple pulmonary metastases fourteen years after amputation for osteochondrogenic sarcoma of tibia; apparent freedom from recurrence two years later. J Thorac Surg. 1953;26(5):544–9. Epub 1953/11/01.
6. Thomford NR, Woolner LB, Clagett OT. The surgical treatment of metastatic tumors in the lungs. J Thorac Cardiovasc Surg. 1965;49:357–63. Epub 1965/03/01.
7. Potter DA, Glenn J, Kinsella T, Glatstein E, Lack EE, Restrepo C, et al. Patterns of recurrence in patients with high-grade soft-tissue sarcomas. J Clin Oncol. 1985;3(3):353–66. Epub 1985/03/01.
8. Pastorino U, Buyse M, Friedel G, Ginsberg RJ, Girard P, Goldstraw P, et al. Long-term results of lung metastasectomy: prognostic analyses based on 5206 cases. J Thorac Cardiovasc Surg. 1997;113(1):37–49. Epub 1997/01/01.
9. Putnam JB Jr, Roth JA. Prognostic indicators in patients with pulmonary metastases. Semin Surg Oncol. 1990;6(5):291–6. Epub 1990/01/01.
10. Mery CM, Pappas AN, Bueno R, Mentzer SJ, Lukanich JM, Sugarbaker DJ, et al. Relationship between a history of antecedent cancer and the probability of malignancy for a solitary pulmonary nodule. Chest. 2004;125(6):2175–81. Epub 2004/06/11.
11. Roth JA, Pass HI, Wesley MN, White D, Putnam JB, Seipp C. Comparison of median sternotomy and thoracotomy for resection of pulmonary metastases in patients with adult soft-tissue sarcomas. Ann Thorac Surg. 1986;42(2):134–8. Epub 1986/08/01.
12. Younes RN, Gross JL, Deheinzelin D. Surgical resection of unilateral lung metastases: is bilateral thoracotomy necessary? World J Surg. 2002;26(9):1112–6. Epub 2002/06/05.
13. Veronesi G, Petrella F, Leo F, Solli P, Maissoneuve P, Galetta D, et al. Prognostic role of lymph node involvement in lung metastasectomy. J Thorac Cardiovasc Surg. 2007;133(4):967–72. Epub 2007/03/27.
14. Szoke T, Kortner A, Neu R, Grosser C, Sziklavari Z, Wiebe K, et al. Is the mediastinal lymphadenectomy during pulmonary metastasectomy of colorectal cancer necessary? Interact Cardiovasc Thorac Surg. 2010;10(5):694–8. Epub 2010/02/23.
15. Pfannschmidt J, Klode J, Muley T, Dienemann H, Hoffmann H. Nodal involvement at the time of pulmonary metastasectomy: experiences in 245 patients. Ann Thorac Surg. 2006;81(2):448–54. Epub 2006/01/24.
16. Loehe F, Kobinger S, Hatz RA, Helmberger T, Loehrs U, Fuerst H. Value of systematic mediastinal lymph node dissection during pulmonary metastasectomy. Ann Thorac Surg. 2001;72(1):225–9. Epub 2001/07/24.
17. Eckardt J, Licht PB. Thoracoscopic or open surgery for pulmonary metastasectomy: an observer blinded study. Ann Thorac Surg. 2014;98(2):466–9; discussion 469–70. Epub 2014/06/15.
18. Internullo E, Cassivi SD, Van Raemdonck D, Friedel G, Treasure T. Pulmonary metastasectomy: a survey of current practice amongst members of the European Society of Thoracic Surgeons. J Thorac Oncol. 2008;3(11):1257–66. Epub 2008/11/04.
19. Graham AN, Chan KJ, Pastorino U, Goldstraw P. Systematic nodal dissection in the intrathoracic staging of patients with non-small cell lung cancer. J Thorac Cardiovasc Surg. 1999;117(2):246–51. Epub 1999/01/27.
20. Rami-Porta R, Wittekind C, Goldstraw P. Complete resection in lung cancer surgery: proposed definition. Lung Cancer. 2005;49(1):25–33. Epub 2005/06/14.

21. Garcia-Yuste M, Cassivi S, Paleru C. Thoracic lymphatic involvement in patients having pulmonary metastasectomy: incidence and the effect on prognosis. J Thorac Oncol. 2010;5(6 Suppl 2):S166–9. Epub 2010/06/05.
22. Suzuki K, Nagai K, Yoshida J, Ohmatsu H, Takahashi K, Nishimura M, et al. Video-assisted thoracoscopic surgery for small indeterminate pulmonary nodules: indications for preoperative marking. Chest. 1999;115(2):563–8. Epub 1999/02/23.
23. Sortini D, Carrella G, Carcoforo P, Pozza E, Sortini A. Sonographic evaluation for peripheral pulmonary nodules during video-assisted thoracoscopic surgery. Surg Endosc. 2004;18(3):563; author reply 4. Epub 2004/04/30.
24. Ichinose J, Kohno T, Fujimori S, Harano T, Suzuki S. Efficacy and complications of computed tomography-guided hook wire localization. Ann Thorac Surg. 2013;96(4):1203–8. Epub 2013/07/31.
25. Powell TI, Jangra D, Clifton JC, Lara-Guerra H, Church N, English J, et al. Peripheral lung nodules: fluoroscopically guided video-assisted thoracoscopic resection after computed tomography-guided localization using platinum microcoils. Ann Surg. 2004;240(3):481–8; discussion 488–9. Epub 2004/08/21.
26. Watanabe K, Nomori H, Ohtsuka T, Kaji M, Naruke T, Suemasu K. Usefulness and complications of computed tomography-guided lipiodol marking for fluoroscopy-assisted thoracoscopic resection of small pulmonary nodules: experience with 174 nodules. J Thorac Cardiovasc Surg. 2006;132(2):320–4. Epub 2006/07/29.
27. Nomori H, Horio H, Naruke T, Suemasu K. Fluoroscopy-assisted thoracoscopic resection of lung nodules marked with lipiodol. Ann Thorac Surg. 2002;74(1):170–3. Epub 2002/07/18.
28. Sancheti MS, Lee R, Ahmed SU, Pickens A, Fernandez FG, Small WC, et al. Percutaneous fiducial localization for thoracoscopic wedge resection of small pulmonary nodules. Ann Thorac Surg. 2014;97(6):1914–8; discussion 1919. Epub 2014/04/15.
29. Bellomi M, Veronesi G, Trifiro G, Brambilla S, Bonello L, Preda L, et al. Computed tomography-guided preoperative radiotracer localization of nonpalpable lung nodules. Ann Thorac Surg. 2010;90(6):1759–64. Epub 2010/11/26.
30. Endo M, Kotani Y, Satouchi M, Takada Y, Sakamoto T, Tsubota N, et al. CT fluoroscopy-guided bronchoscopic dye marking for resection of small peripheral pulmonary nodules. Chest. 2004;125(5):1747–52. Epub 2004/05/12.
31. Iwasaki Y, Nagata K, Yuba T, Hosogi S, Kohno K, Ohsugi S, et al. Fluoroscopy-guided barium marking for localizing small pulmonary lesions before video-assisted thoracic surgery. Respir Med. 2005;99(3):285–9. Epub 2005/03/01.
32. Jaklitsch MT, Mery CM, Lukanich JM, Richards WG, Bueno R, Swanson SJ, et al. Sequential thoracic metastasectomy prolongs survival by re-establishing local control within the chest. J Thorac Cardiovasc Surg. 2001;121(4):657–67. Epub 2001/03/30.

Lung Transplantation

5

Mike Mulligan

Abstract

It is our belief that a successful outcome following single- or double-lung transplant is based on proper donor assessment and management, appropriate donor-recipient matching, and performing a technically sound surgery. Therefore, this chapter will discuss some of the "tips" and "tricks" regarding lung transplantation aimed at the practicing surgeon beginning with both donor and recipient assessment and management as well as conduct of the recipient operation.

At our institution, the majority of patients undergo bilateral lung transplant for which our preferred approach is via clamshell incision. Due to our geographic location and relatively limited donor pool, our wait list is longer than at other institutions, and our recipients are frequently quite ill with high lung allocation scores (LAS) at the time of transplant. We, therefore, frequently use cardiopulmonary bypass to perform our transplants. Thus, our discussion of the transplant procedure itself will be reflective of our patient population.

Keywords

Lung transplant · Clamshell incision · Donor management · Cardiopulmonary bypass · Tips · Tricks

5.1 Introduction

Lung transplant is an accepted treatment for end-stage lung disease and for many with advanced lung disease is the only meaningful way of improving their quality of life and survival. Since the first successful single-lung transplant was performed

M. Mulligan
University of Washington, Seattle, WA, USA
e-mail: msmmd@u.washington.edu

D. Parikh, P.B. Rajesh (eds.), *Tips and Tricks in Thoracic Surgery*,
https://doi.org/10.1007/978-1-4471-7355-7_5

in 1983, there has been a steady increase in the number of patients undergoing transplant with over 4000 lung transplants being performed annually since 2013 [1]. The most common indications for lung transplant are chronic obstructive pulmonary disease (COPD), idiopathic pulmonary fibrosis (IPF), cystic fibrosis (CF), emphysema due to alpha-1 antitrypsin deficiency, and pulmonary arterial hypertension (PAH) which account for 85% of the lung transplant procedures performed annually worldwide. The major limitation to the number of lung transplants being performed is the shortage of suitable lung donors, as less than 20% of cadaveric donors are found suitable for lung donation based on currently accepted criteria. As a result of the paucity of donors, the median waiting list times for lung transplant have increased, as have the number of deaths on the waiting list [2–4]. In an effort to increase the number of donors, the use of marginal donors or "extended" donor criteria has been suggested which when applied selectively has been shown to have results similar to ideal donors when used in recipients that are listed for COPD [5]. Advances in both perioperative management and surgical technique have resulted in improved outcomes in both mortality and morbidity following transplant with reported ISHLT registry 1-, 3-, and 5-year survival rates of 78%, 55%, and 48%, respectively, and median survival in adult lung transplant recipients of 5.7 years.

5.2 Donor Assessment and Management

The criteria for the ideal donor have been well established by the ISHLT as a donor less than 55 years old, with a pAO2 > 300, clear chest radiograph, no evidence of infection or aspiration on bronchoscopy, no significant chest trauma or prior thoracic surgery, and a smoking history of less than 20 pack-years. Unfortunately, not all donors fit these criteria, in which case aggressive donor management is of utmost importance to optimize the potential donor and maximize the donor pool.

Pulmonary edema: Pulmonary edema is one of the most common causes of suboptimal pAO2 in a potential donor and can be potentiated by brain death. Neurogenic pulmonary edema is a known phenomenon and is caused by a systemic inflammatory response secondary to brain death due to the release of cytokines and catecholamines which lead to capillary leak and subsequent interstitial edema [6]. Fluid resuscitation and resultant hypervolemia in the setting of traumatic donor death and hemorrhagic shock also play a role.

Tip: Upon further investigation, donors are frequently volume overloaded at the time of initial evaluation regardless of what the electronic medical record may indicate. In the case of pulmonary edema related to hypervolemia or neurogenic pulmonary edema, it is our preference to initiate bolus dose intravenous furosemide followed by a furosemide infusion which allows for consistent, steady diuresis. Challenge arterial blood gases with FiO2 100% and PEEP 5, and tidal volume of 8–10 cm^3/kg should be checked at minimum every 4 h to evaluate for changes or improvement.

Abnormal CXR findings**:** Up to 12% of potential lung transplant donors are declined based on CXR findings alone [7]. The most common findings are pulmonary consolidation or contusion followed by pleural effusion.

Tip: When CXR does not demonstrate a clear etiology for ongoing suboptimal pAO2, CT with pulmonary angiogram can help elucidate other causes for hypoxia such as pulmonary embolism, underlying lung disease, contusion, or pneumonia. It is our preference that flexible bronchoscopy be performed for all potential lung donors, and we routinely initiate empiric, broad-spectrum antibiotics for any positive gram stain regardless of whether signs or symptoms of a clinical pneumonia are present. Moderate-large effusions should be treated with tube thoracostomy to promote lung expansion and relieve any compressive atelectasis.

Extended donor criteria: In an effort to expand the lung donor pool, the use of "extended donor criteria" or "marginal" donors has been advocated. Extended donor criteria include those with abnormal CXR findings, age > 55 years old, smoking history >20 pack-years, prolonged mechanical ventilation, and positive sputum or BAL gram stain. The literature has consistently demonstrated that the use of marginal donors does not have a significant impact on postoperative morbidity or mortality when used selectively [5, 8].

Tip: When considering marginal donors, an experienced procurement surgeon and careful donor-recipient matching are crucial. In the setting of suspected aspiration or pneumonia, a careful characterization of the quality and quantity of donor secretions is key. If purulent secretions are encountered and limited to the segmental or even lobar level but do not re-accumulate with suctioning, it is feasible to treat through a mild pneumonia for a double-lung recipient with COPD or emphysema. When a donor has a significant smoking history, it is also important to not be fooled by adequate oxygenation and a clear chest radiograph. In this setting, auto-PEEP can result in a falsely reassuring pAO2; CT chest should be obtained to evaluate for signs of emphysema which cannot be appreciated on radiograph.

Donor-recipient matching: Successful donor-recipient matching is multifactorial and is of paramount importance to prevent subsequent pleural space problems or undue postoperative complications. In addition to ABO and size matching, one must also consider the etiology of the recipients underlying pulmonary disease. This becomes important because the expected postoperative management challenges for a patient with cystic fibrosis or severe pulmonary hypertension are very different than that of a patient with COPD or interstitial lung disease. It is imperative to identify these potential management issues preoperatively when able.

Tip: Generally speaking, size differences of 15% are acceptable. Where one can run into trouble is with combining size discrepancies with other donor characteristics such as oversized donor allografts from a male into a female recipient with interstitial lung disease or undersized donor allografts into a male recipient with COPD. When assessing for size, in addition to looking at lung height, chest width, and predicted total lung capacity, evaluation of additional morphometric measurements such as chest circumference serves as a helpful adjunct which can be performed easily at the time of evaluation for both the donor and intended recipient.

Tip: When matching donors to recipients with a high LAS, suppurative lung disease, or right ventricular dysfunction, our aim is to choose the optimal donor, that is, a donor without evidence of edema, infection, or contusions that could potentially complicate recipient management postoperatively. It is our thought that these recipients, who are already the sickest of the sick, have such little physiologic reserve that no chances can be taken with donor allograft dysfunction postoperatively. Thus, for donors whose volume status, oxygenation, or possibility of infection is unclear at the time of procurement, we will frequently call in a backup recipient should the donor lung(s) be deemed marginal quality at the time of procurement.

5.3 Operative Technique

Recipient pneumonectomy: Depending on the diagnosis of the recipient, pneumonectomy of the native lung can be straight forward or prove to be very challenging. Dissection in patients with suppurative disease or chronic infection and resultant adhesions or lymphadenopathy can be particularly difficult. Additionally, in patients with interstitial lung disease, visualization of the hilum and inferior pulmonary ligament and vein can be obscured by an elevated diaphragm.

Tip: For patients with pleural symphysis or dense adhesions due to chronic infection, it is prudent to focus initial dissection on isolation of the hilar vessels rather than mobilization of the lung as this will often result in both parenchymal and chest wall bleeding. Additionally, by avoiding tears in the lung parenchyma which often result from a difficult dissection, you can avoid the subsequent air leaks and increase the likelihood of staying off bypass for dissection. This will also avoid undue blood loss from the chest wall and lung itself while performing the contralateral hilar dissection prior to arrival of the donor lung allografts. Once the donor lung has arrived and the hilar vessels are ligated, the native lung can be removed, and hemostasis can be achieved with an argon beam coagulator.

Trick: In patients who are not tolerating single-lung ventilation during dissection of the hilum, if the assistant maintains adequate lateral retraction on the lung during re-expansion, it is possible to carry on with hilar dissection while the ipsilateral lung is being ventilated.

Tip: Excessive lymphadenectomy should be avoided as these nodes are usually well vascularized and can result in significant bleeding. Bleeding within the posterior mediastinum can be mitigated by performing a mass ligation of the posterior mediastinal pleura to effectively tamponade these bleeding tissues. Care must be taken to avoid taking deep bites so as not to risk injury to the oesophagus.

Tip: When controlling bleeding of the lymphatic vessels and bronchioles near the bronchus, avoid using clips as these may cause erosion into the airway over time.

Trick: Retention sutures placed in the membranous aponeurosis of the diaphragm and brought out through the chest wall can be placed early in the dissection to aid in visualization of the inferior pulmonary ligament and vein. This thoracostomy incision can then be used for a chest tube at the end of the case.

Division of hilar vessels: The ease of donor allograft implantation can be improved by attention to a few small details while performing the pneumonectomy of the native lung and dividing the pulmonary vein and artery.

Tip: When performing the staple ligation of the inferior and superior pulmonary vein, one should attempt to ligate the vessels in parallel and in the same plane. By paying attention to this small detail, you will ensure that when the staple line is subsequently resected, the pulmonary vein cuff will be symmetric. Similarly, from time to time when performing the right donor pneumonectomy, it is necessary to divide the truncus anterior branch and interlobar pulmonary artery separately; these should also be divided in the same plane and in parallel to each other.

Trick: In the case of an early takeoff of the truncus anterior branch, it may be necessary to perform the pulmonary artery anastomosis to the inter lobar PA. If this is the case, be sure to ligate the truncus at its origin to prevent stasis and potential thrombus formation.

Recipient implantation: The key to implantation of the donor lung allograft is in the setup. We have already discussed the use of a retention suture in the diaphragm to aid in visualization which helps not only the native lung pneumonectomy but also with implantation.

Tip: We currently employ a hard-shell venous reservoir which allows for improved drainage while on cardiopulmonary bypass as well as vacuum assistance for drainage when necessary.

Trick: Placement of a pulmonary artery vent is also easily performed to augment drainage.

Trick: Although more easily utilized in the setting of median sternotomy, addition of an SVC cannula can also improve drainage when a two-stage venous cannula is simply not enough.

Tip: In the setting of a large or leftward displaced heart, visualization of the left hilum can be improved with elevation of the heart apex out of the pericardium. This will allow for further retraction of the pericardium upward and medially which will allow for better visualization of the pulmonary veins.

Trick: Placement of a pericardial retraction suture a fingerbreadth above the sternotomy and halfway between the free edge of pericardium and the phrenic nerve on the left is ideal for this exposure. The suture should be retracted across the chest, so it can be used to support the heart in this elevated position.

Tip: A warm folded sponge should be placed between the heart and the cut edge of the sternum and any retraction sutures to prevent injury to the left ventricle or occlusion of the coronary arteries.

Tip: One must be careful when elevating the heart as this may cause the venous cannula to be pushed deeper into the IVC, and drainage may suffer. This can usually be remedied by gentle cephalad traction on the venous cannula to ensure adequate positioning within the right atrium.

Bronchial anastomosis: Proper technique and sound completion of the bronchial anastomosis are of utmost importance in order to minimize the risks of anastomotic complication postoperatively. Avoiding devascularization of both the donor and recipient bronchial stumps is common knowledge.

Trick: Avoid excessive dissection along the donor and recipient bronchi, and leave some of the peribronchial fascia and soft tissue investments in place. This provides a small "flap" of tissue that can be deliberately placed between the bronchial and arterial anastomosis.

Tip: Be sure to take generous bites of the donor and recipient membranous airways with each stitch as this will create a more resilient anastomosis. Small bites are more sensitive to tension and subsequent ischemia which can potentiate dehiscence. Our preference is to complete the posterior membranous airway anastomosis with a running 4-O PDS®, followed by the cartilaginous airway which is completed with multiple figure of eights [9].

Tip: The figure-of-eight sutures should be pulled taut at the same time which will help to avoid distortion of the airway and allow the natural lie of the bronchial anastomosis to develop without buckling. Intentional telescoping is not routinely performed unless there is a size difference, in which case the smaller bronchi are allowed to intussuscept into the larger airway.

Inadequate vessel length: Occasionally one finds that the recipient atrial cuff or pulmonary artery stump is inadequate to perform an appropriate anastomosis. This may be due to overzealous donor cardiectomy or foreshortening secondary to significant hilar scarring.

Tip: When a short donor atrial cuff or pulmonary artery cannot be augmented by the recipient, sewing a strip of donor pericardium to the donor's atria or artery can be performed. It may be that only onc portion of the vessel needs augmentation.

Vessel injury: Iatrogenic injury can also occur if care is not taken when applying the clamp to the atria and pulmonary artery. Additionally, poor tissue quality, aggressive retraction on the vessel, or tearing upon placement of each stitch can compromise the anastomosis.

Tip: When poor tissue quality or vessel length prevents completion of the anastomoses with the clamp on, it is possible to remove the clamp and perform the anastomosis in an open fashion. When removing the clamp from the pulmonary artery anastomosis, it may be necessary to place a pulmonary artery vent to aid with visualization. When removing the clamp for the atrial anastomosis, the key is to allow for adequate de-airing via both the anastomosis and an aortic root vent.

Tip: When applying the clamp to the left atrium in preparation for the pulmonary vein anastomosis, watch your ECG tracing for ST elevations. A clamp placed too proximally may compromise the left circumflex coronary artery.

Hemostasis: Achieving satisfactory hemostasis during a lung transplant is highly variable and can largely be predicted preoperatively based on the recipient's underlying disease and whether they had prior chest surgery.

Tip: The easiest way to prevent bleeding is to not cause it in the first place. All too commonly, those who are new to transplant are overly aggressive in their retraction of the donor allograft after implantation while assessing for chest wall bleeding or atelectasis. Undue torque and tension on the hilar structures can lead to bleeding by pulling on the anastomoses and propagation of needle holes or areas of tenuous intimal apposition.

Trick: When retracting the lung, it is easiest for the assistant on the contralateral side of the table to retract the lung medially using an open palm which is used to cradle the lung and gently roll the lung toward the hilum. This allows the surgeon to lift the lung edge posteriorly and inspect both the posterior hilum and the chest wall.

Trick: Once off bypass, it is our practice to inject Floseal® around the anastomoses. This is most effectively done by inserting the tip of the applicator in between the pulmonary artery and vein and injecting it. This allows delivery of the Floseal® posterior to the anastomosis which is not otherwise easily reached or visualized.

Tip: Cauterize the free edge of donor pericardium and any remaining tissue along the inferior pulmonary ligament prior to lung re-expansion.

Tip: Have an argon beam coagulator available for cases expected to have a large volume raw surface area.

Chest closure: Closing of a clamshell incision can be a surgery unto itself especially in the wee hours of the morning.

Trick: Prior to closing the chest, liberal application of a fibrin-based sealant to the hilum and mediastinum can help seal small lymphatics that may contribute to ongoing chest tube drainage and also improves hemostasis.

Tip: We routinely suture ligate the cut edges of the internal mammary vessels prior to chest closure to prevent delayed bleeding.

Tip: For patients with suppurative disease, the use of absorbable pericostal sutures is preferred as it decreases the likelihood of developing a suture site infection in the future.

Tip: When the sternal wires are in place and ready to be closed, hold the pericostal sutures taut to re-approximate the chest wall and take tension off of the sternal wires before twisting/cinching them down.

Trick: In patients demonstrating outward subluxation of the cut sternal edges or poor bone quality, a titanium plate can be used to bolster the sternal closure and help distribute tension. Rather than using screws, we use cables which are passed down through the holes of the plate, through the sternum and then back through the plate again. The cables can then be secured with a grommet in the usual fashion. The plate can then be fastened in place with additional screws.

Trick: In female recipients with large, pendulous breasts, a skin staple placed at the superior and inferior cut edge of the skin halfway along the incision on either side of the sternotomy can help with proper re-approximation at the end of the case.

Tip: In cases where there is a significant amount of ongoing blood loss due to coagulopathy which will require ongoing correction postoperatively, place a large, fluted silicone drain along the length of the posterior chest wall to help evacuate blood. The long channels of the fluted drain are more effective than the short segment of perforations in PVC tubes at evacuating blood.

Trick: In cases when primary graft dysfunction or bleeding secondary to coagulopathy requires that the chest be left open, a closed suction system can be easily and quickly fashioned out of surgical towels and GORE-TEX®. Chest tubes are placed along the diaphragm and anterior mediastinum and posteriorly along the chest wall as if the chest was being closed. Then a sheet of 2 mm GORE-TEX® is placed over the lung and tucked under the rib cage. This is then covered with a

Empyema Thoracis

6

Dakshesh Parikh

Abstract

Empyema Thoracis is collection of purulent material within the pleural cavity as a result of pneumonia or by secondary infection of the pleural cavity. The pathogenesis of empyema is a continuum. The presentation is dependent on host immune responses to type and virulence of bacterial infection and management instituted. Necrotic pneumonia is increasingly encountered and is the cause of bronchopleural fistula. Radiological diagnosis is achieved with ultrasonography, however, CT scan gives more accurate delineation of pleural collection, lung and mediastinal pathology.

Inadequate management of empyema can lead to necrotic pneumonia in collapsed consolidated lung. Clinical presentation is related to lower respiratory tract infection with decreased air entry, pyrexia and varying degree of respiratory compromise depending on the size of pleural collection and lobar lung consolidation. The principle aim in empyema management should be adequate drainage in order to achieve full expansion of the lung. Failure to recognise inadequate management strategy results in progression of empyema disease process into organizational state. Active monitoring of the management strategy, early recognition of failure to re-expand the lung and continuing infection avoids morbidity and occasionally mortality associated with empyema thoracis.

Various management strategies are employed depending on the institutional experience. Many published outcomes are biased toward institutional experience. Insertion of ultra-sound guided intercostal pig-tail catheter and fibrinolytic instillation may play a role in the management of empyema, however, it should be actively monitored and any failure should be referred for surgical intervention. Many recent studies have shown early intervention using

D. Parikh, MBBS, MS, FRCS (Ped.), MD
Department of Pediatric Surgery, Birmingham Women's and Children's Hospital NHS FT, Birmingham, UK
e-mail: dakshesh.parikh@nhs.net

D. Parikh, P.B. Rajesh (eds.), *Tips and Tricks in Thoracic Surgery*,
https://doi.org/10.1007/978-1-4471-7355-7_6

thoracoscopic techniques have shown improved outcomes and reduced hospital stay. Complicated empyema associated with bronchopleural fistula should be managed with early intervention with decortication and insertion of an appropriate muscle flap onto the fistula. The chapter discusses the management of bilateral empyema, secondary empyema and tuberculous empyema.

Keywords
Empyema thoracis · Pneumonia · Necrotic pneumonia · Bilateral empyema · Pneumatocele · Broncho-pleural fistula · Urokinase · Fibrinolytic instillation · Thoracoscopic debridement · Decortication · Serratus anterior digitation flap · Tuberculous empyema

6.1 Introduction

Thoracic empyema is collection of purulent material within the pleural cavity most commonly as a result of bacterial lobar pneumonia. Secondary infection of pleural cavity also occurs following penetrating injury, traumatic contusion and haemothorax, post thoracotomy and lobectomy, iatrogenic or accidental injury to the oesophagus and secondary infection of sympathetic effusion of acute pancreatitis or subphrenic abscess. Infection in congenital or malignant lung lesion and rupture of amoebic lung abscess or hydatid cyst are other rare causes of empyema [1].

Despite pathological descriptions of distinctive three phases in empyema, its pathogenesis is a continuum. The pathological presentation is not time dependent but on the virulence and type of bacterial infection, host immune responses and treatment received [1]. Increasingly in Western world, associated necrotising pneumonia is seen in association with empyema and is the cause of spontaneous bronchopleural fistula either at presentation or during its management [2, 3].

The principle aims in empyema management should be directed towards adequate drainage in order to achieve full expansion of the lung. Inadequate drainage and failure to recognise continuing infection inevitably result in progression of the empyema disease process into the organisational stage. Active monitoring, recognition and intervention of the failures of any empyema management strategy can avoid the morbidity and occasional mortality.

6.2 Technical Tips and Tricks of Video-Assisted Thoracoscopic Debridement of Empyema

The adequate drainage of empyema and full expansion of the lung are achieved by early intervention and administration of intravenous appropriate antibiotics. Thoracoscopic debridement accomplishes the debridement under vision and achieves the drainage of the empyema cavity [4]. Once diagnosis is made either by ultrasound or CT scan with IV contrast, the insertion of thoracoscope is best performed after making a pleural window.

6.2.1 Review the Radiologic Evidence

1. Optimum perioperative medical management should be an integral component of a successful management strategy of childhood empyema (viz. intravenous antibiotics, adequate hydration, nutrition, antipyretics, analgesia and respiratory physiotherapy). Humidified oxygen should be administered to maintain oxygen saturations above 95%.
2. The best place to insert first port is in the intercostal space from which pus can be aspirated freely. Alternatively, pleural window needs to be created in the presence of thickened pleural rinds by open dissection, and then port is inserted through the incision and fixed. If the port was to be inserted without creating a pleural window, it may enter into the adherent lung parenchyma with a resultant air leak. Blind port insertion without creating pleural space should be avoided.
3. Inserting a second port preferably along the same intercostal space and using Yohan forceps break down all loculations. Repeated warm saline irrigations help loosen the adhesions as well as improve vision by sucking and draining blood and purulent material. Insufflation of CO_2 at low pressures and approximately 2 L/min allows adequate exposure to remove thickened fibropurulent materials and constricting membranes covering the lung.
4. Yohan forceps holding the membrane and twisting it from outside help peel the fibropurulent membrane effectively.
5. Generally two ports are adequate if empyema is intervened early. In the presence of thick fibrous membranes, a third port may be required in order to achieve release of compressed lung from the constrictive pyogenic fibropurulent membrane or rinds.

   After achieving adequate debridement and seeing the expanding trapped lung, port sites are closed leaving behind intercostal drain/drains.

6.3 Tips and Tricks to Avoid and Deal with Intraoperative Anticipated and Unanticipated Complications

1. Bleeding: Bleeding is related to inflammatory ooze after removal of the pyogenic material; this generally stops as the lung expands. Bleeding from the intercostal vessels will require actions and can be effectively stopped either by direct control with coagulation diathermy or bipolar diathermy device. Arterial bleeding spurter needs careful identification and stopped before intercostal tube drainage and closure of port sites.
2. Air leak: During the thoracoscopic debridement, it is best not to disturb the necrotic-looking areas on the surface of the lung as it may result in air leak that may be difficult to contain thoracoscopically. Occasionally spontaneously air leaks are seen that are usually peripheral alveolar leaks due to breach of visceral pleura and do not require operative intervention. In the presence of significant air leak, the VATS is best converted, and the infective bronchopleural fistula can be dealt with by bringing in the pedicled muscle flap [1, 2, 5]. In the presence of significant necrotic pneumonia, air leak can be anticipated (Fig. 6.3b).

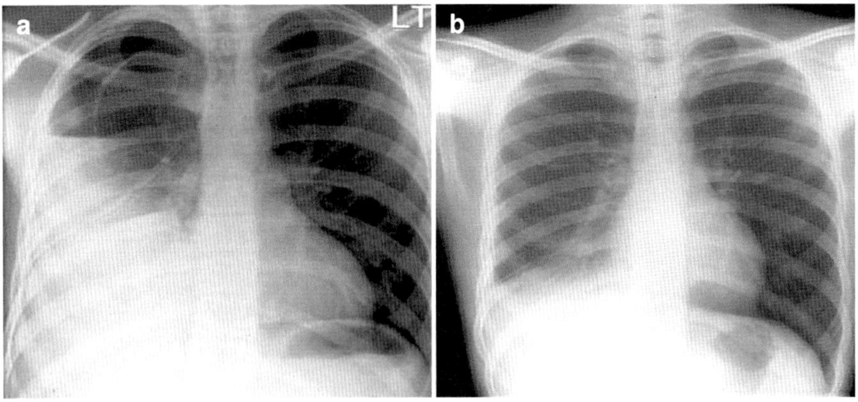

Fig. 6.1 Failed urokinase therapy. (**a**) Intercostal chest drain placed with multiple urokinase instillations: failure to re-expand underlying the lung, continuing infective process and spontaneous bronchopleural fistula and pyopneumothorax. (**b**) Chest radiograph following an open operation with insertion of a serratus anterior digitation flap

3. Inability to safely achieve adequate debridement: This could be related to failure of adequate vision, excessive bleeding, thick organised pleura or significant air leak. Saline irrigations and CO2 insufflations under minimal pressure usually help improve vision to a certain extent. Thick fibrous pleural rinds can be dissected with VATS techniques rather than purely thoracoscopic debridement. Use of blunt dissections with the help of tissue-dissecting forceps through a small intercostal incision.
4. Previous operations and inadequate drainage and persistent collections: Insertion of previous intercostal drain or drains, use of urokinase and previous thoracoscopy and/or thoracotomy may make subsequent debridement/decortication more difficult (Fig. 6.1a, b). This could be due to fibrous adhesions, trapped lung and bleeding caused by anticoagulation effect of urokinase. The insertion of primary port must be done with utmost care to avoid injury to adherent lung parenchyma. Carefully create plural window that may require an open technique. In the presence of large loculation, aspiration of pus with a needle and insertion of first port in the collection may help port insertion without open dissection. Subsequent port can be inserted by creating adequate plural space by swiping action of the scope in order to increase the pleural space. Occasionally the bleeding, fibrosis and air leaks from the trapped lung may lead to conversion to open thoracotomy for adequate debridement or decortication.
5. Excessive air leak may result inadequate oxygenation through positive-pressure ventilation and would lead to a conversion to open thoracotomy, decortications and muscle flap insertion onto the leaking bronchopleural fistula.

6.4 Alternative Methods of Empyema Management

1. In children and sometimes in adult empyema, insertion of small-bore pigtail catheter and instillations of urokinase have been carried out in many centres. The urokinase in appropriate doses are instilled twice a day and then clapped for half

an hour before connecting the drain to a low-pressure suction. Advantages include: it is performed under ultrasound guidance with a small-bore drain. It is found to be effective in a multicentre randomised trial from the UK [6, 7]. However the results have been disputed by other trials and adult studies [8–10]. The disadvantages of this method include requirement of anaesthesia mainly in young children, possibility that it may not result in adequate drainage, requires active monitoring and is not effective in later stages of empyema.

2. Mini-thoracotomy: Mini- or lateral thoracotomy sometimes can be achieved by sparing muscle approach in order to perform debridement and decortication. This still remains the gold standard in instances where thoracoscopic techniques are not available and in cases where other therapies have failed. Open method should allow reasonable exposure and allow dissection of layers fibrous visceral pleural covering to achieve decortications and full expansion of underlying lung parenchyma. There is more chance of bleeding and requirement of intensive care postoperatively in an open technique. In contrast, thoracoscopy requires expertise and team that is used to this form of operative technique. While conversions are always a possibilities and insertion of additional muscle flap can only be achieved by an open method, minimally invasive technique achieves the same objective with reduced requirement of pain relief and morbidity of open operation.

6.5 Variations and Complex Presentations

6.5.1 Failed Urokinase Therapy

The early insertion of muscle flap onto a bronchopleural fistula along with a limited decortication allows early resolution of and re-expansion of the lung as described in 2004 [5] and was subsequently audited with a longer-term outcome [2]. It is effective in children as it occupies less intrathoracic space compared to bulky muscles and is easily available along the thoracotomy incision. Not all failures of urokinase will require open operation; most can be adequately managed by thoracoscopic technique achieving adequate drainage/debridement/decortications and expansion of the underlying collapsed lung. Previous urokinase instillation is likely to cause more bleeding compared to primary thoracoscopy.

6.5.2 Failure of Thoracoscopy to Adequately Manage Empyema Debridement

It is possible during thoracoscopy that all the loculations may not have been broken down and the debridement was not complete. This in addition to administration of inappropriate antibiotics may not result in full postoperative lung expansion (Fig. 6.2). Any empyema management strategy should be appropriately monitored postoperatively so that principle aims of management can be achieved. Adequate analgesia, physiotherapy and appropriate antibiotics should be continued postoperatively after any empyema strategy. In case there is evidence of continuing sepsis and

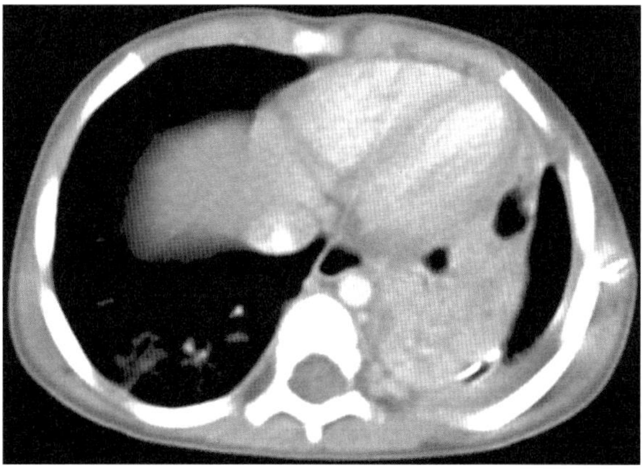

Fig. 6.2 Failed thoracoscopic debridement. CT scan with IV contrast with continuing collapsed lung left lower lobe (*arrow*). There is residual pneumothorax

demonstration of collection within pleural cavity in association with collapsed underlying lung parenchyma, the intervention to deal with this recurrence should be carried out. In an expert hand, repeat VATS drainage and decortication can be achieved. However this should be evaluated carefully, and open decortication may be required if the objective cannot be achieved through VATS techniques.

6.5.3 Pyopneumothorax and Necrotic Pneumonia

Spontaneous tension pneumothorax and pyopneumothorax can be present from the outset and will require urgent management, as it can be a life-threatening emergency (Fig. 6.3a). Additionally, if the patient requires positive-pressure ventilation, the preferential leakage of oxygen through the bronchopleural fistula and intercostal drain results. In this situation selective intubation of contralateral bronchus or alternatively high-frequency oscillatory ventilation is required to achieve adequate oxygenation. This situation is fortunately rare but requires careful medical and surgical management in order to successfully treat bronchopleural fistula, empyema and possibly underlying necrotic pneumonia.

Empyema associated with necrotic pneumonia is associated with morbidity even after successful management of empyema. The diagnosis of underlying necrosis within the consolidated lung can only be accurately defined using computed tomography with intravenous contrast. Prolonged antibiotic treatment may be required in this group of cases. In the presence of significant lung parenchymal damage, ventilatory support may be necessary in the pre- and postoperative period.

Resectional surgery advocated by some including pneumonectomy is significant and radical step to undertake and is associated with significant postoperative morbidity and even mortality [11, 12]. It is very difficult to distinguish and identify recoverable lung parenchyma from consolidated and collapsed lung. Therefore, it is prudent not to undertake resection in acute stage but merely carry out adequate empyema debridement/decortications and then contemplate resection if required. In most children as suggested by our experience, resection of necrotic pneumonia is not necessary (Fig. 6.3b). However, despite good medical management,

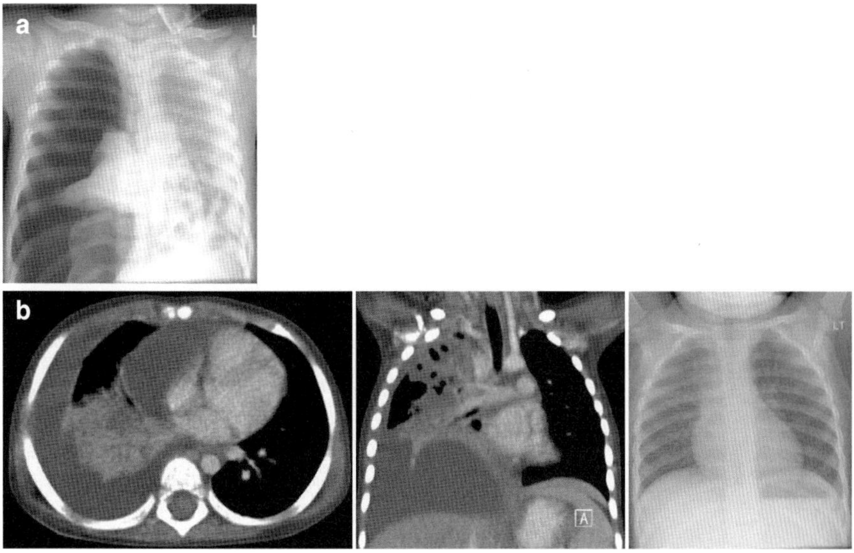

Fig. 6.3 Pyopneumothorax. (**a**) Chest radiograph showing tension pneumothorax. (**b**) Pyopneumothorax: CT scan with IV contrast showing the pyopneumothorax and necrotic pneumonia. Chest radiograph showing outcome following lateral thoracotomy and insertion of serratus anterior digitation flap successfully containing the bronchopleural fistula

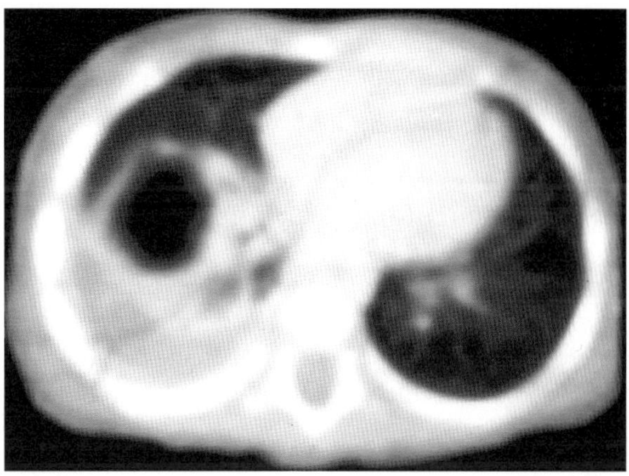

Fig. 6.4 Residual pneumatocele following debridement of empyema. CT scan showing pneumatocele in a consolidated lung

resection of the affected lung in the underdeveloped country may become a life-saving surgery [12].

6.5.4 Pneumatocele in Consolidated Lung

The outcome of empyema associated with pneumatocele depends on adequate post-operative lung expansion and appropriate antibiotic therapy. Pneumatoceles will generally resolve after debridement or decortication of the empyema (Fig. 6.4).

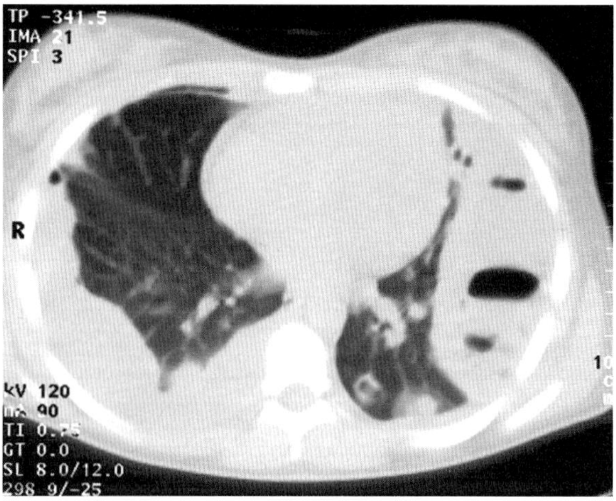

Fig. 6.5 Bilateral empyema. CT scan with IV contrast showing bilateral empyema and multiple abscesses

6.5.5 Bilateral Empyema

Bilateral empyema can be a complication of necrotising mediastinitis following oesophageal injury related to dilatation of its stricture. Bilateral empyema is occasionally encountered in infants, immunocompromised patients and bulimic adolescents with recurrent aspirations. Bilateral empyema has been successfully managed with VATS debridement. Multiple lung abscesses as seen in the CT scan were successfully managed with VATS debridement and appropriate antibiotics and antifungal (Fig. 6.5).

6.5.6 Tuberculous Empyema

This Asian girl with a history of tuberculosis contact and spiking temperature required thoracoscopic drainage and pleural biopsy to achieve the diagnosis of tuberculosis (Fig. 6.6). In most tuberculosis cases, the associated pleural effusion gets secondarily infected causing empyema. In these instances the empyema is managed in a usual way.

6.5.7 Secondary Empyema: Ruptured Oesophagus Following Balloon Dilatation

Oesophageal injury following stricture dilatations (balloon or rigid Savary-Gilliard bougies) can result in mediastinitis and leakage of saliva and food content in the pleural cavity resulting in empyema (Fig. 6.7a, b). In children button battery and accidental ingestion of corrosive agents such as bleach may result in oesophageal rupture. Descending mediastinitis from injury in the neck or penetrating chest

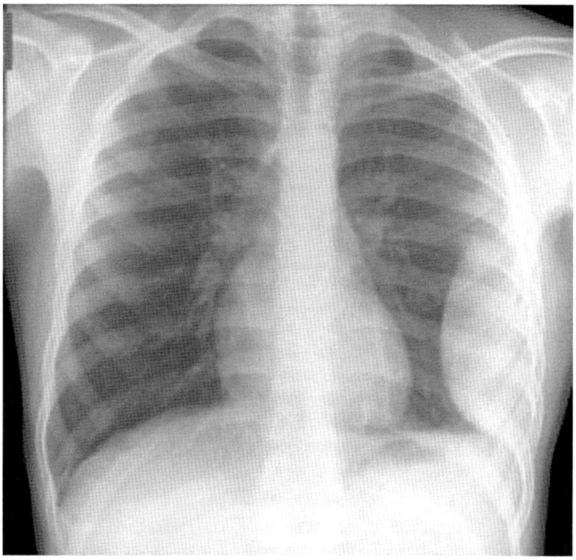

Fig. 6.6 Tuberculous empyema. Chest radiograph showing an effusion in an Asian child with TB contact

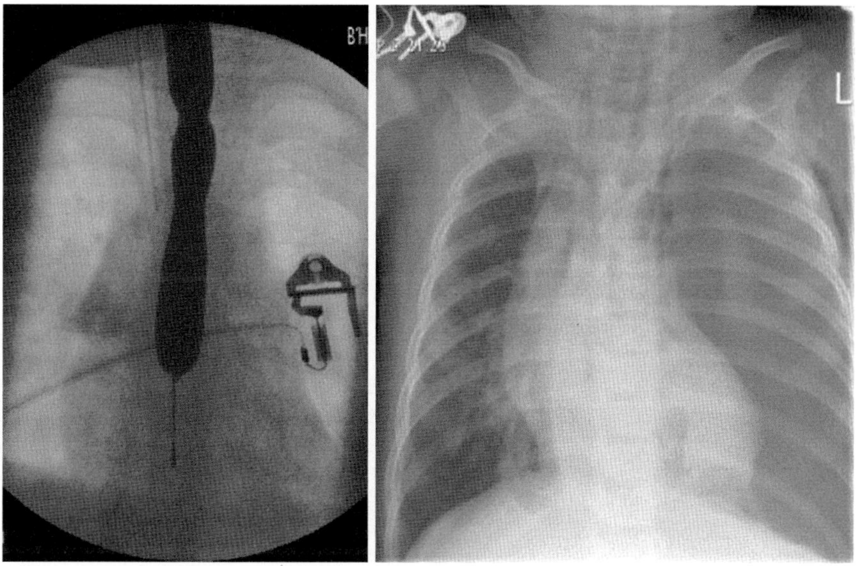

Fig. 6.7 Secondary empyema. Balloon dilatation performed under fluoroscopic control and subsequent chest radiograph showing pleural effusion containing milk and saliva

injuries is also recorded to cause empyema. Early detection and institution of appropriate management are the keys to the outcome of the oesophageal injury and secondary infection from penetrating injury. Post-blunt traumatic lung contusion and secondary infection have resulted in empyema. These cases should be managed by early detection and debridement of pleural cavity by VATS.

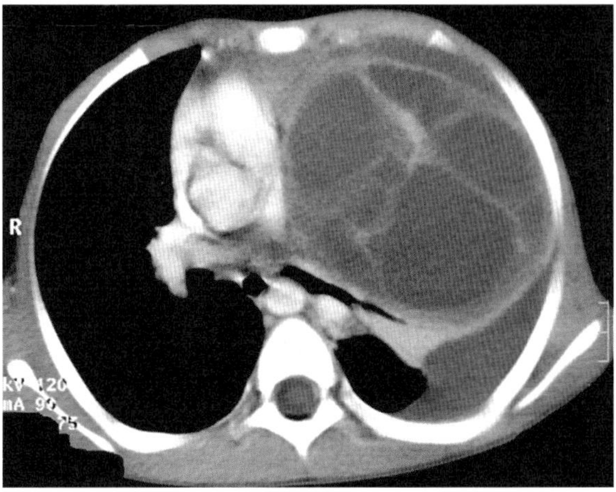

Fig. 6.8 Thoracic tumours presenting as empyema. CT scan with IV contrast showing a mediastinal teratoma and empyema

6.5.8 Thoracic Tumours, Congenital Lung Lesions and Other Conditions Presenting as Empyema

Many thoracic tumours, infection in congenital lung lesions and bacterial infection in parasitic lesions may be presented as empyema [1, 13]. The clinical features, inflammatory parameters and plain radiography are indistinguishable from empyema. CT scan with intravenous contrast is the only preoperative investigation that may be able to identify underlying pathology [14] (Fig. 6.8). The strategy to solely rely on ultrasound to diagnose empyema before intervention carries risk of missing the lung parenchymal and mediastinal pathology. Infected congenital lung lesion can look similar radiologically on preoperative CT scan and is not possible to differentiate it from consolidated lung with cavitatory lesions. These pathological lesions in first instance should be left alone in acute infective stage unless it is very early and inflammation is minimal. Persistence of cavitary lesions in the follow-up radiology would be an indication for their resection.

A biopsy should be taken if solid mass is encountered during empyema management for the histological diagnosis. The figure shown above was a benign teratoma with empyema at the same time that was resected in an open operation. Due to the cystic nature of the mediastinal tumour, biopsy was thought not to be a prudent decision and complete resection was carried out.

Conclusions

Adequate drainage of the empyema and re-expansion of collapsed lung remain the fundamental principles of empyema management. Despite controversy probably related to lack of evidence and number of studies trying to reinvent the past experience, the best management strategy should focus on the final outcome. It is not always possible to rationalise one strategy suitable to all pathological stages of empyema. However, early VATS debridement tends to produce very good results and very few complications. The insertion of ultrasound-guided pigtail catheters and instillation of fibrinolytics may play a role in the early stages of empyema, but these patients must be monitored and referred for surgical intervention if the response is less than adequate.

References

1. Parikh DH. Empyema thoracis. In: Parikh DH, Crabb DCG, Auldist A, Rothenberg S, editors. Pediatric thoracic surgery. London: Springer; 2009. p. 109–27.
2. Jester I, Nijran A, Singh M, Parikh DH. Surgical treatment of bronchopleural fistula in paediatric empyema: efficacy of the serratus anterior digitation flap. J Pediatr Surg. 2012;47(7):1358–62.
3. Ramphul N, Eastham KM, Freeman R, Eltringham G, Kearns AM, Leeming JP, et al. Cavitatory lung disease complicating empyema in children. Pediatr Pulmonol. 2006;41:750–3.
4. Bishay M, Short M, Shah K, Nagraj S, Arul S, Parikh D, Jawaheer G. Efficacy of video-assisted thoracoscopic surgery in managing childhood empyema: a large single centre study. J Pediatr Surg. 2009;44(2):337–42.
5. Hallows MR, Parikh DH. Surgical management of children with pyopneumothorax: serratus anterior digitation flap. J Pediatr Surg. 2004;39(7):1122–4.
6. Thomson AH, Hull J, Kumar MR, Wallis C, Balfour-Lynn IM. Randomised trial of intrapleural urokinase in the treatment of childhood empyema. Thorax. 2002;57:343–7.
7. Balfour-Lynn IM, Abrahamson E, Cohen G, et al. BTS guidelines for management of pleural infection in children. Thorax. 2005;60(Suppl 1):i1–21.
8. Avansino JR, Goldman B, Sawin RS, Flum DR. Primary operative versus nonoperative therapy for pediatric empyema: a meta-analysis. Pediatr. 2005;115(6):1652–9.
9. Maskell NA, Davies CWH, Nunn AJ, Hedly EL, Gleeson FV, Miller R, et al. UK controlled trial of intrapleural streptokinase for pleural infection. N Engl J Med. 2005;352(9):865–74.
10. Heffner JE. Multicenter trials of treatment for empyema after all these years. Editorials. N Engl J Med. 2005;352(9):926–7.
11. Hacimustafaoglu M, Celebi S, Sarimehmet H, Gurpinar A, Ercan I. Necrotizing pneumonia in children. Acta Paediatr. 2004;93:1172–7.
12. Ayed AK, Al-Rowayeh A. Lung resection in children for infectious pulmonary disease. Pediatr Surg Int. 2005;21(8):604–8.
13. Parikh DH. Empyema thoracis. In: Burge DM, Griffiths DM, Steinbrecher HA, Wheeler RA, editors. Paediatric surgery. 2nd ed. London: Hodder Arnold; 2005. p. 283–9.
14. Sharif K, Alton H, Clarke J, Desai M, Morland B, Parikh DH. Paediatric thoracic tumours presenting as empyema. Pediatr Surg Int. 2006;22(12):1009–14. Epub 13 Oct 2006.

Bronchiectasis

7

Rajan Santhosham

Abstract

Incidence of Broncheictasis in the developing world is still significant. The emergence of bacterial resistance to antibiotics, immunocompromised patients, hospital- and community-acquired pneumonia and suppurative lung diseases and re-emergence of tuberculosis are the main causes of bronchiectasis. Better understanding of the disease process, early diagnosis and good medical management may avoid surgery and its associated complications. Surgery in localized bronchiectasis in association with good pulmonary reserve produces low morbidity and good long-term outcome. Preoperative preparations with good anaesthetic considerations are essential components of successful surgical outcome. Video-assisted thoracoscopic surgery (VATS) resection in bronchiectasis requires advanced thoracoscopic skills.

Keywords

Bronchiectasis · Recurrent chest infections · Pneumonia · Tuberculosis Lobectomy · Bronchoscopy · Physiotherapy

7.1 Introduction

The term bronchiectasis is derived from a Greek word and basically describes an abnormal and permanent dilatation of bronchi. In the past, prior to antibiotic era, suppurative lung disease and tuberculosis were significant cause of mortality, and the survivors suffered from its resultant sequelae, bronchiectasis. Improvement in healthcare, immunization programme, understanding of the disease process and

R. Santhosham
Santosham Chest Hospital, Chennai, India

D. Parikh, P.B. Rajesh (eds.), *Tips and Tricks in Thoracic Surgery*,
https://doi.org/10.1007/978-1-4471-7355-7_7

administration of bacterial pathogen-specific antibiotics have resulted in significant reduction in complications of lower respiratory tract infections. There is recorded increase in community-acquired pneumonia and empyema in western countries; however, the incidence of bronchiectasis has remained low [1, 2]. In developing countries various factors such as inappropriate management of lower respiratory tract infections, malnutrition, tuberculosis, HIV, poverty and overcrowding are responsible for pleuropulmonary suppurative diseases and bronchiectasis [3].

Tracheobronchial tree has natural mucociliary and other immune defence mechanisms that protect against inhaled bacterial pathogens. Recurrent chest infections cripple the defences and result in breach and subsequent destruction of bronchial wall and scarring. Destruction of elastic and muscular component of bronchial wall generally starts from segmental bronchi as the lower branches of bronchial tree have least amount of cartilaginous support resulting in bronchial dilatation and stasis of mucous. As the bronchial dilatation and the cilia loss from respiratory tract lining continue, the respiratory lining is replaced with cuboidal and squamous epithelium; hypertrophy of bronchial glands, lymphadenitis and vascular inflammation occur. These changes cripple the airway defences further and promote recurrent bacterial invasion resulting in vicious cycle of ongoing infection. Depending on the area of involvement, the resultant bronchiectasis may be either localized or diffuse.

Recurrent respiratory tract infection, excessive and foul smelling sputum production and haemoptysis are the most common clinical features. Bronchiectasis may arise from various aetiologies that can either be genetic, congenital or acquired. Increase in immunocompromised cases from transplantation or cancer therapy, emergence of antibiotic-resistant organisms, drug abuse, increasing incidence of tuberculosis and HIV, migration of people for economic reasons and overcrowding can all lead to recurrent lower respiratory tract infections and bronchiectasis. The reader is advised to read causes of bronchiectasis from thoracic surgery textbooks or review articles. Bronchiectasis after an infective episode is frequently located in basal segments of lower lobes and middle lobe; in contrast, bronchiectasis associated with congenital or genetic causes is likely to be diffuse and bilateral. Bronchiectasis caused by bronchial obstruction external (TB lymph node) or endobronchial (unrecognized inhaled FB) is limited to the affected lobe [4].

7.2 Classification

Pathological classifications are academic interest as these descriptive anatomical variations have very little associations with clinical symptoms.

1. Dry: bronchiectasis sicca – post-tubercular bronchiectasis with symptom of haemoptysis. This is commonly seen in India.
2. Wet
   - Cylindrical or fusiform – bronchi are uniformly dilated and have regular outline.

- Saccular – extensive damage peripheral bronchi are dilated forming cystic spaces. Occasionally air-fluid level is also visible on x-ray.
- Mixed/varicose – varying degree of irregular beaded appearance of bronchi.

Lady Windermere syndrome refers to bronchiectasis with centrilobular nodules, eventual scarring and volume loss affecting the middle lobe and lingula. This syndrome is described in infection caused by *Mycobacterium avium complex* (MAC).

The medical and surgical management are based on clinical symptoms, and the extent surgical resection is based on anatomical distribution of bronchiectasis.

Resections should not be carried out only on radiological images alone.

Bronchiectasis is often progressive without management.

Temporary dilation of airway is with collapse of adjacent parenchyma, is sometimes called "pseudobronchiectasis" or "prebronchiectasis" and is fully recoverable, but on occasion it may progress to permanent changes [5, 6]. These changes are much more common in Pediatric practice.

Early symptoms may be non-specific but with recurrent chest infections associated with chronic cough with productive sputum often worse in the morning with relative symptom-free periods.

Breathlessness on exertion can suggest widespread disease. Haemoptysis and chest pain can be encountered and sometimes are the presenting symptoms. Clinical signs are characteristically non-specific, malnourishment, failure to thrive, finger clubbing, bronchial breathing and coarse crepitation on auscultation. Mild, moderate and severe disease can be classified as per clinical symptomatology and may be more relevant.

Investigations are directed towards diagnosis of the causative aetiology and assess the extent and severity of the bronchiectasis by means of high-resolution CT scanning (HRCT). Chest x-rays are of limited value and non-specific such as changes of atelectasis, compensatory hyperinflation, tramlining suggestive of dilated bronchi or ring-shaped cystic spaces as honeycomb are suggestive of bronchiectasis.

Bronchography is rarely performed. Bronchoscopy is useful in children to diagnose inhaled FB and allow bacteriological specimen for effective antibiotic therapy. Upper gastrointestinal contrast study to diagnose either achalasia or gastro-oesophageal reflux is indicated if suspected as the cause of bronchiectasis. Ventilation perfusion scans are useful for determining the function prior to consideration of localized disease and preserving the functioning parenchyma.

7.3 Medical Management

In mild disease, although the bronchiectatic disease is seen radiologically, the symptoms are minimal and can easily be controlled with medical management with postural physiotherapy and antibiotics during acute exacerbations.

In moderate disease the clinical symptoms are significant and affect the quality of life and interfere with daily life style. Aggressive medical management with specific antibiotics and postural physiotherapy to improve drainage of secretion and reduce recurrent lower respiratory tract infections is mainstay of controlling symptoms [7]. However, in cases where no improvement is noticeable, and recurrent overflow infections to other unaffected lobes, surgery should be considered.

In severe disease symptoms are not controllable with conservative aggressive management, and surgical option is considered in localized disease preserving less affected areas.

Underlying aetiology should be fully investigated as its effective management can reduce episodes of acute exacerbations. If effective, the bronchiectasis may remain static and have prolonged asymptomatic periods and can be monitored in outpatient review with occasional radiology. In order for the postural drainage to be effective, patients and, in the case of children, parents should be educated and trained.

Antibiotics for acute lower respiratory tract infections based on sputum cultures or upper respiratory secretions in high and prolonged courses can reduce the progress further courses of broad-spectrum oral antibiotics for several weeks are known to clear secretions and bacterial overgrowths. Some physicians routinely prescribed prophylactic antibiotics during winter months to prevent infections progressing to lower respiratory tract. Immunization is mandatory to avoid viral and pneumococcal infections. The mucolytic agents and aerosolized recombinant deoxyribonuclease are beneficial in patients with cystic fibrosis [8]. Bronchodilators are useful in presence of bronchospasms.

7.4 Surgical Management

Before embarking on surgical resection in bronchiectasis: The surgeon should make sure all the underlying aetiology has been fully investigated, the bronchial damage is irreversible and there is no active infection. The symptoms are affecting the patient's life style, schooling, growth; as it is not just the radiological diagnosis and medical management has been given adequate time. It is important for surgeon to make sure the disease is resectable as delineated by HRCT [9].

- Surgical resection should remove bronchiectatic segment or lobe safely, preserve reasonable functioning lung parenchyma and not compromise pulmonary reserve.
- Patients with localized bronchiectasis are most likely to benefit from surgical resection.
- Surgical resection is beneficial in children with recurrent symptoms despite adequate and intensive medical management.
- Surgery is essential to manage the aetiology such as inhaled FB, gastro-oesophageal reflux and achalasia cardia causing chronic recurrent aspiration pneumonia.

7.4.1 Preoperative Considerations

A thorough and guideline-based preoperative preparations are essential and are known to reduce intraoperative and postoperative complications. Intensive preoperative intravenous culture-specific antibiotics, preoperative bronchoscopy if considered essential to suck out as much secretion from bronchiectatic segment and physiotherapy are essential components to improve preoperative status.

7.4.2 Anaesthetic Considerations

Intubation should be performed in semi-supine position especially in patients with significant secretions.

Double-lumen tubes or bronchial blockers are essential and must be used in order to avoid contamination of contralateral lung during surgery. In young children it is not feasible to use a double-lumen tube in which blockage can be achieved by flexible bronchoscopy selectively Fogarty catheter insertion and inflating its balloon in the bronchiectatic lobe. Selective intubation of right side bronchus is possible if the left side needs surgery in children.

Prior to intubation bronchoscopy, it is essential to clear the secretions as much as possible making sure that if a FB is seen that is not disturbed as its removal may cause flooding of purulent secretions in the tracheobronchial tree.

Pre-emptive analgesia with thoracic epidural prior to surgical incision is shown to allow postoperative coughing and reduce postoperative atelectasis.

7.4.3 Surgical Technical Tips and Tricks

Examine preoperative HRCT so as to be familiar with segmental or lobar anatomy prior to resection.

The incision and entry into the chest has to be decided according to the site of the lesion and size of hemithorax. Sometimes the entire hemithorax can be grossly contracted. Fissures have to be carefully dissected with minimal air leak. The involved lung may be very adherent, grossly atelectatic and contracted. Chest wall adhesions should be carefully dissected.

Dissection in inflamed and indurated hilum: Vessels should be painstakingly dissected free from inflamed and sometimes matted lymph nodes. It may be necessary to dissect vessels underneath their adventitia. Good haemostasis while dissecting inflamed lymph nodes should be carried out with judicious use of bipolar diathermy. Large vessels should be doubly ligated. In presence of large lymph nodes that are difficult to dissect off the hilar vessels, more distal intra-parenchymal subdivisions can be identified and divided between ligatures. Specific attention should be paid to significantly large bronchial vessels as bleeding from them can be significant if retracted. The bronchus is thin and could tear easily; therefore, a careful interrupted suturing should be done in order to avoid postoperative complications. Excessive devascularization or trauma caused by aggressive use of diathermy is the main cause of postoperative bronchopleural fistula. Excessive sutures can also lead to devascularization and may result in fistula formation. Stapled closure of bronchus is appropriate, if applied making it sure not to include surrounding vessels.

VATS resection of bronchiectatic lobe or segment requires advanced minimally invasive techniques. Magnified vision, less postoperative pain and reduced handling and manipulation of the lung are the main reasons for undertaking thoracoscopic resections.

7.5 Postoperative Complications

Prolonged air leak: Air leaks from raw fibrotic or consolidated adjoining lung parenchyma are common in segmental resection. Careful checking prior to chest closure is vital in bronchiectasis surgery. Visceral pleura closure of adjoining parenchyma is known to reduce these annoying leaks. In lobectomy if the bronchus is closed with care, bronchopleural fistula is unlikely occurrence. However, if significant in immediate postoperative phase, it is prudent to reoperate in order to contain the leak with primary suturing if the bronchial stump is healthy. If the bronchial stump is thin and necrotic, it may be necessary to bring a vascularized pedicled muscle flap appropriate to resection carried out, size of the thoracic cavity, the capacity of the residual lung to re-expand and pulmonary reserve. Post-lobectomy empyema should be avoided. If the remaining lung is also severely affected and patient with poor respiratory reserve, it may be necessary to bring in a large pedicled muscle flap to occupy the residual thoracic cavity.

Bleeding: The sutures from the ligated vessels may come off during postoperative coughing fit or related to raised pressures or inappropriate ligatures. The bleeding in this instant is significant and requires immediate surgical intervention to identify the source of bleeding and ligating it securely. In certain instance it may be necessary to trace the main vessel inside the pericardium by opening it and then securely ligating uninflammed vessel.

Inflammatory bleeding from minor vessels can be defined and securely sutured with fine suture ligation.

Postoperative atelectasis: Avoiding contamination of the contralateral lung during surgery should prevent this complication. However, in some instances in patients with poor respiratory reserve, ineffective coughing in presence of pain may result in atelectasis due to retained secretions. Postoperative physiotherapy with administration of effective pain relief helps re-expand the collapsed lung. In patients with poor lung reserve, positive pressure ventilation may be required to re-expand the lung parenchyma and achieve adequate oxygenation.

Conclusion

Efforts should be directed towards the prevention of suppurative lung disease and bronchiectasis. However, unlikely in many parts of the world, poverty, overcrowding, tuberculosis, HIV infection and emergence of bacterial resistance to known antibiotics are causing a significant concern. It is possible that overall incidence of bronchiectasis in years to come may rise. Therefore, it is essential to maintain adequate surgical skills to resect or perform lobectomy in infective conditions. Surgical skills to deal with infected lung parenchyma require good understanding and experience to reduce associated morbidity and mortality. Further research is necessary to introduce a new generation of antibiotics against emerging bacterial resistance are also essential.

References

1. Rees JH, Spencer DA, Parikh DH. Increase in incidence of childhood empyema in West midlands. Lancet. 1997;349:402.
2. Byrington CL, Spencer LY, Johnson TA, et al. An epidemiological investigation of a sustained high rate of pediatric parapneumonic empyema: risk factors and microbiological associations. Clin Infect Dis. 2002;34:434–40.
3. Karakoc GB, Yilmaz M, Altintas DU, et al. Bronchiectasis still a problem. Pediatr Pulmonol. 2001;32:175–8.
4. Hewitson JP, Von Oppell UO. The role of thoracic surgery for childhood tuberculosis. World J Surg. 1997;21:468–74.
5. Gillard EA, Carty H, Heaf D, et al. Reversible bronchial dilatation in children: comparison of serial high-resolution computer tomography scans of the lung. Eur J Radiol. 2003;47:215–20.
6. Spencer DA. From hemp seed to porcupine quill to HRCT. Advances in the diagnosis and epidemiology of bronchiectasis. Arch Dis Child. 2005;90:712–4.
7. Jones AP, Rowe BH. Bronchopulmonary hygiene physical therapy in chronic obstructive pulmonary disease and bronchiectasis (Cochrane Review). The Cochrane Library 1988; 3.
8. Dinwiddie R. Pathogenesis of lung disease in cystic fibrosis. Respiration. 2000;67(1):3–8.
9. Hewitson JP. Bronchiectasis. In: Pediatric thoracic surgery. Eds. Parikh DH, Crabbe DCG, Rothenbergh S, Aldist A. London: Springer; 2009; 169–178.

Fungal Infections: Current Role of Thoracic Surgeons in Cases of Pulmonary Aspergillosis

8

Masaaki Sato and Hiroshi Date

Abstract

Among pulmonary fungal infections, aspergillosis poses a major challenge to thoracic surgeons. Aspergilloma classically arises in preexisting cavitary lesions secondary to previous tuberculosis; more recently, they have also been linked to other underlying lung diseases such as sarcoidosis, bronchiectasis, and emphysema. Because the effect of systemic antifungal agents is usually limited, life-threatening hemoptysis and/or deterioration of a patient's general condition often necessitates surgical intervention. Surgical strategies for pulmonary aspergillomas range from radical pulmonary resection and semi-radical cavernostomy with or without muscle-flap transposition and thoracoplasty to conservative intracavitary instillation of antifungal agents. To select an optimal strategy, it is important to understand the nature of the patient's aspergilloma—noninvasive or invasive (chronic necrotizing pulmonary aspergillosis), simple or complex—in association with the underlying pulmonary condition.

Acute invasive pulmonary aspergillosis, which usually arises in immunocompromised patients, may also necessitate surgical resection in selected cases, such as those involving lesions that are contiguous with the chest wall, great vessels, or pericardium.

Lung transplantation is another area in which pulmonary aspergillosis is a significant challenge. Preexisting aspergillomas elevate the risk associated with lung transplantation, mandating careful patient selection, and cautious surgical and medical management. Posttransplant aspergillosis can manifest as invasive bronchial aspergillosis, typically at healing bronchial anastomoses, or as acute invasive pulmonary aspergillosis followed by diffuse pneumonia. Both conditions remain the important causes of graft dysfunction and patient death.

M. Sato, M.D., Ph.D.
Department of Thoracic Surgery, The University of Tokyo, Tokyo, Japan
e-mail: satomasa@kuhp.kyoto-u.ac.jp

H. Date, M.D., Ph.D. (✉)
Department of Thoracic Surgery, Kyoto University, Kyoto, Japan
e-mail: hdate@kuhp.kyoto-u.ac.jp

D. Parikh, P.B. Rajesh (eds.), *Tips and Tricks in Thoracic Surgery*,
https://doi.org/10.1007/978-1-4471-7355-7_8

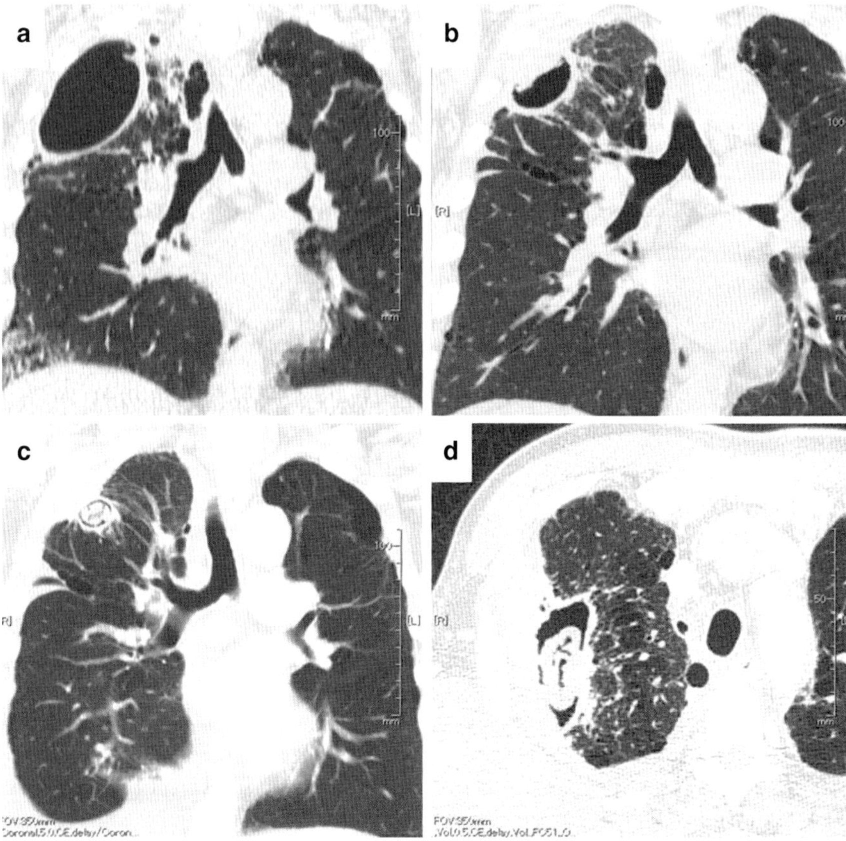

Fig. 8.2 Pulmonary aspergilloma arising in a preexisting cavitary lesion secondary to pulmonary emphysema. (**a**) Bullous lesion in the right upper lobe. (**b**) Thickening of the bulla wall accompanied with mild fever and systemic inflammatory responses. (**c**, **d**) Formation of an aspergilloma in the cavity

opposed to the colonization of a preexisting cavity seen with the latter, CNPA represents a focally invasive form of aspergillosis that eventually undergoes central necrosis and cavitation, forming its own cavity. The finding of tissue invasion distinguishes CNPA from a more common noninvasive aspergilloma.

Acute invasive aspergillosis is commonly called "invasive pulmonary aspergillosis" or angioinvasive aspergillosis, and it usually arises in immunocompromised patients (e.g., transplant recipients, patients undergoing chemotherapy). A halo sign—a macronodule ≥1 cm in diameter that is surrounded by a perimeter of ground-glass opacity—is often an early indicator of acute invasive aspergillosis (Fig. 8.4a) [5]. Without effective medical treatment, this form of pulmonary aspergillosis tends to rapidly advance into diffuse pneumonia (Fig. 8.4b). Although antifungal agents are the mainstay of treatment for acute invasive aspergillosis, selected cases necessitate surgical intervention (as discussed later).

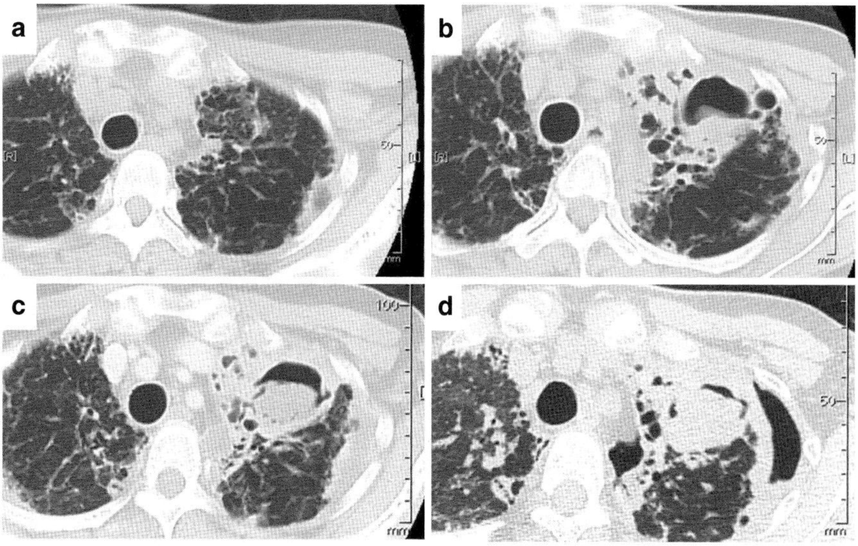

Fig. 8.3 Case of chronic necrotizing pulmonary aspergillosis (CNPA) arising in the presence of underlying pulmonary fibrosis. (**a**) Focally invasive pulmonary aspergillosis in the left upper lobe (note that there is no preexisting cavity). (**b**) Aspergillosis that has undergone central necrosis. (**c**) Formation of an aspergilloma secondary to central necrosis. (**d**) Chronic progression of necrosis into the surrounding lung tissue. The process from (**a**) to (**d**) took 1.5 years, illustrating the semi-invasiveness of CNPA. Although the end result at a given time point, such as at (**c**) or (**d**), is indistinguishable from that associated with a noninvasive type of aspergilloma, the time course enables their distinction, which is potentially important in selecting optimal surgical intervention

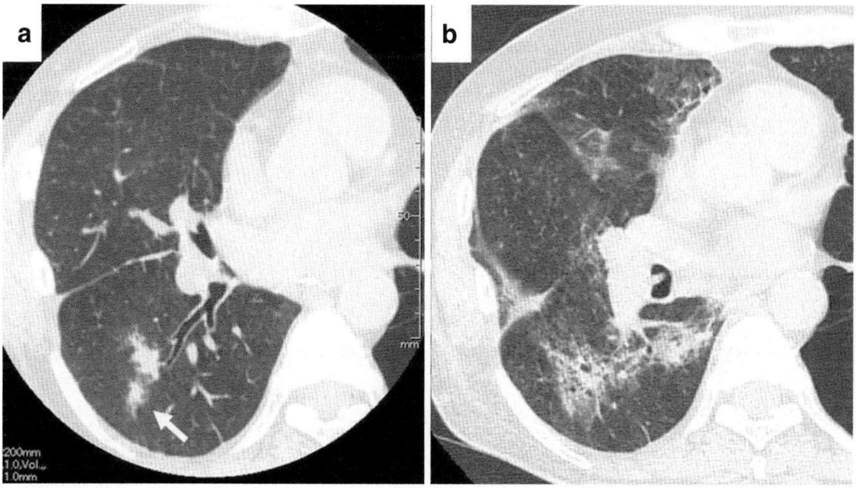

Fig. 8.4 Case of acute invasive pulmonary aspergillosis that occurred after lung transplantation. (**a**) A halo sign (arrow) was observed in association with multiple, newly emerged pulmonary nodules. The patient showed a mild fever and respiratory distress. (**b**) A week later, the disease process rapidly progressed into diffuse pneumonia that resulted in a fatal outcome

8.2.2 Classification of Aspergillomas

Aspergillomas are the most frequent targets of surgical intervention. In addition to categorizing them according to the invasiveness of the underlying aspergillosis, another useful classification is that proposed by Belcher and Plummer: simple and complex [6]. *Simple aspergillomas* are thin-walled cysts with little surrounding parenchymal lung disease. *Complex aspergillomas* are thick-walled cavities with substantial surrounding parenchymal disease and/or associated infiltrates, often connected to the thoracic wall by thick and extremely vascularized adhesions (Fig. 8.1). Complex aspergillomas often overlap with CPNA, representing a more invasive type of aspergilloma. Distinguishing between simple and complex forms is important in determining whether surgical management, such as resection, or more conservative management is indicated for a given aspergilloma; as discussed below, this distinction also aids in selecting the extent of pulmonary resection to be performed when surgery is required.

8.3 Surgical Management of Aspergillomas

Although there is controversy concerning the optimal management of aspergillomas, the role of medical management (antifungal agents) is limited. Because neither the size of the aspergilloma nor the associated clinical features predict the development of life-threatening hemoptysis, an aggressive approach is justified independent of the patient's symptoms [1]. Babatasi and colleagues, in a 39-year series of 80 patients, concluded that pulmonary resection is the best option whenever the diagnosis of aspergilloma has been confirmed and the patient is a suitable candidate for the operation [7]. However, in reality, many patients have limited pulmonary reserve, and pulmonary resection is often not optimal. In such cases, more conservative options should be considered (Fig. 8.5).

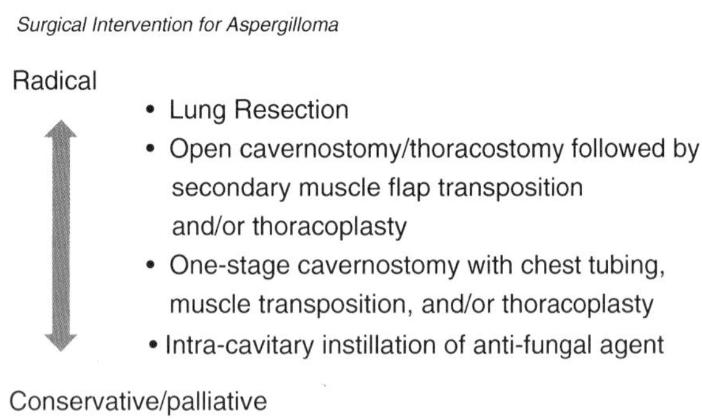

Fig. 8.5 Schematic diagram of surgical interventions for pulmonary aspergillomas. The optimal intervention for a given case should be selected based on the patient's pulmonary reserve and general condition

8.4 Technical Tips and Tricks for Lung Resection for Aspergilloma

The goals of lung resection performed for pulmonary aspergillomas are similar to those associated with resections performed for lung cancer: to completely resect the disease and to preserve pulmonary function as much as possible. The functional reserve of patients with pulmonary aspergillomas, especially complex aspergillomas, is usually limited secondary to the underlying pulmonary disease. Residual *Aspergillus* infection in the lung tissue can cause recurrence of the disease and contamination of the thoracic cavity (i.e., *Aspergillus* empyema). Each type of resection has its advantages and disadvantages. For example, limited resections, such as wedge resection or segmentectomy, may leave infected lung tissue behind, especially if the disease is invasive as with CNPA. Limited resection also necessitates stapling or dissection of the diseased lung, which tends to result in prolonged air leakage and ultimately in empyema. Conversely, major resections, such as lobectomy and pneumonectomy, are detrimental to pulmonary function and leave a large space in the chest. Particular attention should be paid to the fact that the diseased lung tends to expand poorly after lung resection, further aggravating the problem of the space left in the chest postoperatively [1]. Because bronchial fistula is a life-threatening complication, the use of buttress sutures and/or one-stage muscle-flap transposition is encouraged for reinforcing the bronchial stump [1].

In general, patients with complex aspergillomas are more prone to postoperative complications, as mentioned above [8]. The mortality rate of lung resection for aspergilloma has been reported to range from 0 to 44% [1]. In high-risk patients with chronic fibrosis and severe pleural-mediastinal adhesions, the mortality rate may exceed 25%, and complications related to hemorrhage, bronchopleural fistulas, and empyema may affect 60% of the patients [9]. However, in the last 20 years, a decrease in tuberculosis also reduced the incidence of complex aspergilloma, which has lessened operative challenges and led to significant decreases in postoperative mortality and morbidity. Despite this, some patients and types of operations remain extremely challenging. Pneumonectomy and pleuropneumonectomy should be avoided whenever possible because of the high associated morbidity and mortality [1]; pneumonectomy should be reserved for patients whose entire lung is destroyed (Fig. 8.6), and pleuropneumonectomy should only be applied in cases with severe, diffuse pleural adhesions and/or a contaminated pleural space.

8.5 Two-Stage Cavernostomy

Two-stage cavernostomy, i.e., open cavernostomy followed by secondary closure in combination with muscle-flap transposition and/or thoracoplasty, is a "semi-radical" procedure that may achieve eradication of the infection together with complete healing [10]. The first stage of the operation is essentially the same as that performed in an open thoracotomy for empyema in combination with cavernostomy:

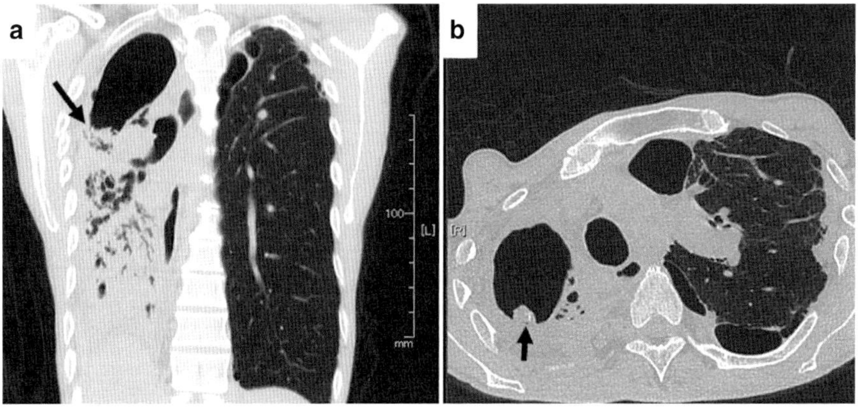

Fig. 8.6 Case of an aspergilloma accompanying a destroyed lung. The patient showed progressive destruction of the right lung from repetitive bronchopneumonia with multidrug-resistant *Pseudomonas aeruginosa*. Eventually, an aspergilloma developed in a cavitary lesion. Progressive weight loss and deterioration of the patient's general condition necessitated right pneumonectomy. Despite the latissimus dorsi muscle transposition onto the right main bronchial stump, the patient developed a bronchial fistula and contralateral pneumonia with *Pseudomonas*, which resulted in the patient's death

the pleura and the lung parenchyma over the cavitary lesion are dissected, the fungus ball is removed, and the cavity is cleaned as much as possible. Daily packing with gauze is performed for weeks to months, followed by the second stage of the operation, in which muscle-flap transposition and/or thoracoplasty are conducted to eliminate the space in exactly the same manner as in the second stage of the operation for empyema.

Because the second operation is electively conducted when eradication of the fungal infection is confirmed and the cavity is sufficiently cleaned, this procedure is considered semi-radical and potentially curative for *Aspergillus* infection.

There are several points to consider.

1. The pleura needs to be tightly adherent around the cavity when leaving it open; otherwise, the procedure may contaminate the pleural space, resulting in empyema. If limited adhesion is anticipated (e.g., in the presence of pleural fluid accumulation as in Figs. 8.2c, d), concurrent drainage with a chest tube is effective in eliminating the pleural space and excluding preexisting *Aspergillus* empyema.
2. The point of cavernostomy needs to be accurately predicted on the pleural surface; virtual 3D imaging, preoperative CT marking, and/or intraoperative ultrasound may help to facilitate this procedure.
3. Administration of an antifungal agent is recommended between the stages of the operation and for at least few weeks following closure of the thoracotomy.

After the first stage of the operation, a bronchial fistula often exists in the open space. Because the persistence of a bronchial fistula at the second operation is likely

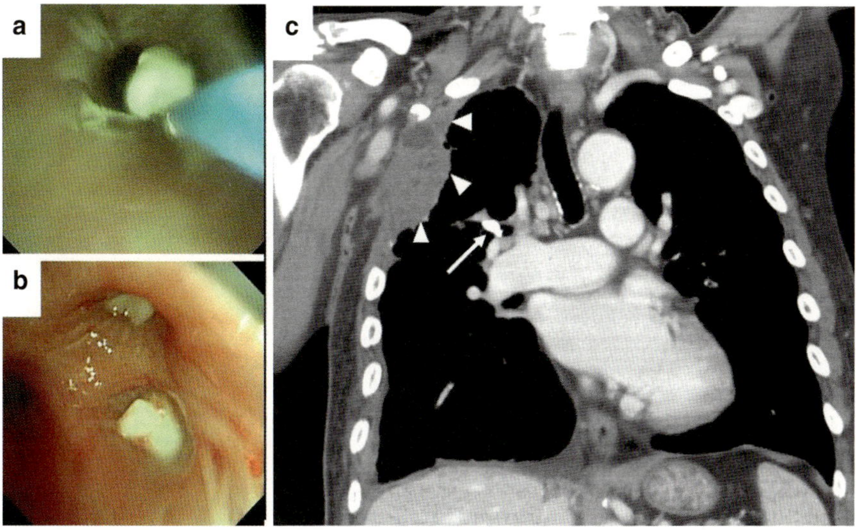

Fig. 8.7 Application of endobronchial Watanabe spigots (EWSs) during the interval between the operations in two-stage cavernostomy for aspergilloma. (**a**) Bronchoscopic placement of EWS using a bronchoscopic forceps in the right upper lobe bronchus after open cavernostomy/thoracotomy in the same patient shown in Fig. 8.2. (**b**) Two EWSs were placed in the subsegment bronchi of the right upper lobe. This procedure significantly reduced air leakage into the cavity. (**c**) CT scan after the second operation, in which the pectoralis major muscle flap was transpositioned into the cavity and fixed with nonabsorbable sutures (arrowheads). The arrow indicates an endobronchially implanted EWS

to increase its failure rate, we elect to transbronchially close such fistulas by bronchoscopically applying endobronchial Watanabe spigots [11] a few weeks before the planned second operation. This procedure eliminates direct air leakage from the bronchi even if minor air leakage from the pulmonary parenchyma persists (Fig. 8.7).

Unlike lung resection for aspergillomas, however, two-stage cavernostomy only eliminates the fungus ball, leaving the surrounding lung tissue behind; thus, if an active invasive component of the disease exists, the efficacy of this procedure would be limited. In other words, this procedure is only indicated for treating noninvasive aspergillomas that arise in a preexisting pulmonary cavity lesion or for CNPA that is controlled with antifungal medication.

8.6 One-Stage Cavernostomy

Although two-stage cavernostomy is a semi-radical strategy that avoids pulmonary resection, the procedure usually necessitates long-term hospitalization of the patient and strenuous involvement of thoracic surgeons. If a more palliative approach is appropriate or such lengthy surgical treatment is not affordable, one-stage cavernostomy is an option that may enable long-term control of *Aspergillus* infection [12]. Essentially, the cavernostomy is conducted in the same manner as described for the two-stage procedure. However, the chest wall is manipulated appropriately for one-stage muscle-flap transposition and/or thoracoplasty [12, 13]. One-stage cavernostomy can also be completed by leaving a chest tube in the cavity even without muscle-flap transposition or thoracoplasty [14]. Although the reported incidence of recurrence is relatively high, this option is considered acceptable by many palliative patients and surgeons.

8.7 Intracavitary Administration of Antifungal Agents

The direct intracavitary administration of amphotericin B, miconazole, micafungin, and other agents has been reported via either a percutaneously placed catheter or a bronchoscope. This conservative management has been reported to control hemoptysis in the short term [15] and may even achieve disappearance of the aspergilloma in more than half of the patients by some reports [16]. Because high hemoptysis recurrence rates have also been reported [15, 16], this conservative management should be reserved for inoperable, high-risk patients.

8.8 Role of Surgery in Acute Invasive Aspergillosis

The mainstay of treatment in cases of invasive aspergillosis is antifungal medications such as voriconazole and liposomal amphotericin B [17]. However, surgical resection of lung tissue invaded by *Aspergillus* may be useful in selected patients. Surgical resection of lesions that are contiguous with the great vessels or pericardium may prevent the erosion of pulmonary lesions into the great vessels and pericardial space. Additionally, the resection of lesions invading into the chest wall from the contiguous pulmonary area may relieve pain and prevent pleurocutaneous fistulas [17].

Hemoptysis is a life-threatening complication of invasive pulmonary aspergillosis; it is classically caused by erosion of the bronchial arteries. Embolization of involved blood vessels and cauterization can reduce hemorrhage and stabilize patients, but recurrence of bleeding is relatively frequent because of the complex network of neovascularized blood vessels typically involved. Because life-threatening hemoptysis is most frequently reported in patients already receiving antifungal chemotherapy, surgical resection may be the only option for successfully eradicating the focus [17].

8.9 Special Considerations Regarding Aspergillosis and Lung Transplantation

8.9.1 Indications for Lung Transplantation in a Patient with Aspergillosis

Although colonization with highly resistant or highly virulent fungi is a relative contraindication for lung transplantation, colonization with *Aspergillus* per se is not considered a contraindication for lung transplantation [18]. However, there is limited information available regarding the outcomes of lung transplantation in patients with pulmonary aspergillosis. Hadjiliadis et al. reported the outcomes of nine patients

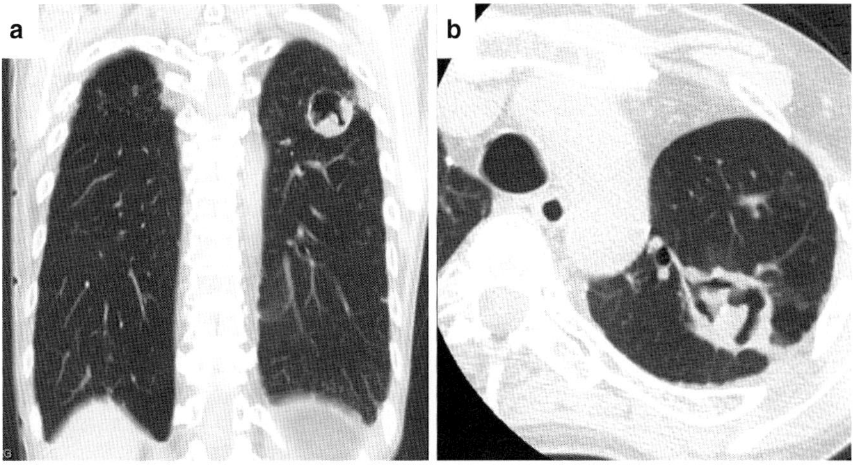

Fig. 8.8 Case of lung retransplantation for bronchiolitis obliterans syndrome in a patient whose first transplant was compromised by a pulmonary aspergilloma. Complete resection of the lung and perioperative antifungal prophylaxis resulted in successful long-term survival of the patient after the second bilateral lung transplant

whose explanted native lungs contained aspergillomas [19]. The underlying pulmonary diagnoses were sarcoidosis (six patients), emphysema, idiopathic pulmonary fibrosis, and pneumoconiosis. Four patients (44%) died in the first month after transplantation. Notably, however, only one of these four patients had received aggressive prophylaxis and had limited disease, suggesting that acceptable posttransplant survival is possible in carefully selected patients with sufficient pretransplant management [19]. Vadnerkar et al. also reported relatively poor outcomes for patients with pretransplant bronchopulmonary aspergillosis [20]. However, only one of the patient deaths in this study was attributed to invasive aspergillosis; the majority of mortality was considered to be a consequence of patients' comorbidities and associated secondary infections such as other fungi [20]. In our personal experience, lung transplantation has been successful in selected patients with aspergillomas (Fig. 8.8).

Taken together, the data suggest that pulmonary aspergillosis is not an absolute contraindication for lung transplantation. Selection criteria for lung transplant recipients with *Aspergillus* infection should include patient tolerance of aggressive pre- and posttransplant prophylaxis (ideally, sterilization of the airway culture would be achieved before transplantation), a radiographically localized disease process that can be removed during transplantation and minimal comorbidities. In addition, single-lung transplantation may not achieve adequate removal of fungal organisms and should probably be avoided.

8.9.2 Posttransplant Bronchopulmonary Aspergillosis

Lung transplant recipients are vulnerable to bronchopulmonary aspergillosis in three main forms: airway colonization, bronchial aspergillosis (usually at the bronchial anastomosis), and invasive pulmonary aspergillosis.

Clinically silent *airway colonization* may occur in up to 30% of patients within 6 months after transplantation [21] and has been suggested to increase the incidence of invasive aspergillosis and chronic lung allograft dysfunction. Because of the significant potential sequelae of airway colonization, monitoring of sputum culture (with or without measurement of serum galactomannan and precipitated antibodies) and prophylactic treatment with antifungal agents are generally recommended.

Bronchial aspergillosis tends to grow at healing bronchial anastomoses, leading to endobronchial complications such as necrosis, dehiscence, bronchoarterial fistulas, and/or excessive granulation and bronchial stenosis [21]. Conversely, abnormal bronchial healing processes at anastomoses, such as ischemia, necrosis, and dehiscence, make these sites vulnerable to *Aspergillus* infection. Close monitoring and preemptive antifungal therapy are recommended for patients with bronchial airway mechanical abnormalities [21]. Most bronchial anastomotic infections occur within 3 months of transplantation. In a previous study, although the early mortality of patients with bronchial anastomotic aspergillosis did not significantly differ from patients without aspergillosis, the patients with aspergillosis experienced reduced long-term survival [22]. Although the resulting airway stenosis is often treated by airway dilatation with or without stenting, surgical intervention is not usually indicated for the *Aspergillus* airway infection itself; medical management that includes systemic and topical antifungal agents (e.g., inhaled amphotericin B) is the treatment of choice.

Invasive or disseminated pulmonary aspergillosis tends to occur during the chronic phase after lung transplantation (2.8 years posttransplantation on average) and generally affects severely immunocompromised patients such as the patient shown in Fig. 8.4 [20]. Among lung transplant recipients, the overall incidence of invasive aspergillosis is as high as 17%, and it accounts for up to 9% of deaths in this population [23]. Reducing the intensity of immunosuppression and administering an antifungal agent are the treatments of choice.

8.9.3 Prophylaxis After Lung Transplantation

Given the high mortality associated with invasive aspergillosis and the risk of graft dysfunction following *Aspergillus* colonization among lung transplant recipients, an increasing emphasis has been placed on prophylaxis with antifungals. Accordingly, the majority of the centers performing lung transplantation have adopted universal or targeted antifungal prophylaxis such as months of orally administered voriconazole or itraconazole or the inhalation of amphotericin B (deoxycholate or lipid complex) [24]. However, a recent meta-analysis did not find a significant reduction in either invasive aspergillosis or *Aspergillus* colonization in association with universal anti-*Aspergillus* prophylaxis. The authors caution against over-interpreting these results because of the heterogeneity of the analyzed studies. A multicenter randomized controlled trial is necessary to accurately evaluate the efficacy of antifungal prophylaxis in lung transplant recipients [25].

8.10 Conclusions

Aspergillus infection remains a significant challenge for general thoracic and lung transplant surgeons. A complete understanding of this complex disease process and the multidimensional therapeutic strategies available are important in achieving optimal management of affected patients.

8.11 Pediatric Perspective

In most instances childhood pleuropulmonary opportunistic fungal infection is possible to manage with appropriate antifungal agents. However, surgeon may be asked to provide tissue diagnosis, to rule out malignancy, and to resect diseased lung causing complications such as hemoptysis, pneumothorax, or empyema [26]. The rising incidence of opportunistic fungal infection is reported in children surviving cancer, children with HIV infection, and children undergoing organ transplantation.

Histoplasmosis is endemic in certain parts of the world (Saharan Africa, Australia, Eastern Asia) due to inhalation of fungal spore found in soil and droppings of fowl and bats [26]. Although it assumes a benign course in majority, progressive disseminated histoplasmosis in immunocompromised children should be managed by intensive antifungal treatment. Surgical intervention is required when a persistent solitary pulmonary nodule or a hilar lymphadenopathy causes a diagnostic dilemma.

Aspergillus infection is extensively covered in chapter above. Allergic bronchopulmonary aspergillosis (ABPA) is seen in children with asthma and cystic fibrosis with high levels of IgE and responds well with corticosteroids.

Pulmonary candidiasis is seen in premature infants with prolonged ventilator requirements and receiving repeated and prolonged intravenous antibiotics, in children receiving intensive chemotherapy, and in children having to use central venous catheters for prolonged periods of time.

Coccidioidomycosis and blastomycosis both can cause granulomatous and cavitary lesions and may have similar presentation as aspergillosis and require surgical intervention for diagnosis and lung resection for complicating lesions.

References

1. Passera E, Rizzi A, Robustellini M, Rossi G, Della Pona C, Massera F, et al. Pulmonary aspergilloma: clinical aspects and surgical treatment outcome. Thorac Surg Clin. 2012;22(3):345–61.
2. Barnes PD, Marr KA. Aspergillosis: spectrum of disease, diagnosis, and treatment. Infect Dis Clin North Am. 2006;20(3):545–61.
3. Rafferty P, Biggs BA, Crompton GK, Grant IW. What happens to patients with pulmonary aspergilloma? Analysis of 23 cases. Thorax. 1983;38(8):579–83.
4. Nam HS, Jeon K, Um SW, Suh GY, Chung MP, Kim H, et al. Clinical characteristics and treatment outcomes of chronic necrotizing pulmonary aspergillosis: a review of 43 cases. Int J Infect Dis. 2010;14(6):e479–82.

5. Greene RE, Schlamm HT, Oestmann JW, Stark P, Durand C, Lortholary O, et al. Imaging findings in acute invasive pulmonary aspergillosis: clinical significance of the halo sign. Clin Infect Dis. 2007;44(3):373–9.
6. Belcher JR, Plummer NS. Surgery in bronchopulmonary aspergillosis. Br J Dis Chest. 1960;54:335–41.
7. Babatasi G, Massetti M, Chapelier A, Fadel E, Macchiarini P, Khayat A, et al. Surgical treatment of pulmonary aspergilloma: current outcome. J Thorac Cardiovasc Surg. 2000;119(5):906–12.
8. Kim YT, Kang MC, Sung SW, Kim JH. Good long-term outcomes after surgical treatment of simple and complex pulmonary aspergilloma. Ann Thorac Surg. 2005;79(1):294–8.
9. Chen JC, Chang YL, Luh SP, Lee JM, Lee YC. Surgical treatment for pulmonary aspergilloma: a 28 year experience. Thorax. 1997;52(9):810–3.
10. Regnard JF, Icard P, Nicolosi M, Spagiarri L, Magdeleinat P, Jauffret B, et al. Aspergilloma: a series of 89 surgical cases. Ann Thorac Surg. 2000;69(3):898–903.
11. Kurihara M, Kataoka H, Ishikawa A, Endo R. Latest treatments for spontaneous pneumothorax. Gen Thorac Cardiovasc Surg. 2010;58(3):113–9.
12. Grima R, Krassas A, Bagan P, Badia A, Le Pimpec Barthes F, et al. Treatment of complicated pulmonary aspergillomas with cavernostomy and muscle flap: interest of concomitant limited thoracoplasty. Eur J Cardiothorac Surg. 2009;36(5):910–3.
13. Ono N, Sato K, Yokomise H, Tamura K. Surgical management of pulmonary aspergilloma. Role of single-stage cavernostomy with muscle transposition. Jpn J Thorac Cardiovasc Surg. 2000;48(1):56–9.
14. Iuchi K, Tanaka H, Shirahasi K, Okura E, Katsura H, Matsumura A, et al. Cavernostomy and simultaneous removal of fungus ball of pulmonary aspergilloma. Nihon Kokyuki Gakkai Zasshi. 2001;39(12):903–9. [In Japanese].
15. Kravitz JN, Berry MW, Schabel SI, Judson MA. A modern series of percutaneous intracavitary instillation of amphotericin B for the treatment of severe hemoptysis from pulmonary aspergilloma. Chest. 2013;143(5):1414–21.
16. Giron J, Poey C, Fajadet P, Sans N, Fourcade D, Senac JP, et al. CT-guided percutaneous treatment of inoperable pulmonary aspergillomas: a study of 40 cases. Eur J Radiol. 1998;28(3):235–42.
17. Walsh TJ, Anaissie EJ, Denning DW, Herbrecht R, Kontoyiannis DP, Marr KA, et al. Treatment of aspergillosis: clinical practice guidelines of the Infectious Diseases Society of America. Clin Infect Dis. 2008;46(3):327–60.
18. Orens JB, Estenne M, Arcasoy S, Conte JV, Corris P, Egan JJ, et al. International guidelines for the selection of lung transplant candidates: 2006 update—a consensus report from the Pulmonary Scientific Council of the International Society for Heart and Lung Transplantation. J Heart Lung Transplant. 2006;25(7):745–55.
19. Hadjiliadis D, Sporn TA, Perfect JR, Tapson VF, Davis RD, Palmer SM. Outcome of lung transplantation in patients with mycetomas. Chest. 2002;121(1):128–34.
20. Vadnerkar A, Clancy CJ, Celik U, Yousem SA, Mitsani D, Toyoda Y, et al. Impact of mold infections in explanted lungs on outcomes of lung transplantation. Transplantation. 2010;89(2):253–60.
21. Solé A, Salavert M. Fungal infections after lung transplantation. Transplant Rev (Orlando). 2008;22(2):89–104.
22. Hadjiliadis D, Howell DN, Davis RD, Lawrence CM, Rea JB, Tapson VF, et al. Anastomotic infections in lung transplant recipients. Ann Transplant. 2000;5(3):13–9.
23. Husain S, Paterson DL, Studer S, Pilewski J, Crespo M, Zaldonis D, et al. Voriconazole prophylaxis in lung transplant recipients. Am J Transplant. 2006;6(12):3008–16.
24. Neoh CF, Snell G, Levvey B, Morrissey CO, Stewart K, Kong DC. Antifungal prophylaxis in lung transplantation. Int J Antimicrob Agents. 2014;44(3):194–202.
25. Bhaskaran A, Mumtaz K, Husain S. Anti-Aspergillus prophylaxis in lung transplantation: a systematic review and meta-analysis. Curr Infect Dis Rep. 2013;15(6):514–25.
26. Gupta DK, Sharma S. Chronic pleuro-pulmonary and chest wall infection. In: Parikh DH, Crabb DCG, Auldist AW, Rothenberg SS, editors. Paediatric thoracic surgery. London: Springer; 2009. p. 179–90.

Surgical Management in Pulmonary Tuberculosis

9

Rajan Santosham

Abstract

The anti-tuberculosis medications have changed the perspective of tuberculosis (TB) management, as effective medical management has significantly reduced the need for surgical intervention. However, recently the tuberculosis management in patients that are immunocompromised with HIV infection and poor drug compliance and drug resistance has become a challenge. The human mycobacterium tuberculosis is developing drug resistance, and the need for surgery in developing countries is increasing in multidrug resistance (MDR) and extreme drug resistance (XDR) cases. Modern surgeons will have to learn from the history of surgery in thoracic tuberculosis rather than reinventing the wheel. Surgery in these cases should be planned, and spread of this global disease needs to be curtailed by monitoring and education of the healthcare professionals, patients and their relatives. In Western countries developing countries, TB has varied presentation and can mimic many diseases, and surgery is performed more frequently for its diagnosis. Parenchyma-preserving surgery should be considered in successfully medically managed cases where scarred lung parenchyma needs resection.

Keywords

Tuberculosis · Decortication · Segmental Resection · Thoracoplasty · Balloon Dilatation · Broncopleural Fistula · Pneumonectomy

R. Santosham, M.S., M.Ch., F.R.C.S.
Department of Thoracic Surgery, Santosham Chest Hospital, Chennai, India

D. Parikh, P.B. Rajesh (eds.), *Tips and Tricks in Thoracic Surgery*,
https://doi.org/10.1007/978-1-4471-7355-7_9

9.1 Introduction

With the advent of chemotherapy against tuberculosis (TB) and early diagnosis, the role of surgery has decreased. Surgery has a role to play in some developing countries with complications of active or healed TB and in immunocompromised and drug-resistant cases. As per World Health Organization (WHO), TB is a global public health concern as strains resistant to standard anti-TB chemotherapy are being isolated with increasing frequency [1]. The concern is that the incidence of TB in densely populated countries like India, China, sub-Saharan Africa, Indonesia and Bolivia is increasing [2]. In Western Europe and other developed countries, caseload is 10 per 100,000, while it is much more prevalent in Eastern European countries. The incidence of TB in the UK is noticed to be increasing and reported as 12.9/100,000 population [3].

Before the advent of chemotherapy, TB was treated with sanatorium treatment, fresh air, good nutrition, sunlight and various collapse procedures. The surgical collapse therapy was accidentally discovered as the patient with pneumothorax or pleural effusion did better compared with other forms of pulmonary TB [4]. Historically, the lung collapse was achieved using the following procedures of which thoracoplasty is still useful in selective cases.

1. Phrenic crushing
2. Artificial pneumothorax
3. Pneumoperitoneum
4. Plombage
5. Thoracoplasty
6. Jacobaeus thoracoscope—used to cut pleural adhesions to aid collapse

9.2 Technical Tips and Tricks that Will Enhance Operative Experience and Improve Results

9.2.1 Diagnosis

The bacteriological diagnosis of TB is difficult as yield of isolation of *Mycobacterium* from clinical specimens is low even in optimum conditions.

Newer diagnostic tests that help microbiological investigations from clinical specimens are amplification of nucleic acid using polymerase chain reaction (PCR) and serological diagnosis by employing monoclonal antibody technology using enzyme-linked immunosorbent assay (ELISA) and interferon-Y release assays. Histopathological diagnosis is required in non-endemic areas by either fine-needle aspiration of lymph nodes or pleural or lung biopsy to confirm the diagnosis of TB before commencing the anti-TB chemotherapy.

Radiology: Plain chest X-ray, computed tomography and magnetic resonance imaging are helpful in detecting hilar lymphadenopathy in association with parenchymal pathology. It also helps in monitoring and resolution by the effective treatment.

9.3 Medical Management

- Most tuberculosis cases respond to first line of anti-TB treatment by directly observed treatment short-course (DOTS) therapy: initial intensive phase followed by a continuation phase.
- Clinical resolution at the end of and monitoring during the treatment is essential in order to improve compliance and reduce drug resistance.
- Effective drug regimens prevent not only the development of drug resistance but also the spread of TB with very low risk of adverse side effects.
- The use of corticosteroids is indicated in central nervous system involvement and at times in endobronchial and military TB.
- The surgeon should get the direction of medical management from a specialist in infectious disease or tuberculosis. The difficult cases that are referred to surgeons are invariably from the medical specialist either for diagnosis to obtain histological specimen, in relapse cases to diagnose MDR or progressing disease despite effective medical therapy.

9.4 Surgical Management

Indications for surgery in TB can be varied although not prescriptive which are described in Table 9.1. In carefully selected patients with MDR or XDR TB and having complication of medical treatment, surgical resection can increase cure rate to 90%.

- A thorough preoperative radiological evaluation is mandatory.
- Preoperative bronchoscopy is indicated to evaluate the extent, document the endobronchial disease and predict operative difficulty and the status of the contralateral lung.
- Surgical resection can reduce bacterial burden especially in MDR cases and help medical management. Resection of bronchiectatic segment controls the symptoms.
- Compression of lymph nodes can cause stridor in children and may necessitate a surgical decompression to relieve symptoms. Decompression of lymph nodes by evacuating its content should be performed and is preferable to its excision, which may cause damage to the airway.
- Pleural effusion may require drainage or decortication in order to improve lung expansion.

9.4.1 Avoiding Complications of TB Surgery

- Surgery should be performed after adequate evaluation, if possible after a period of anti-TB therapy, in consultation with other specialists including anaesthetists.

Table 9.1 Indication for surgery in TB [4]

1.	Failure of medical therapy
	• Progressive disease, lung destruction
	• Lung gangrene
	• Aspergillosis complicating treatment
2.	Surgery for diagnosis
	• Pulmonary lesion of unknown cause
	• Suspected carcinoma
	• Mediastinal adenopathy of unknown origin
3.	Complications of scarring
	• Massive haemoptysis
	• Cavernoma
	• Tracheo- or broncho-oesophageal fistula
	• Bronchiectasis
	• Airway obstruction by tuberculous lymph nodes
	• Endobronchial narrowing
4.	Extra-pulmonary thoracic disease
	• Constrictive pericarditis
	• Cold abscess and osteomyelitis of the chest wall
	• Pott's disease
5.	Pleural TB
	• Pleural effusion/empyema
	• Bronchopleural fistula
6.	Infections with mycobacteria other than tubercle bacilli (MOTT)
7.	Complications resulting from previous surgery

- Single-lung anaesthesia with either double-lumen tube or bronchial blockers is essential in the surgery of pulmonary TB.
- Preoperative bronchoscopy and aspiration of secretions will reduce intraoperative contamination of contralateral normal lung.
- It is vital to improve patient's nutrition, as many are malnourished. Postural drainage, physiotherapy in high sputum-producing patients, is essential to reduce postoperative complications.
- Secondary bacterial infection should be managed by appropriate perioperative antibiotics.
- Some surgeons prefer prone position for surgery to prevent contamination of contralateral lung.

9.4.2 Obtaining Tissue for Diagnosis

1. Many a times the diagnosis of TB in Western world is suspect unless there is a family history or history of exposure from an active infected case is obtained and/or the diagnosis from secretions such as sputum, gastric lavage or bronchial lavage is confirmatory of M tuberculosis. This is only possible in approximately 20–50% cases depending on bacterial burden. TB can mimic many known con-

genital anomaly, chronic infective causes, other granulomatous conditions and tumours (see Appendix figures).

2. Tissue diagnosis can either be obtained using thoracoscopic techniques or by open biopsies. A small biopsy taken from specific area is more likely to histologically reveal typical granulomatous lesion, caseating necrosis and with ZN stain or PCR for M tuberculum or other forms of granulomatas. Thoracoscopy allows an access to mediastinal nodes or all surfaces of lung parenchyma without thoracotomy.
3. Bronchoscopic tissue diagnosis can be achieved if an inflammatory polyp or a white/yellow nodule is seen (see Appendix figures).

9.4.3 Surgical Management of Pleural Disease

1. Aspiration of pleural effusion and continuing anti-TB therapy sometimes are sufficient
2. Insertion of intercostal drain is required for recurring effusion.
3. Secondarily infected or chronic multiloculated pleural disease trapping the lung requires decortication as described in Empyema chapter.
4. On occasion with significant lung disease or bronchopleural fistula, either parenchyma resection with muscle flaps or thoracoplasty may be required. Continuation and monitoring of anti-TB medical therapy are mandatory.
5. Rarely in chronic recurring empyema cases, thoracostomy may be required.

9.4.4 Technique of Decortication

- The adherence to the pleural peel to the underlying lung cannot be judged preoperatively, and by a combination of blunt by the finger and sharp dissection, decortication should be completed with minimal air leak.
- In areas where there is puckering and unhealthy granulation tissue, it is better to avoid peeling of the visceral pleura, as it will inevitably result in air leak and bronchopleural fistula.
- VATS is a good option for early cases of empyema with reasonably good peel that can release the trapped lung effectively.

9.5 Surgery for Pulmonary Tuberculosis

With effective chemotherapy healed and healing tuberculous lesions started giving problems like massive haemoptysis, aspergilloma, destroyed lung and MDR-TB where the role of surgery has been re-established. Drug resistance is so extensive that there is high chance of relapse or failure. Disease is sufficiently localized preoperatively that resection can be done and mycobacterial burden can be reduced for subsequent medical therapy.

The parenchyma-preserving surgery should be considered in order to preserve all functioning lung parenchyma especially if the tuberculosis is not effectively medically managed. The destroyed lung parenchyma related to scarring in previously medically well-managed tuberculosis is to perform lobectomy or segmental resection in scarred bronchiectatic segment to prevent future infective complications.

Tips and tricks for pulmonary resection that will avoid and deal with intra-op anticipated and unanticipated complications:

9.6 Surgical Techniques

- Meticulous haemostasis.
- Avoid using diathermy near the bronchus.
- Extra-pleural approach if necessary when there are severe vascular adhesions.
- Segmental resection with fingers.
- Bronchial closure with staplers/sweets technique (it is a method of clamping the bronchus and cutting proximal to the clamp little by little and using interrupted sutures for closure. It is done before the advent of double-lumen endotracheal tube for single-lung ventilation).
- Re-inforce bronchus with muscle flap/omentum.
- Success of any pulmonary surgery depends on maintaining minimal/no air leak.

9.6.1 Segmental Resection

- Inflammatory lesions are common in the apical and posterior segments of the upper lobes and superior segments of the lower lobes.
- These segments have independent pulmonary artery, vein and bronchus.
- Ideally the artery and vein are ligated and the bronchus clamped and ligated and peeled off by finger-fracture technique.
- The correct plane is determined by the presence of inter-segmental vein and minimal air leak.
- In my opinion using staplers for segmental resection should be avoided because it interferes with the uniform expansion of the lung.

9.6.2 Tips and Tricks to Deal with Postoperative Complications

- Bronchopleural fistula (early/late)
  Bronchopleural fistula is managed initially with intercostal drains and anti-TB drugs. If the fistula is large, once the infection is under control, it has to be closed/contained using omentum or intercostal muscle pedicle or other large muscle flaps in order to occupy post-lobectomy space.
- Post-lobectomy empyema
  This invariably is related to persisting infection that is not effectively managed either by the correct specific antibiotics, inadequate drainage, failure of expan-

sion of the trapped or scarred remaining lung or undiagnosed bronchopleural fistula from the sutured stump. This should be managed by muscle thoracoplasty bringing a large muscle on its pedicle to occupy the space after its debridement.
- Pleural space problems:
  - Benign—no fever/toxicity
  - Malignant—fever/toxicity

9.6.3 Thoracoplasty

The rationale of thoracoplasty is to relax the walls of the cavity to allow healing by fibrosis and collapse of the cavity. In developing countries, there is still significant role for thoracoplasty for salvaging sick patients not fit for resection.

9.7 Indications of Thoracoplasty

- Drug-resistant cavitatory disease with endobronchial TB
- Haemoptysis with poor respiratory reserve
- Empyema post-TB/pyogenic
- Bronchopleural fistula
- Post-pneumonectomy infections

9.8 Thoracoplasty in Tuberculous Cavities

- Functioning underlying lung.
- Done as a stage procedure—not removing more than five ribs at a stage.
- TB cavities are usually present in the apico-posterior segments of upper lobes and superior segments of lower lobes.
- Costo-transversectomy and apicolysis are essential.

9.9 Thoracoplasty for Post-pneumonectomy Empyema

- No functioning underlying lung
- Done in single sitting
- Window thoracostomy done in very ill patients followed by completion thoracoplasty if necessary

9.9.1 Surgery in Aspergilloma

- Aspergilloma is most commonly present in healed tubercular cavity in a diabetic individual.
- In recurrent haemoptysis the bronchial artery embolization has limited role.

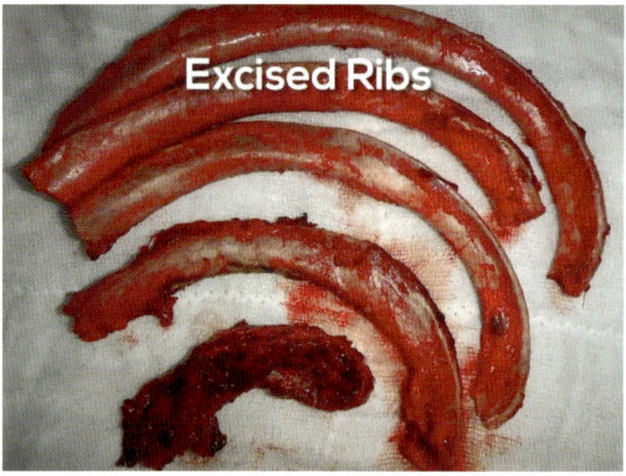

Excised ribs

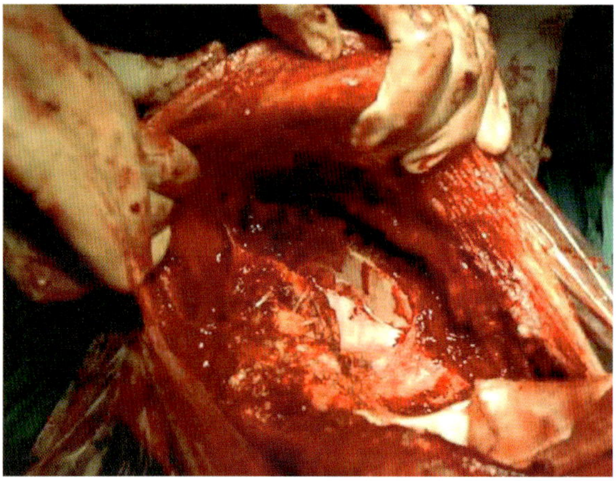

Thoracoplasty – complete collapse of pleural tent. First rib seen

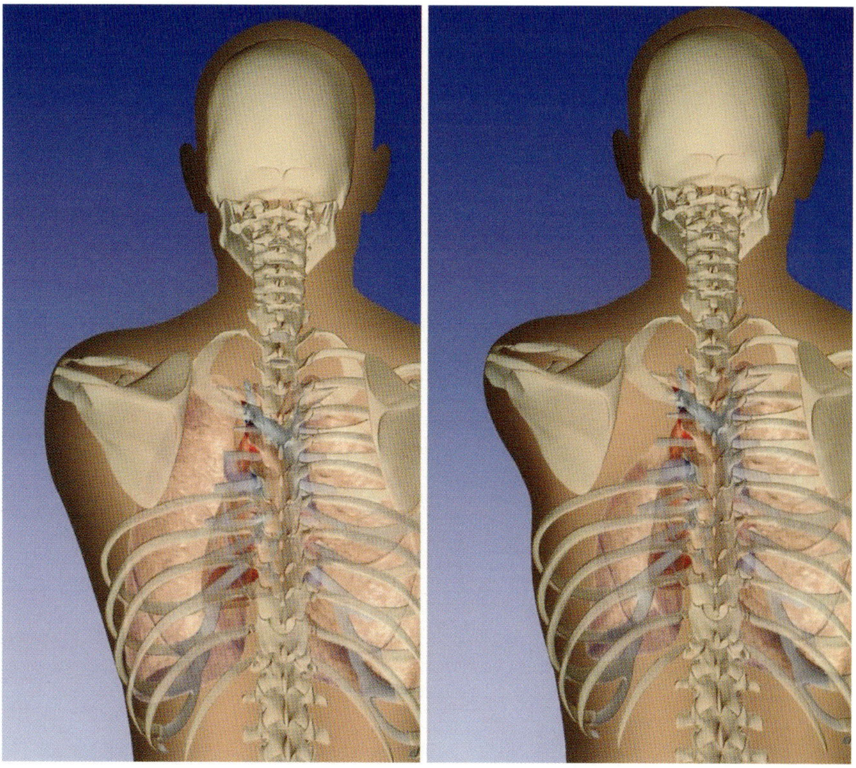

Showing collapse of the lung after thoracoplasty

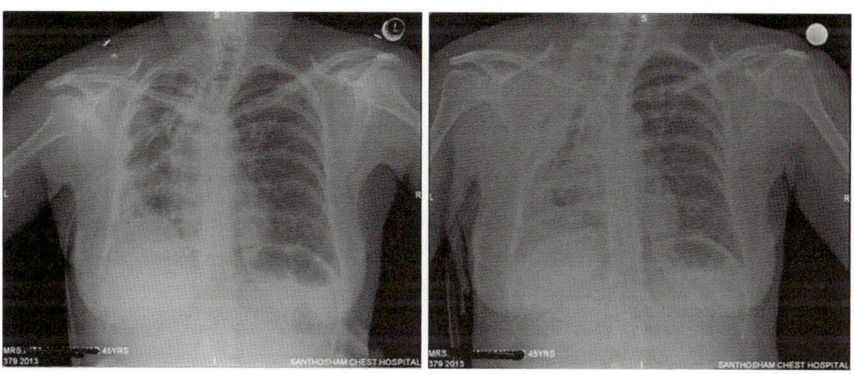

Pre- and post-thoracoplasty

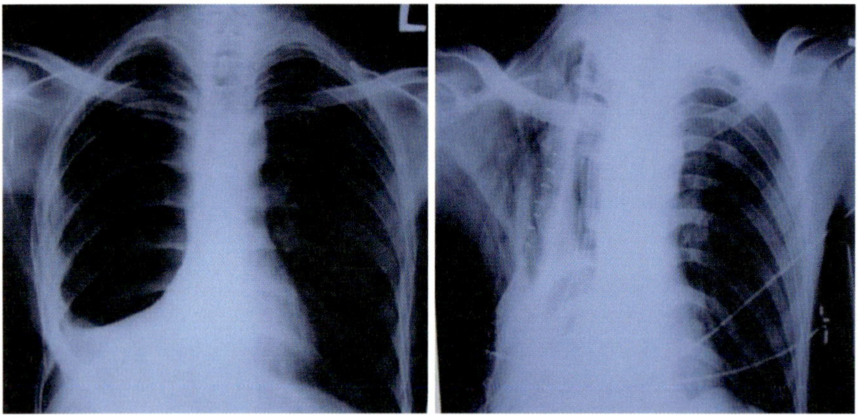

Post-pneumonectomy empyema (pre-op and post-thoracoplasty)

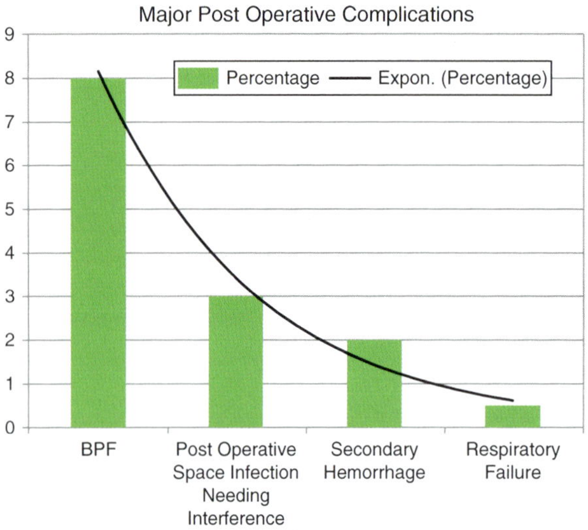

Major postoperative complications

Disclosure Statement No Disclosures.

References

1. Busillo CP, Lessnau KD, Sanjana V, et al. Multi-drug resistant Mycobacterium tuberculosis in patient with immunodeficiency virus infection. Chest. 1992;102:797.
2. Global Tuberculosis control—surveillance, planning, financing. WHO Geneva. 2007. http://www.who.int/tb/publications/global_report/en/

3. Wright A, Atkinson P, Maguire H. Communicable disease surveillance in London 2000. London: Communicable Disease Surveillance Centre; 2001.
4. Parekh P. Pulmonary tuberculosis. In: Parikh DH, Crabbe DCG, Rothenberg S, Auldist A, editors. Pediatric thoracic surgery. London: Springer; 2009. p. 129–43.
5. STOP TB partnership. The global plan to stop TB 2006-2015. The executive summery available at: www.stoptb.org/globalplan/assets/documents/GP_ES_Eng.pdf. Full document available at http://www.who.int/tb/publications/global_plan_to_stop_tb/en/index.htm/

Lung Abscess

10

Dragan Subotic

Abstract

Pulmonary/lung abscess is encountered either as result of primary necrotising lower respiratory tract infections or secondary infection within metastasis, congenital or acquired lung lesions, tuberculous cavities or traumatic lung contusion. With the advent of antibiotics and good early medical supportive management, need for surgery is rare in immunocompetent individuals. However, due to increase of the bacterial resistance rate, of the number of immunocompromised patients, due to still high HIV incidence and need to achieve diagnosis of lung cancer, surgical resection may be required. Surgical resection should preserve as much parenchyma as possible as likely chance of subsequent infection is significant. Surgery in patients with poor pulmonary reserve and generalised parenchymal involvement is associated with significant morbidity and mortality. Patient selection and adequate preoperative preparations are vital to the outcome.

Keywords

Pulmonary abscess · Necrotising pneumonia · Chronic lung abscess · Fungal infection · Lung cancer · Inhaled foreign body · Bronchiectasis · Lobectomy Pneumonectomy · Post-lobectomy and post-pneumonectomy empyema

D. Subotic, M.D., F.C.C.P.
Clinic for Thoracic Surgery, Clinical Center of Serbia, University of Belgrade School of Medicine, Belgrade, Serbia

D. Parikh, P.B. Rajesh (eds.), *Tips and Tricks in Thoracic Surgery*,
https://doi.org/10.1007/978-1-4471-7355-7_10

10.1 Introduction

Lung/pulmonary abscess is a localised collection of pus within lung parenchyma mostly related to necrotising lung infection [1]. Although rare indication for surgery, the diversity of causes, radiographic manifestations and selection of the appropriate surgical procedure, together with perioperative anaesthesiological problems, make a lung abscess a challenging surgical problem, even for experienced teams.

Great deal of lessons can be learned by studying the history of lung abscess surgery as modern surgeons are encountering increasing bacterial antibiotic resistance and cases with necrotising pneumonia with abscess formation especially in immunocompromised patients that cause difficult and challenging scenarios. Once the surgery and anaesthesia were considered uniformly fatal, the dedicated work of number of innovators over the years improved its outcome. Historically Lilienthal in 1910 was the first to undertake an open thoracotomy using an intra-tracheal general anaesthesia in a 55-year-old man [2] and then in 1914 successfully performed right lower lobectomy for a lung abscess, after ineffective drainage in a small boy with an inhaled nut [3]. Neuhof introduced a new concept of a one-stage open drainage procedure, which became widely accepted as it decreased morbidity and mortality. The principle was based on precise location of abscess with respect to the chest wall, exposure in order to evacuate its suppurative content and then packing the cavity with gauze. The subsequent bronchopleural fistula if encountered was allowed to take the natural course of healing by open drainage. Neuhof's one-stage procedure decreased mortality as reported in his personal series as well as reported in other centres [4–6].

The survival and mortality of acute lung abscess improved significantly during the antibiotic era, as medical management became standard and surgical management was reserved for non-responding chronic abscess [5, 7]. This trend has continued in modern era; resectional surgery was reserved for chronic persistent abscess and when underlying cancer could not be ruled out [8–10]. In recent years with increasing bacterial resistance and aggressive necrotising pneumonia with putrid abscess formation, the Neuhof's procedure is being rejuvenated.

10.2 Classification, Differential Diagnosis

Pulmonary abscesses are classified as primary, occurring in otherwise healthy individuals, and secondary, complicating some pre-existing conditions such as lung cancer or systemic diseases with most frequently.

Primary pulmonary abscess is most frequently a consequence of the aspiration pneumonia. Endobronchial obstruction (lung cancer, foreign body) is the most common cause of secondary abscess. Pre-existing lung cavities, subject to secondary infection, are not true abscesses but may have an identical clinical course and similar radiographic features (Table 10.1).

Table 10.1 Differential diagnosis of the pulmonary abscess

Infectious diseases
Aspergillosis, histoplasmosis, nocardiosis, cryptococcosis, coccidioidomycosis, tuberculosis, atypical mycobacterial disease, necrotising bacterial pneumonia, loculated empyema
Neoplasms
Bronchogenic carcinoma, metastatic carcinoma, lymphoma
Inflammatory diseases
Wegener's granulomatosis, rheumatoid nodule
Miscellaneous
Pulmonary infarct, pneumatocele, sarcoidosis (rare), silicosis
Developmental lesions
Bronchogenic cyst, pulmonary sequestration, cystic adenomatoid malformation, diaphragmatic hernia

According to symptom duration, lung abscess may be acute (symptoms less than 4–6 weeks) and chronic, with longer symptom duration. According to some earlier classifications, abscesses were considered as acute, subacute and chronic, if the symptom duration was <4, 4–8 or >8 weeks, respectively.

10.3 Diagnosis

Clinical history of a copious purulent sputum expectoration and pyrexia is similar to severe lower respiratory infections/pneumonia with decreased air entry, and bronchial breathing leads a clinician to perform a chest x-ray. The round shadow with or without fluid level suggests the development of a lung abscess. However, it is important to identify the underlying causes that led to its development.

Computerised tomography (CT) with intravenous contrast is not routinely done in patients with typical chest x-ray appearance but nevertheless extremely useful. In our experience, lung abscess location by means of CT scan is mandatory and may help diagnose underlying predisposing lesions. Care should be taken of the patient position while performing a CT scan, because in some patients with large abscesses, copious expectoration may occur in the supine position.

Bronchoscopy should always be done, both to exclude endobronchial obstruction and to collect secretion for microbiological analysis. It is important not to dislodge foreign body as it may flood the tracheobronchial tree with purulent material. A good suction device is essential while undertaking bronchoscopy in this situation.

10.4 Management of Acute Lung Abscess

Medically, culture-specific appropriate antibiotic therapy constitutes the mainstay in the management of an acute lung abscess. Other supportive therapies such as physiotherapy, antipyretics and analgesia, oxygen, adequate hydration and nutrition as required help recovery from infection. Surgery or other forms of interventional drainage are now necessary in only 11–21% of patients who have not responded to antimicrobial therapy [11, 12].

- Empirical intensive intravenous antibiotics should be commenced suspecting Gram-positive as causative organisms.
- It is essential to consult hospital microbiologist (if available) to ration multiple combination antibiotics, in immunocompromised patients, and if resistant organisms are identified in either blood culture or bronchoscopic lavage specimens.
- Culture-specific antibiotic is better than broad-spectrum antibiotics, and efforts should be made to obtain specimen prior to the start of antibiotics. This is mandatory especially in immunocompromised and transplant patients.
- There are numerous antibiotics available for both Gram-positive and Gram-negative and antibiotic-resistant organisms. It is essential for everyone involved in the management in septic patients to be aware not to be overzealous with antibiotics. Antibiotic stewardship is mandatory in order to avoid drug resistance.
- Regular clinical assessments, haematological septic markers and radiology as deemed necessary are required to monitor clinical progress.
- Treatment duration is determined by the response, host factors and bacterial resistance and monitoring of the patient. Usually at least 6–8 weeks of antibiotic management is required. Cavity closure generally takes at least 4 weeks, sometimes several weeks [13, 14]. Resolution of surrounding infiltrates may take around 8 weeks.
- Patients who are previously healthy generally recover faster than those with secondary abscesses with underlying predisposing aetiology.

10.4.1 Surgical Management

Surgical intervention is seldom necessary. However, in acutely septic patient with tense pulmonary abscess, aspiration drainage with the help of interventional radiologist may be required. Either aspiration or a pigtail catheter drainage of a tense or unresponsive abscess may help improve respiratory compromise. If a patient remains seriously ill, and/or clinical condition deteriorates despite appropriate antibiotics, then as a last resort, external drainage procedure must be considered. It is proven that interventional drainage performed by a radiologist dramatically relieves symptoms, improves wellbeing and enhances the recovery. Radiological percutaneous drainage is proven to be more effective and associated with fewer morbidities than traditional open drainage. In patients with ineffective cough, significant immunodeficiency where internal drainage may be more hazardous, early decision should be made for an external drainage. Success rate with conservative external drainage with antibiotics in resolving lung abscess is in range of 90%.

Investigations should be carried out concomitantly to diagnose underlying cause.

In patients with acute lung abscess and associate empyema, adequate drainage of empyema and release of the trapped lung parenchyma are essential. Continuing antibiotics and re-expansion of the lung lead to resolution of the associated lung abscess. The contained lung abscess should not be disturbed while managing empyema as it may lead to prolonged broncho-pulmonary fistula. In patients with pyopneumothorax with ruptured abscess into the pleural cavity, again adequate empyema drainage/decortication and insertion of muscle flap onto the ruptured cavity may be required rather than resectional surgery in presence of acute infection. The reader is directed to the Empyema chapter, which deals with the associated lung abscess.

Surgical resection is seldom necessary in acute pulmonary abscess but should be considered in some patients resistant to all conservative measures.

Indications for resection include:

- Large/tense cavities not responding to conservative measures
- Massive haemorrhage
- Obstructive neoplasms or foreign bodies
- Infections caused by multiresistant bacteria or fungi

Survival rates after lung resection range from 89 to 95%.

10.5 Management of Chronic Lung Abscess

The optimal duration of conservative management after the diagnosis of a lung abscess under antimicrobial therapy is not clearly defined, but it should not be shorter than 4–6 weeks, unless the patient's condition is deteriorating rapidly. Even the lesions with a significant cavity size at presentation, and unlikely to respond, may significantly decrease after 4–6 weeks of antibiotic treatment, as presented in Fig. 10.1.

The described clinical course and radiographic resolution represent the major clinical challenge and dilemma, especially if the patient has good general health. It is difficult to reliably determine the type of the persisting lung lesions, as there is always a possibility of underlying malignancy. In a patient presented in Fig. 10.1, because of the solid lesion that was visible on (Fig. 10.1c) bronchoscopy with biopsy under fluoroscopy or CT guided would also be an appropriate course of action, despite the evident response to medical treatment. In conservatively managed cases, it is, therefore, mandatory to perform follow-up radiology and confirm

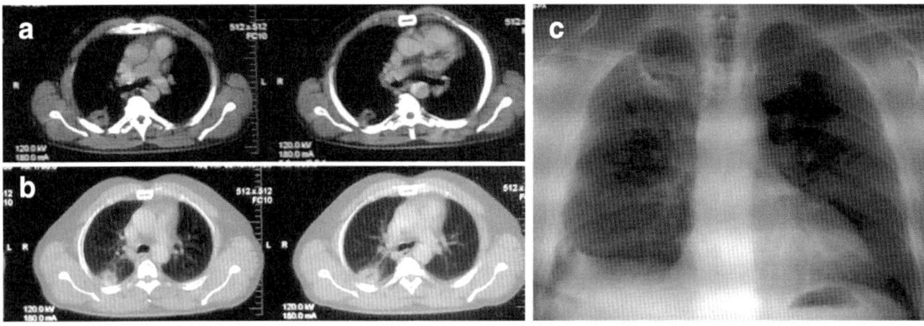

Fig. 10.3 (**a**–**c**) Male, 54 years, with no previously well presented with 3 weeks history of non-productive cough, slight dyspnoea, one episode of high spiking pyrexia (up to 40 °C) that improved after 2–3 days of antibiotic treatment. The thoracic CT after 1 week of antibiotic therapy revealed a 4 × 3-cm-thick-walled cavitation in the posterior segment of the right upper lobe (**a**). Bronchoscopy: normal with nonspecific inflammation. A persisting ovoid lesion of similar size was identified on chest radiography 2 weeks later (**b**). Right thoracotomy, ex tempore biopsy of the lesion was benign. Resection of the posterior segment of the right upper lobe was carried out to diagnose chronic abscess on pathology. He had an uneventful recovery (**c**)

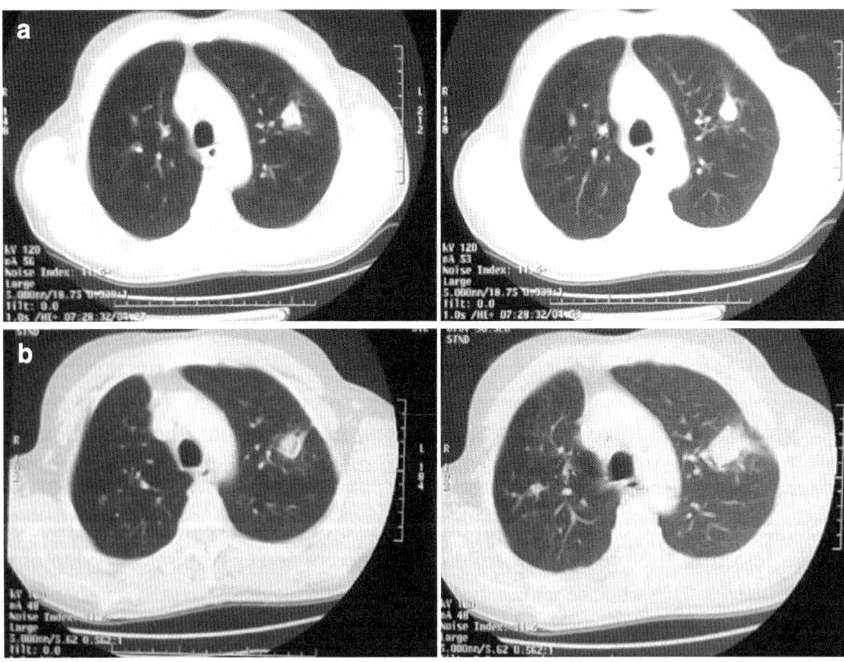

Fig. 10.4 (**a**, **b**) In a 64-year-old man, a right middle lobectomy was performed for a persistent right middle lobe infiltration after a CT scan. The histopathology diagnosed bronchiectasis. The preoperative CT also revealed a synchronous ovoid left upper lobe lesion (**a**, upper row). This increased in size on a follow-up without any specific symptoms suggestive of infection (**b**, lower row). Therefore, a second thoracotomy was performed on the left side to diagnose the underlying pathology. This on pathology also showed features of bronchiectasis and ruled out underlying malignancy

rises to 33% in patients older than 45 years [15]. In practice, it is not always easy to distinguish a benign infective cavity from secondarily infected in carcinomatous necrotic pulmonary abscess. The plain chest x-ray can only diagnose the presence of a cavitatory lesion and is difficult to suspect associated malignancy (Fig. 10.5a, b). Two radiological signs on CT scan can suggest underlying lung cancer: (1) an irregular cavity wall that is more likely to be malignant than benign cavitatory lesions (Fig. 10.5c) and (2) associated hilar density close to the lung cavity (Fig. 10.5d) [16].

Patients with cavitatory lesions without histological confirmation of the underlying disease may represent a diagnostic dilemma, especially in the presence of incomplete response to treatment and persistent radiological shadow (Fig. 10.6). It may be a clinician who may decide to manage with an expectant approach with close follow-up. In case of persisting lesion after more than a month after initial regression, as presented on Fig. 10.6, surgery would be a reasonable option, but that decision can be postponed in the presence of significant co-morbidity.

Some patients may have radiographic and clinical features suggestive of acute abscess at presentation associated with systemic sepsis, and at the same time, malignancy cannot be excluded. In some instances a pneumonectomy may be considered as life-saving procedure in rapidly deteriorating sepsis in debilitating and immune-compromised patients (patient 4 as discussed in Fig. 10.7).

In patients where the infection and pulmonary abscess occurred in the lobe of obstructed bronchus, the diagnosis of cancer was achieved on diagnostic bronchoscopy. Management plan should be tailored as dictated by patient's condition and possibility of controlling sepsis. Medical management if successful with culture-specific antibiotics can reduce the extent of surgery and postoperative morbidity. Surgical resection in the presence of acute sepsis is fraught with on-table complications of bleeding due to friable vascular inflamed tissue and bronchial stump breakdown with bronchopleural fistula and post-lobectomy empyema.

In a large study containing 1148 patients that underwent pneumonectomy in an 8-year period, intraoperative infection from the pre-existing lung infection occurred in 4/76 (5.3%) patients. Postoperative pleural empyema occurred in 76 (6.65%) patients with bronchopleural fistula as a cause of empyema in ¾ of these patients [17].

Lung abscess or bronchial obstruction with retained infected secretions is a common cause of fever in patients with primary bronchial cancer, with a reported incidence of 21.1% [18, 19]. Imaging techniques are unreliable in differentiating idiopathic infection from necrotic cavitating lung tumours. Ultrasound-guided biopsy and aspiration from the cavity help both diagnosis and obtaining material for culture and antibiotic sensitivity [19]. The culture-specific antibiotics in responding patient will reduce the need for emergency surgery and associated postoperative complications. Bronchoscopy is mandatory in patients with lung abscess as it helps diagnose intra-bronchial obstructive tumour of foreign body and collection of bronchial lavage materials for cytology and culture [16].

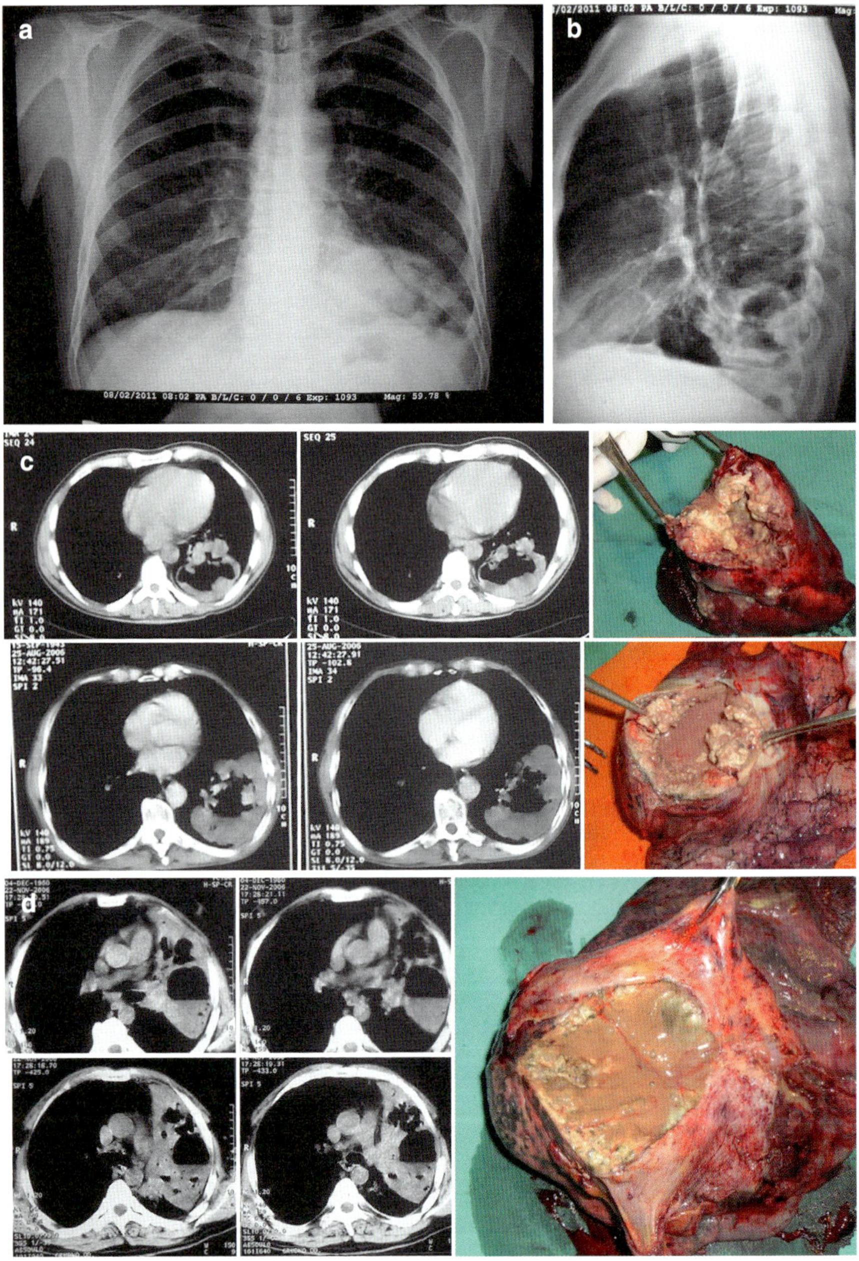

Fig. 10.5 Left lower lobe cavitation diagnosed on chest x-ray PA (**a**) and lateral views (**b**). Irregular cavity wall on chest CT, suggestive of lung cancer, operative specimen showing intracavitatory solid lesion confirming lung cancer on pathology (**c**). Hilar density associated with the lung cavitation can also suggest lung cancer (**d**)

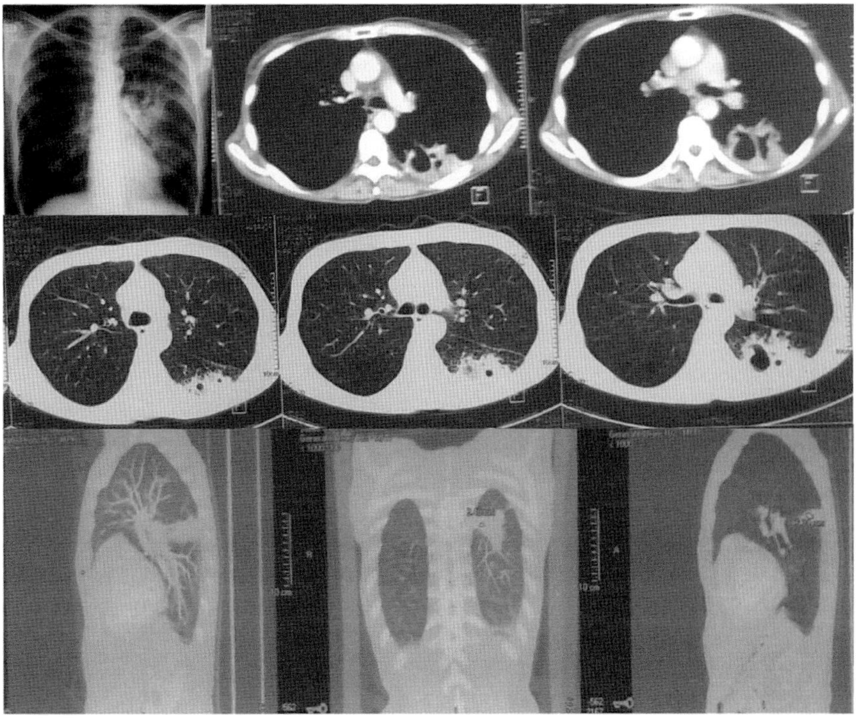

Fig. 10.6 Left lung cavitation—incomplete response to treatment. Upper two rows, before treatment; lower row, after treatment

10.6.2 Necrotic Lung Cancer Can Mimic an Acute Lung Abscess or a Parasitic Infection

This is aptly presented by a clinical case shown in Fig. 10.8. Chronic hydatid cyst can also get infected and present as abscess. Empyema is known to occur, and either pericystectomy or lobectomy may be required.

10.6.3 Human Immunodeficiency Virus (HIV) Infection and Lung Abscess

Increase in number of HIV-infected patients both in underdeveloped and Western-developed countries is a significant cause of pulmonary sepsis with unusual organisms. Administration of antiretroviral therapy has led to substantial decrease in opportunistic pneumonia in community with access to therapy. Although abscess formation is rare with opportunistic organisms as generally

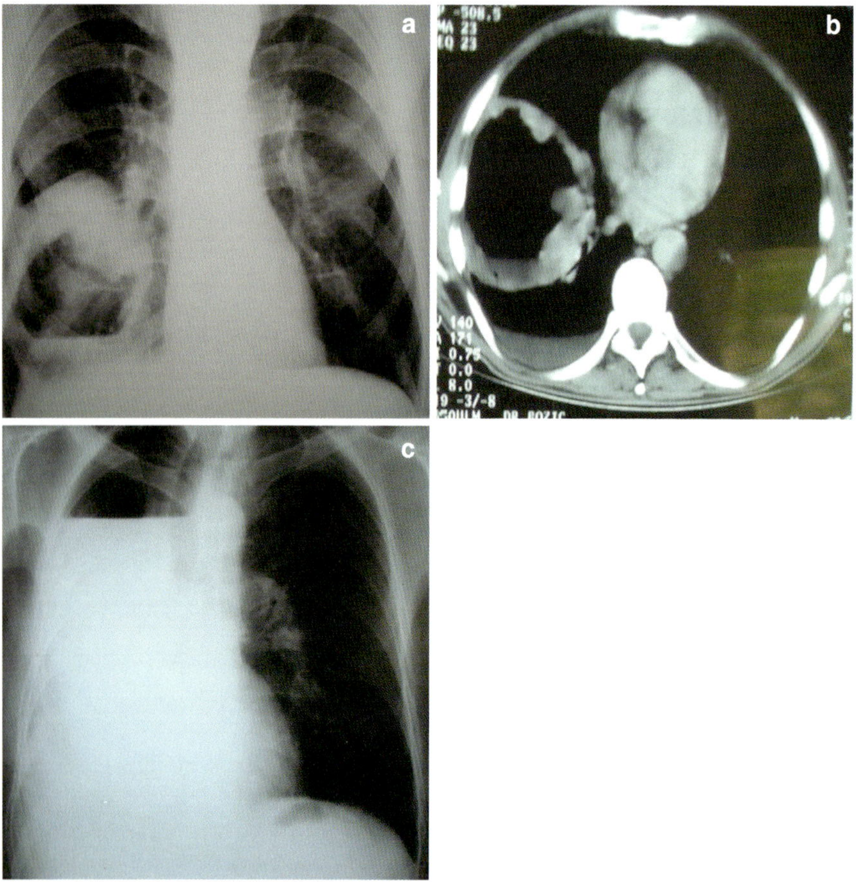

Fig. 10.7 (**a**–**c**) Patient 4. In a 60-year-old man, a lung abscess was diagnosed and managed with antibiotics after his presentation with high temperature and productive cough (**a**). Bronchoscopy performed showed submucosal neoplastic growth extending up to the level of the intermediate bronchus (biopsy pathology-squamous cell carcinoma). The thoracic CT revealed a 12 cm cavity with irregular wall, partly filled with liquid associated with a small pleural effusion (**b**). Clinical condition of the patient continued to deteriorate, despite receiving culture-specific antibiotic therapy. Surgery was considered the only available option to control the sepsis, but in the presence of a right lower lobe bronchus tumour invading the middle lobe and intermediate bronchus, together with a poor quality, emphysematous upper lobe pneumonectomy was performed. This resulted in control of sepsis, improvement in patient general condition and uneventful postoperative course (**c**)

they are slow growing and cause pneumonia rather than abscess formation. Combination with pneumocystis and other invasive pathogens such as *Streptococcus pneumoniae* may cause abscess formation. These should be managed in the same way as the other patients with lung abscess. Because sepsis can spread rapidly in immunocompromised patient, it may be necessary to consider early surgical drainage procedure, at the same time providing culture-specific antibiotics, adequate nutrition and hydration and postural physiotherapy. It is

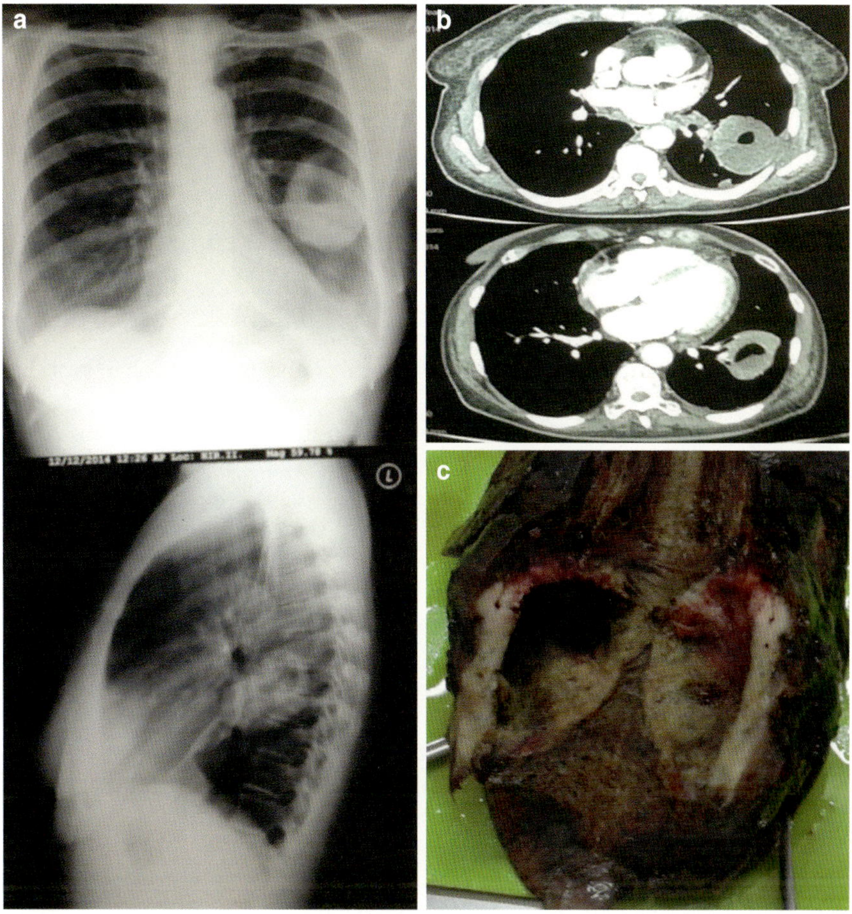

Fig. 10.8 (**a**–**c**) Patient 5. A preoperative chest x-ray (**a**) in a woman who had a history of acute weight loss living with many animals in the house showed an irregular cavity with fluid level. CT scan performed showed left lower lobe fluid and air-containing irregular cavity that lead to a suspicion of hydatid disease (**b**). At operation while opening the cyst cavity to evacuate hydatid, it was discovered that this was not hydatid disease. The cyst was closed, and lobectomy was performed to diagnose squamous cell carcinoma on pathology (**c**)

essential to get an advice from HIV specialist regarding administration of hyperactive antiretroviral therapy.

10.7 Tips and Tricks to Avoid and Deal with Intraoperative Anticipated and Unanticipated Complications

In the lung abscess surgery, the treatment outcome depends equally on both the quality of anaesthesia and surgery. The role of the anaesthesiologist can never be overstressed in this type of surgery.

10.7.1 Anaesthesiological Considerations

The best way to prevent intraoperative complications in lung abscess surgery is to avoid contamination of the healthy lung especially in patients with abundant purulent expectoration or major haemoptysis:

- Preoperative consultation with the anaesthetist.
- Good preoperative physiotherapy postural drainage and if necessary appropriate antibiotics
- Preoperative flexible or rigid bronchoscopy in patients with poor respiratory reserve and with thick purulent expectoration and haemoptysis.
- Consider bronchial blockers and isolate either the main or lobar bronchus (Fig. 10.9).
- During surgery lobar manipulation may result in sudden copious purulent expectoration or major haemoptysis drainage into main airways causing a life-threatening emergency. Therefore, the use of a double-lumen tube (DLT) or some type of blockers is mandatory [20]. Both surgeon and anaesthetist should be aware of this emergency situation and be prepared for the emergency bronchoscopy and suctioning of the airway to allow adequate oxygenation.

1. Should the lung separation be achieved with the patient in the sitting or semi-sitting position?
   - We recommend both rigid or flexible bronchoscopy and aspiration prior to surgery and insertion of double-lumen tube (DLT) for anaesthesia should be undertaken in semi-sitting position and reposition as required after muscle relaxation. Further ventilation should be avoided until the DLT is positioned and the bronchial cuff inflated [21].

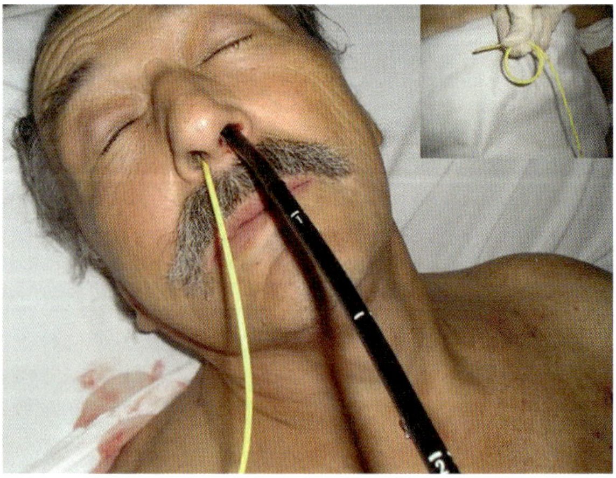

Fig. 10.9 Use of the Fogarty catheter for temporary isolation of the main bronchus

2. What is the preferred way of DLT placement?
   - Besides the usual DLT placement with a patient in the supine position, some teams also suggest to induce anaesthesia with the patient sitting on the horizontal lower half of an operating table that is broken at the mid-point, with the patient's thorax reclining, abscess-side dependent, against the steeply angulated upper half. Once asleep and paralysed, the patient can be maintained abscess-side dependent, and the head-up tilt could have been reduced if necessary to facilitate bronchoscopy and intubation.
3. How to protect the operated lung, as well as the healthy lung from infective material?
   - A standard recommendation is a frequent removal of secretions during surgery by suction via the DLT lumen on the diseased side.

Furthermore, keeping the abscess-bearing lung non-ventilated is also considered beneficial. If a single-lung ventilation is applied before the chest is opened and before the non-ventilated lung is able to collapse, ambient air and nitrogen enter the non-ventilating lung. But, if the airway of the non-ventilated lung is connected to an ambient-pressure oxygen reservoir, the aforementioned scenario will be prevented [22]. In that case, the oxygenation of the shunted pulmonary blood flow will be good but without carbon dioxide elimination once the Pco_2 of gas in the reservoir bag has equilibrated with that of the mixed venous blood. So, in case of delay in opening the chest and in lung collapse, the minute volume ventilation should be guided by arterial blood gases.

10.7.2 Surgical Considerations

From the surgical standpoint, there are three major concerns in the lung abscess surgery: (1) to avoid opening the abscess cavity, (2) maximal preservation of the remaining lung and (3) prevention and safely dealing with eventual vascular injuries.

The best way to achieve the first two goals is the upfront extrapleural dissection above the cavity whenever necessary, guided by the cavity location on CT scan. As major adhesions may be located above the unaffected lobe(s) as well, one should not hesitate with some extension of the extrapleural dissection whenever necessary.

Related to the third concern, on the left side, the main pulmonary artery should be secured first in case of difficult interlobar dissection, especially in case of absent or poorly defined fissures. On the right side, one should not hesitate with intrapericardial isolation of the main pulmonary artery in case of dense perivascular fibrosis or firmly adherent lymph nodes. It may be life saving in case of the vascular injury in the fissure.

As some hilar retraction and pericardial adherence may also exist, great care should be taken to identify both pulmonary veins before vessel ligation. This is because severe inflammation may cause overlooking of the eventual common confluence of both veins that may be of the same size and have the usual anatomic position either of the upper or lower pulmonary vein (Fig. 10.10).

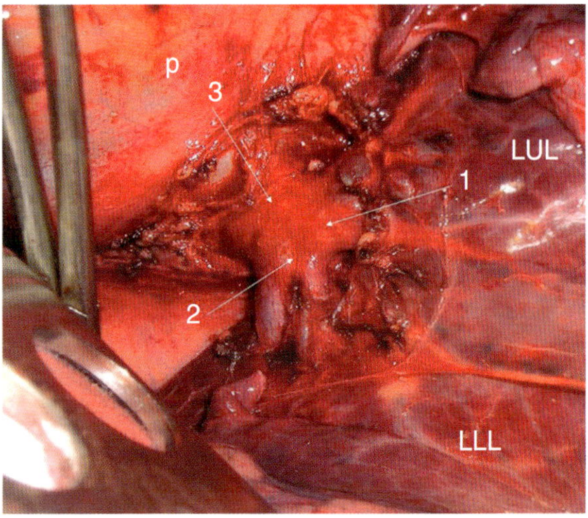

Fig. 10.10 Common pulmonary vein. *LUL* left upper lobe, *LLL* left lower lobe; 1, upper lobe vein; 2, lower lobe vein; 3, common vein; *p* pericardium

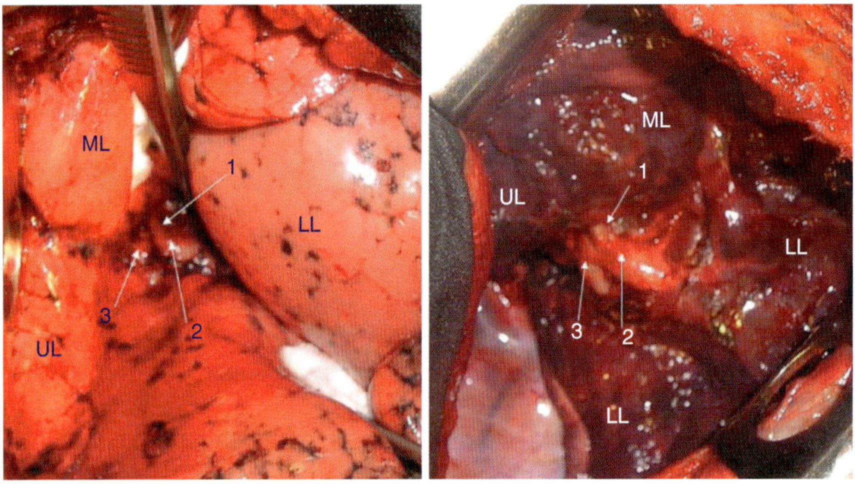

Fig. 10.11 Variation of the middle lobe artery origin (left, inflated lung; right, lung excluded from ventilation): *LL* lower lobe, *UL* upper lob, *ML* middle lobe; 1, middle lobe artery; 2, basal segment artery; 3, artery for the VI segment

Similarly, dissection of the sufficient length of the fissures may be difficult because of the inflammation. In this situation, insufficient length of the fissure liberation bears some important risks. On the right side, the artery for the VI segment may be significantly retracted backwards, which may cause the posterior border of the basal segments artery to be mistakenly considered as the VI segment artery. Similarly, in the presence of severe inflammation, the middle lobe artery as a branch of the basal artery or two separate middle lobe arteries may also be overlooked (Fig. 10.11). On the left side, variation of the lingular artery position may also be

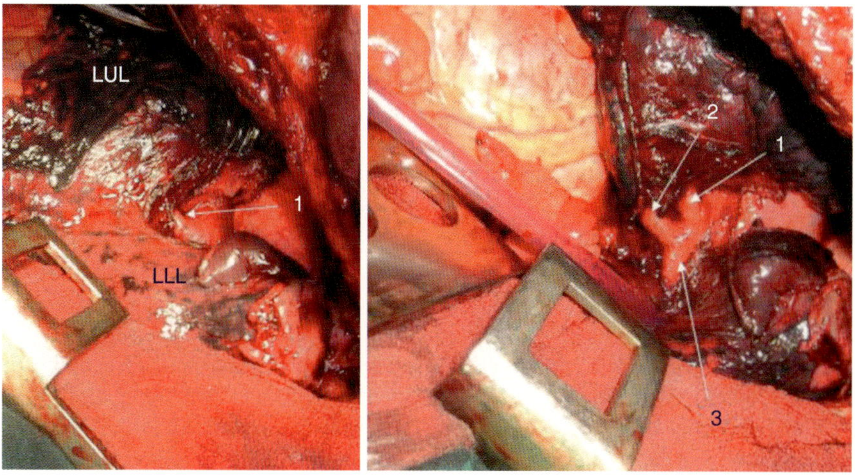

Fig. 10.12 Variation of the lingular artery. Left, fissure partially developed; right, fissure fully developed; 1, first lingular artery; 2, second lingular artery; 3, artery for the basal segments

overlooked in case of the insufficient fissure liberation (Fig. 10.12). All these problems may also exist in patients with diseases other than lung abscess, but in the latter patients, because of associated inflammation, they should be always taken into account.

10.8 Alternative Ways of Operative Management: Advantages and Disadvantages

As already mentioned, lung resection is a usual option after the failure of medical treatment. In some patients, percutaneous transthoracic drainage or endoscopic abscess drainage can be considered as alternatives.

10.8.1 Percutaneous Transthoracic Drainage

Based on the recent review of 21 studies with 124 cases (14 patients with secondary and 110 with primary pyogenic abscesses), percutaneous drainage can be indicated in several situations:

1. In severely ill patients who cannot tolerate lobectomy.
2. In the presence of the homogeneous ovoid lesion representing the abscess cavity without an air-fluid level.
   In this situation, some tension may exist within the cavity, with the risk of sudden, potentially fatal endobronchial decompression [23].

3. In patients with a lung abscess and massive haemoptysis, if the patient is unfit for lobectomy. In this situation, drainage enables prompt evacuation of the abscess contents and stops further growth of the cavity [24].
   This condition was described in one of the seven cases reported by Weissberg et al. [25]. In addition, the efficacy of PTD in the treatment of both sepsis and massive haemoptysis was also confirmed in a review article recently published by Wali [26].
4. In patients on mechanical ventilation in the intensive care unit or in debilitated patients with ineffective cough and inadequate spontaneous drainage of the abscess content.

The main advantage of this kind of treatment is a prompt clinical recovery, as reported by Weissberg et al. (see [26]) on seven patients and by Shim et al. [27] on four patients. Furthermore, avoidance of potential complications associated with conservative and prolonged treatment is also important and supported by vanSonnenberg et al. [28] reporting a 100% cure rate in 19 unresponsive patients with CT-guided percutaneous drainage and average duration of drainage was 9.8 days. Ha and colleagues reported complete abscess resolution in four of six patients treated with small catheters and the mean drainage duration being 15.5 days [29].

A reported high complication rate is a main disadvantage of this procedure as reported by Yunus on 19 patients [30] with 79% success rate and 60% complication rate. In the series of Hirshberg and colleagues, the procedure was technically successful in 8/11 patients only, five of whom died [31]. There is always a concern of soiling the pleural space with the abscess contents in the case of PTD.

Factors that may lead to failure of PTD may include:

Secondary lung abscess
Co-morbid diseases
Highly virulent organisms
Multiloculation
Poor definition of the cavity
Thickened wall cavity that may not collapse

10.8.2 Endoscopic Drainage

Endoscopic drainage is an alternative to percutaneous drainage. Initially reported by Metras and Chapin in 1954 [32], only 4 additional reports have been published consisting of a total of 49 cases with 9 treatment failures [33–36].

This procedure may be justified in the following situations:

- In patients with coagulopathies
- In patients with central abscess, where a percutaneous drainage could be dangerous because of the amount of lung tissue that needs to be traversed in order to reach the cavity, or in patients in whom anatomic structures (usually scapula) impede the access to the cavity

Endoscopic drainage should also be considered if the CT clearly demonstrates the airway leading to the abscess, or if the confirmed endobronchial obstruction prevents the abscess drainage.

Conclusion

Pulmonary abscess can be a surgical challenge even in the hands of experienced surgeon. Increasing number of patients with HIV infection, haematological malignancy, cancer chemotherapy and organ transplantation are the main aetiological factors in developed countries and cause significant management challenge. Although surgery is seldom necessary, it is important when required adequate preparations and surgery are undertaken so that minimum morbidity and good outcome can be achieved. Lung cancer with parenchymal necrosis in adult can get secondarily infected causing diagnostic dilemma, and therefore, in the absence of resolution and persisting radiological shadow, resectional surgery is required. Percutaneous drainage is a good management option in severely ill septic patients with poor respiratory reserve.

References

1. Bartlett JG. Lung abscess. In: Baum GL, Wolinsky E, editors. Textbook of pulmonary diseases. 5th ed. Boston: Little Brown; 1994. p. 607–20.
2. Lilienthal HIV. The first case of thoracotomy in a human being under anaesthesia by intratracheal insufflations. Ann Surg. 1910;52:30–3.
3. Lilienthal HIX. Pulmonary abscess and bronchiectasis: a clinical report. Ann Surg. 1914;59:855–83.
4. Neuhof H, Hurwitt E. Acute putrid abscess of the lung: VII (Relationship of the technic of the one-stage operation to results). Ann Surg. 1943;118:656–64.
5. Schweppe HI, Knowles JH, Kane L. Lung abscess (An analysis of the Massachusetts General Hospital cases from 1943 through 1956). N Engl J Med. 1961;265:1039–43.
6. Shaw RR. Pulmonary abscess: value of early one-stage drainage. J Thorac Surg. 1942;11:453–66.
7. Neuhof H, Touroff AS, Aufses AH. The surgical treatment, by drainage, of subacute and chronic putrid abscess of the lung. Ann Surg. 1941;113:209–20.
8. Shaw RR, Paulson DL. Pulmonary resection for chronic abscess of the lung. J Thorac Surg. 1948;17:514–22.
9. Myers RT, Bradshaw HH. Conservative resection of chronic lung abscess. Ann Surg. 1950;131:985–93.
10. Waterman DH, Domm SE. Changing trends in the treatment of lung abscess. Dis Chest. 1954;25:40–53.
11. Merritt RE, Shrager JB. Indications for surgery in patients with localised pulmonary infection. Thorac Surg Clin. 2012;22:325–32.
12. Athanassiadi K, Jakovic R, Siafakas N. Abscess of the lung: current therapeutic options. Eur Res Mono. 2013;61:81–9.
13. Davis B, Systrom DM. Lung abscess: pathogenesis, diagnosis and treatment. Curr Clin Top Infect Dis. 1998;18:252–73.
14. Hood MR. Bacterial diseases of the lung. In: Shields TW, editor. General thoracic surgery. 4th ed. Philadelphia: Lea and Febiger; 1989. p. 751–71.
15. Wallace RJ Jr, Cohen A, Awe RJ, Greenberg D, Hadlock F, Park Carcinomatous SK. lung abscess. Diagnosis by bronchoscopy and cytopathology. JAMA. 1979;242(6):521–2.

Thoracic surgeons in Western Europe and North America rarely encounter hydatid disease cases due to travel and migration.

Primary hosts are Canidae family, mostly dogs. Hydatid cyst develops and reproduces in the intestines of the primary host, and worms are released with the feces of the primary host. Intermediate hosts (sheep, goats, swine, etc.) ingest contaminated vegetables, grass, and water and sustain the pathogen, and then larval stage starts. The pathogen is absorbed through gastrointestinal tract via portal venous system or lymphatic circulation. Once in the organ mainly liver or lungs, it develops into typical hydatid cysts. The liver is the most common site for hydatid disease (60–80%) and followed by lungs (10–30%). The disease manifests most commonly in the right side and particularly in lower lobes bilaterally [2, 3]. 75–90% of the disease is solitary. Contrary to adults, pulmonary hydatid disease is more common than hepatic hydatid disease in pediatric patients [4].

The hydatid cyst is composed of cyst wall and hydatid fluid (Fig. 11.1). The wall has three layers. These layers aid for the nutrition and constitute integrity of the cyst. The hydatid fluid is odorless, clear fluid. The rupture of the cyst can be inside the pericystic membrane or into the pleura, adjacent organ, bronchus, or vessels. Cystic rupture can be spontaneous or due to trauma or antihelminthic medications. This complication has different clinical consequences like anaphylactic shock, spread of the disease, infection of the cyst, asphyxia, and hemoptysis. Rarely the cyst can be calcified because of infection and usually these cysts are connected with the bronchial tree.

Clinical manifestations vary according to the integrity or rupture of the cyst. Intact cysts do not have any specific symptoms and depend on the size and the localization. In symptomatic patients cough and bloodstained sputum are the most common symptoms. Also some patients have chest pain and feeling of pressure on their chests. In patients with ruptured cysts (Fig. 11.2), symptoms can be different like

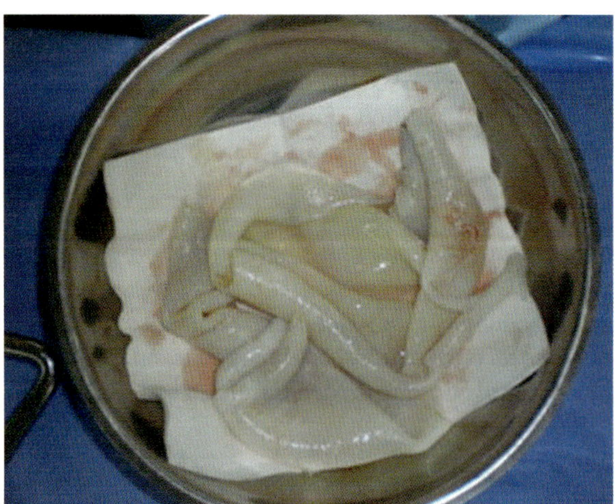

Fig. 11.1 Resected specimen: Membrane of the cyst

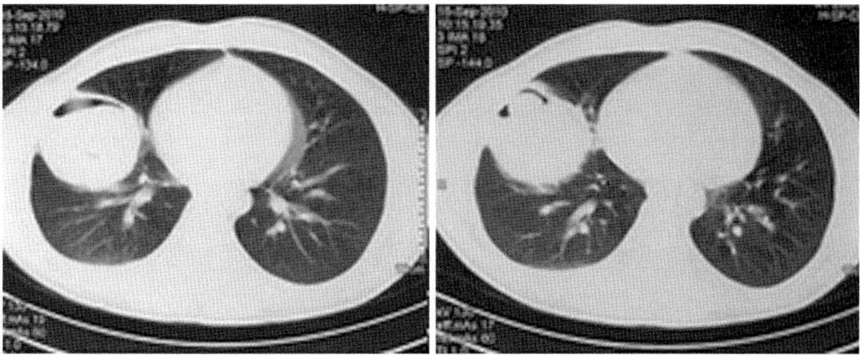

Fig. 11.2 CT showing perforated hydatid cyst

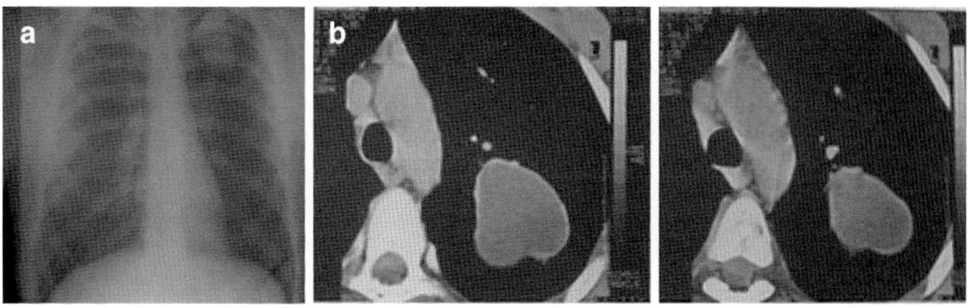

Fig. 11.3 (**a**) Lobulated hydatid cyst of the left upper lobe on X-ray. (**b**) Hydatid cyst of the upper lobe on CT

severe dyspnea, salty sputum containing fragments of the cyst (parasites can be detected microscopically), high fever, pruritus, and hypersensitivity reaction.

Patients can be diagnosed primarily by clinical suspicion and abnormal findings on their routine chest X-rays. Radiologically, cysts are seen like homogenous opacities with definite boundaries (Fig. 11.3). Sometimes cysts cause obstruction on bronchial tree resulting atelectasis and pneumonitis on the imaging modalities. The cysts settled in the central region may cause compression on bronchovascular structures presenting depression at the site of compression. Cysts are mostly located at the right lower lobe and are mostly solitary. Presentation of the ruptured cyst may vary from tension hydropneumothorax to partial loculated hydropneumothorax on radiological modalities. CT scan is also useful in the early diagnosis of the small or ruptured cysts [5]. CT scan also aids for the follow-up of patients who are treated surgically or medically. Further investigations can be done for the evaluation of pericardial/cardiac or hepatic cysts.

Laboratory diagnosis of the disease is supportive to clinical and radiological evaluation. Casoni's intradermal test and Weinberg's complement fixation test are valuable and were used frequently in the past. These test are not preferred nowadays because of their limited diagnostic value. Instead of those tests, new serological tests are improved for the diagnosis. Indirect hemagglutination test and indirect immunofluorescence test are the most common tests. Application of these tests verifies the diagnosis up to 94%. Nevertheless, seronegativity does not exclude the diagnosis but a serological follow-up is necessary after the resection for the detection of recurrences.

Treatment of the pulmonary hydatid disease is basically surgical. Antihelminthic agents like albendazole and mebendazole are used for the medical treatment of the hydatid disease. These agents have a tendency for rupturing the cyst [3, 6].

11.2 Technical Tips and Tricks of Surgical Treatment of Hydatid Disease

Surgical intervention is the main treatment modality for pulmonary hydatid disease.

Most surgeons prefer to spare the lungs so they prefer enucleation of the cyst, cystectomy and capitonnage, or pericystectomy (Perez-Fontana technique) which includes closure of the bronchial openings and capitonnage of the space if needed [7–9]. It is important not to resect lung tissues because atelectatic lung will expand after cystectomy.

In the Preoperative and Perioperative Period

1. Preoperative preparations are similar to any patient undergoing thoracotomy for any reason for uncomplicated hydatid cysts and otherwise healthy individual. Preoperative antibiotics, postural drainage, and other supportive measures should be included in large and suppurative lesions.
2. Bilateral cysts – one or two stages: Indications for two-stage operations are (1) larger number of cysts, (2) requirement for lobectomy, (3) cardiopulmonary reserve limitations, and (4) uncompensated chronic conditions. In two-stage operations, the lung with larger cyst or having numerous cysts should be operated first. Contralateral lesion can be resected 2–4 weeks after the first operation. One-stage resection of bilateral cysts with bilateral thoracotomies or median sternotomy is also advocated by numerous of researchers in uncomplicated cysts and healthy individuals [10, 11] (Fig. 11.4).
3. Double-lumen endotracheal tube is preferred for preventing the cysts to spread into the tracheobronchial tree or the suppurative content to spill over into unaffected lung parenchyma. Posterolateral thoracotomy through fifth or sixth intercostal space is performed. It is important not to rupture the cyst during thoracotomy.
4. In intact cysts, excision of the cysts can be done with or without needle aspiration (Fig. 11.5). Pericystic zone should be carefully separated from the laminated membrane during the enucleation without needle aspiration. It is not difficult to apply this process in small cysts but it is challenging in larger ones. Larger cysts have greater possibility of rupture during separation of the laminated membrane from the pericystic zone. Because of this potential complication, the surgical field must be covered with gauzes steeped in hypertonic

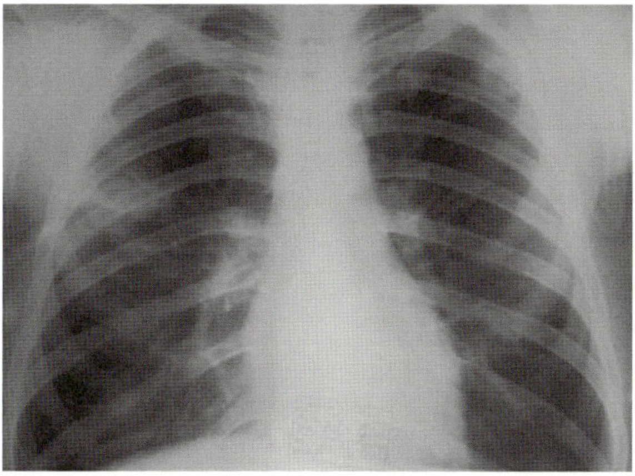

Fig. 11.4 Bilateral hydatid cysts, which are later operated with sternotomy

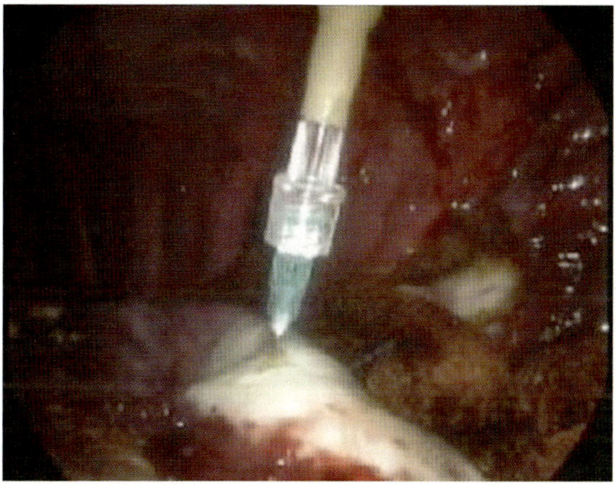

Fig. 11.5 Video-assisted thoracoscopic aspiration of the cyst with needle

saline solutions for preventing contamination of the parasitic material. Despite this preventative measures, hydatid fluid may still contaminate pleural space and trigger an anaphylactic reaction.

5. After isolating the cyst, tissue over it is dissected with extreme care. Cyst is exposed and an incision is performed diagonally on the pericystic zone for creating a space between the laminated membranes.
6. During the separation of the membranes, it is important to lower the airway pressure. This maneuver avoids the laminated membrane to protrude through the opening on pericystic zone and risk rupture of the cyst. After separating the two zones completely, airway pressure is increased in order to remove the cyst.
7. Following removal of the cyst, residual space has to be checked for bronchial openings and air leaks over sewn. Residual pericystic zone has to be folded

with any of the identified techniques. We first close the bronchial openings and then resect the free portion of the pericyst and then capitonnage is performed into the residual space. Finally we suture the edges with a continuous suture.

8. *Capitonnage*: In this method we pack the pleural cavity with gauze pieces soaked in hypertonic saline immobilizing the lobe containing the cyst. The lung is inflated, two suctions system has to be available and ready before aspirating of the cyst with 20-gauge needle. The content of the cyst is aspirated as much as possible followed by excising a small portion of the cyst to allow a suction catheter to aspirate the residual content. While aspirating inside of the cyst, the second suction aspirates any hydatid fluid overflowing from the cyst. During evacuation of all parasitic contents, lung has to be kept inflated for preventing cystic content pass through bronchial openings into the bronchial tree. Finally, laminated membrane is excised. Cavity is again irrigated with hypertonic saline solution and cavity and bronchial openings are closed in the manner described above.
9. An alternative method is to needle aspirate the content of the cyst and refill with scolicidal agents (hypertonic saline) as a precaution to prevent spillage of hydatid fluid into the pleural space. We prefer hypertonic saline solutions over other scolicidal agents as it does not affect tissue healing. The solutions has to be kept in the thorax at least 10 min for optimal efficiency [12, 13].
10. Complicated cyst: If the cyst has ruptured into the bronchus or pleural cavity or infected with secondary bacterial infection, it is defined as complicated cyst. Precautions have to be performed initially for preventing complications resulting from spread of the cystic contents into the tracheobronchial tree and pleural space. Orotracheal suction or bronchoscopy has to be performed for aspirating secretions and cystic contents. After the acute period, the patient has to be operated urgently for the removal of the cystic contents from pleural cavity.
11. In the event the cyst is infected, the cyst is incised carefully taking care not to damage surrounding consolidated parenchyma [14]. The cavity is irrigated many times with hypertonic solutions. Bronchial openings are closed with or without capitonnage according to the surgeon. Complicated cysts can result in fibrosis over parenchyma or pleura so additional procedures may be needed like decortication, segmentectomy, or lobectomy [15].
12. Video-assisted thoracoscopic surgery (VATS) is a novel approach for the resection of pulmonary hydatid cysts [16]. Main surgical principles have to be maintained similar to the open surgical approach mentioned above. Findikcioglu A et al. [17] reported their series of 12 cases without any mortality or recurrence. Parelkar and colleagues [18] had a series of five patients where three cases were managed with VATS and the other two required converted to open surgery.

11.3 Tips and Tricks for Surgical Complications of Hydatid Disease

Postoperative complications can vary and are related to the size and number of cysts, type of operations, and degree of infection. With appropriate care and surgery, the prognosis of the disease is good.

1. The most common complications are pleural infection and prolonged air leak. Aubert and Viard [19] presented a 2.54% pleural infection and 2.19% prolonged air leakage rate in 8384 cases.
2. Mortality and morbidity rates are low. Turkyilmaz and colleagues [20] reported no mortality on their series of pediatric 35 cases and also Topcu et al. [21] had no mortality in 128 pediatric patients, while Solak and colleagues [22] experienced 0.6% mortality and 0.4% recurrence on their series of 460 patients. The recurrence rate is also very low. In a report of 301 cases containing both the pediatric and adult patients, Ibrahim Dincer and colleagues [23] experienced 4.5% recurrence in pediatric group and 4.3% in adult patients, while Ayuso and colleagues [24] reported 2.7% recurrence rate in their series.

Conclusion

Surgical management is the main stay and treatment modality of choice for pulmonary hydatidosis. The Medical therapy supports the healing period and reduces the recurrence of the disease following surgery. Although thoracotomy is the traditional approach, recently VATS has gained popularity in the management of hydatid disease. Hydatid disease has overall good prognosis following surgery and medical supportive treatment with low recurrence rates.

References

1. Orueta A, Fau LF, Montero A, Prieto J, Duarte PG. Surgical treatment of hydatid cysts of the lung. Br J Dis Chest. 1974;68:183–92.
2. Burgos R, Varela A, Castedo E, Roda J, Montero CG, Serrano S, Tellez G, Ugarte J. Pulmonary hydatidosis: surgical treatment and follow-up of 240 cases. Eur J Cardiothorac Surg. 1999;16(6):628–35.
3. Dogan R, Yuksel M, Cetin G, Suzer K, Alp M, Kaya S, Unlu M, Moldibi B. Surgical treatment of hydatid cysts of the lung: report on 1055 patients. Thorax. 1989;44:192–9.
4. Balci AE, Eren N, Eren S, Ulku R. Ruptured hydatid cysts of the lung in children: clinical review and results of surgery. Ann Thorac Surg. 2002;74:889–92.
5. Saksouk FA, Meheddin HF, Ghassan KR. Computed tomography of pulmonary hydatid disease. J Comput Assist Tomogr. 1986;10(2):226.
6. Kurul IC, Topcu S, Altinok T, Yazici U, Tastepe I, Kaya S, Cetin G. One-stage operation for hydatid disease of lung and liver: principles of treatment. J Thorac Cardiovasc Surg. 2002;124(6):1212–5.
7. Ugon CV. Therapy of hydatid cysts of the lungs and their complications. J Int Chir. 1952;12(3):155–78.
8. Barrett NR. The treatment of pulmonary hydatid disease. Thorax. 1947;2:21.
9. Perez-Fontana V. Le traitement des kystes hydatique du poumon. La method Uruguayenne ou extirpation du perikyste. Arch Int Hydatid. 1951;12:469.
10. Cetin G, Dogan R, Yuksel M, Alp M, Ucanok K, Kaya S, Unlu M. Surgical treatment of bilateral hydatid disease of the lung via median sternotomy: experience in 60 consecutive patients. J Thorac Cardiovasc Surg. 1988;36(2):114–7.
11. Petrov DB, Terzinacheva PP, Djambazov VI, Plochev MP, Goranov EP, Minchev TR, Petrov PV. Surgical treatment of bilateral hydatid disease of the lung. Eur J Cardiothorac Surg. 2001;19(6):918–23.
12. Shalabi RIY, Ayed AK, Amin M. 15 years in surgical management of pulmonary hydatidosis. Ann Thorac Cardiovasc Surg. 2002;8(3):131–4.

Blunt Thoracic Trauma 12

Edward J. Caruana and Sridhar Rathinam

Abstract

Blunt thoracic trauma (BTT) accounts for a significant proportion of chest injuries, which may present in isolation or in the polytrauma patient. There are two well-defined groups of patients who present with BTT:

- Patients with high-energy injuries who tend to have multi-trauma and are critically ill. The aim in managing these patients is to identify life-threatening underlying injuries and stabilise them as much as possible prior to referring to thoracic surgery. Occasionally, the need for urgent surgery by a thoracic surgeon is required, but in most cases minor procedures which can be performed in the prehospital setting and emergency department (ED) will suffice to achieve clinical stability. Specific conditions may require the skills of a specialist cardiothoracic surgeon once clinical stability is achieved.
- Patients with isolated low-energy thoracic trauma with rib fractures and some of the underlying complications. The treatment of these patients tends to concentrate on respiratory support and effective analgesia. In patients with significant fractures and flail segments, early surgical fixation of rib fractures should be performed to achieve better analgesia, faster recovery and prevent prolonged ventilation.

This chapter aims to offer an overview on blunt thoracic trauma and outline practical tips and tricks in the surgical management of blunt thoracic trauma.

E.J. Caruana, M.D., M.R.C.S.Ed. • S. Rathinam, FRCSEd(CSiG), FRCSEd(CTh) (✉)
Department of Thoracic Surgery, Glenfield Hospital, University Hospitals of Leicester NHS Trust, Leicester, UK
e-mail: srathinam@rcsed.ac.uk

D. Parikh, P.B. Rajesh (eds.), *Tips and Tricks in Thoracic Surgery*,
https://doi.org/10.1007/978-1-4471-7355-7_12

Keywords
Blunt thoracic trauma · Thoracic · Trauma · Rib fixation · Tractotomy · Diaphragmatic injuries

12.1 Introduction: Epidemiology and Outcomes

Thoracic trauma remains one of the leading causes of presentation and mortality in emergency departments (ED) worldwide. Blunt thoracic trauma (BTT) accounts for the majority of cardiothoracic trauma in civilian practice, with the remainder caused by penetrating trauma. BTT can be an isolated injury or part of the polytrauma spectrum [1].

The standard of care provision varies significantly depending on whether the injuries are isolated or associated with other injuries as well as the presence of comorbidities.

1. Major blunt trauma is caused by road traffic collisions (RTCs), work-related accidents, blast injuries in the military setting or civilian terrorism. The treatment of trauma patients is often multidisciplinary in nature, involving emergency physicians, trauma surgeons and specialist care, i.e. neurosurgery, cardiothoracic surgery, general surgery, interventional radiology and intensivists. RTC remains the most common cause of accidental injuries leading to death. Patient mortality due to trauma follows a tri-modal pattern: [2]
   (a) *Immediate* (prehospital) deaths (0–30 min) are responsible for half of RTA deaths, and the causes are often myocardial rupture or thoracic aorta transection along with high spinal and head injury [3].
   (b) *Early* (30 min–3 h) deaths include treatable causes like pneumothorax, cardiac tamponade, airway obstruction and uncontrolled haemorrhage. These conditions if managed promptly and effectively can save lives. Some thoracic interventions in this cohort can be performed in prehospital and in emergency departments improving the outcomes.
   (c) *Delayed* (hours to days) deaths are caused by multi-organ failure and sepsis. The role of dedicated major trauma centres and early access to such specialised centres are essential in improving the outcome of these patients.
2. Isolated BTT with low-energy mechanisms of injury causes rib fractures, flail segments, pneumothorax, haemothorax and lung contusion. The challenge in these patients is the prevention of life-threatening respiratory complications particularly in elderly patients with multiple rib fractures, pre-existing cardiopulmonary disease and limited physiological reserve.

This chapter outlines the basic assessment and management of BTT and offers tips and tricks in surgical interventions and management of blunt thoracic trauma.

12.2 Mechanisms of Trauma

Blunt thoracic trauma results in organ damage by compression, acceleration or deceleration and shear forces often sustained in RTCs, assaults and falls. However, in the elderly, even minor trauma—for example, a fall from standing—can result in serious injury. These mechanisms are usually divided according to the pattern of injury:

- Direct impact from a seat belt or air bag deployment in a RTC which may cause cardiac contusions, pulmonary contusion, sternal or rib fractures (with or without flail segment) and thoracic spine fractures
- Acceleration or deceleration injury—typically caused by a high-energy RTC or a fall from height, resulting in aortic disruption, major airway injury and diaphragmatic rupture
- Crush and asphyxiation injury caused by sudden severe compressive trauma to the chest and abdomen, lasting 2–5 min and often associated with motorcycle accidents

An understanding of specific mechanisms involved in individual trauma patients is crucial because patterns of injury are produced with significant differences in pathophysiology and clinical course, and often life-threatening injuries without obvious external signs are missed.

12.3 Mechanism of Death After Blunt Trauma

The main consequences of BTT are combined respiratory and cardiovascular failure leading to tissue hypoxia and death. This can be caused by:

- Hypovolaemia resulting from major blood loss, with subsequent hypoperfusion and shock
- Ventilation/perfusion mismatch in pulmonary contusion
- Loss of negative intrathoracic pressure such as in tension pneumothorax or open pneumothorax

Immediate deaths from BTT are usually related to cardiac or aortic disruption.

12.4 Tips and Tricks in Diagnosis and Triage

BTT patients should be managed according to the Advanced Trauma Life Support (ATLS) guidelines of assessment and resuscitation [4], which rely on making diagnosis of life-threatening conditions in a systematic way and offer the necessary interventions simultaneously through the primary and secondary surveys.

Primary survey focuses on the ABCDE approach:

- A—airway maintenance and cervical spine control
- B—breathing and ventilation

- C—circulation and haemorrhage control
- D—disability or neurological status
- E—exposure and environmental control

The main injuries to identify include:

- Airway obstruction
- Tension pneumothorax
- Open pneumothorax
- Flail chest and pulmonary contusion
- Massive haemothorax
- Cardiac tamponade

Secondary survey includes a focused history and top-to-toe examination after initial assessment and treatment of life-threatening injuries. When assessing chest injuries, the mechanism of trauma is invaluable in terms of immediate injury management and eventual outcome. Diagnosis is reliant on accurate history from pre-hospital teams in order to tailor the clinical assessment and investigations to identify and exclude various injuries.

Relevant information like speed of collision, position of colliding vehicles, position of patient in the car, use of seatbelt and extent of vehicle damage (intrusion, windscreen damage, difficulty and length of extrication, air bag deployment) help in diagnosis.

Likewise for falls from a height, height of fall, objects struck (banisters or scaffolding), landing surface, part of body injured and reason of fall (industrial, drugs or alcohol, epilepsy) are all relevant in management decisions [5].

12.5 Tips and Tricks in Imaging

12.5.1 Chest Radiograph

Chest radiography (CXR) is the most frequently performed first-line investigation in thoracic trauma as it can be performed in the resuscitation area whilst actively managing critical patients. Although it offers limited information, it helps in diagnosis and guides further imaging. Injuries to the first two ribs indicate high-velocity trauma and warrant a computed tomography (CT) of the thorax to rule out vascular injuries. Fractures to the lower four ribs are commonly associated with injuries to the abdominal organs which warrants an ultrasound scan or a CT of the abdomen.

A widened mediastinum should lead to suspicion of aortic injury, and a globular heart shadow may indicate the possibility of a pericardial collection. CXR also reveals features suggestive of aortic transection including loss of the aortic knob, displacement of the nasogastric tube to the right of the T4 spinous process, left apical pleural cap, widened paraspinal lines, widened right paratracheal stripe greater than 5 mm and loss of the descending aortic line, although these are not pathognomonic of aortic transection and the only diagnostic sign of aortic rupture is a widened mediastinum >8 cm at the aortic knob [6].

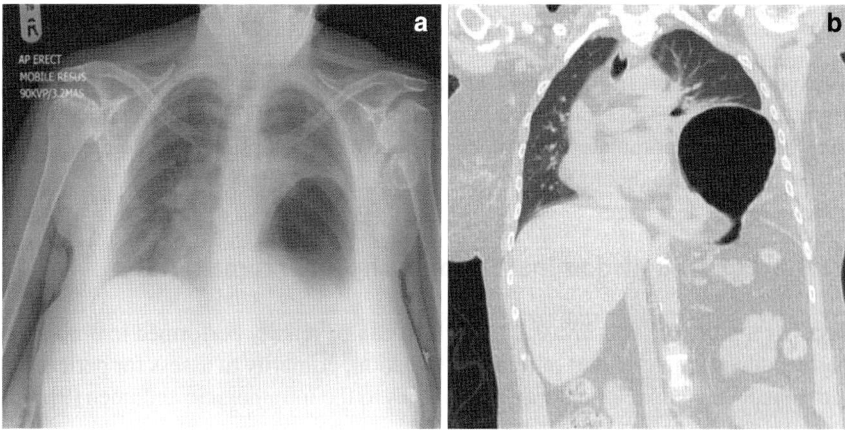

Fig. 12.1 Chest radiograph and CT scan demonstrating diaphragmatic rupture

The presence of pneumomediastinum indicates possible oesophageal perforation or tracheobronchial injury, whilst in diaphragmatic injury, bowel gas shadows may be seen in the chest (Fig. 12.1). Tracheobronchial disruption is confirmed by the 'fallen lung' sign, pneumothorax with the hilum of the collapsed lung situated lower than the normal hilar position. These features need further evaluation with appropriate further imaging.

12.5.2 Computed Tomography (CT)

CT in haemodynamically unstable polytrauma patients has become an integral part of the management of multi-trauma patients. Although once discouraged and historically referred to as 'the doughnut of death', the speed and the quality of this modality offer a wealth of information with regard to the skeletal injuries, pleural collections underlying pulmonary status as well as mediastinal structures. Recent reconstructed CTs offer better visualisation of rib fractures, flail segments and diaphragmatic injuries (Fig. 12.1b). The use of CT does not increase the mortality of haemodynamically unstable patients; meanwhile it prevented unnecessary surgery [7]. Results of the REACT-2 randomised controlled trial which investigated the role of total-body CT scanning compared to those by the 'standard work-up' with selective CT scanning have shown no survival benefit and only modest improvement in detecting relevant incidental findings. The use of routine CT scan to screen for aortic injury will remain debatable as aortography is the gold standard in aortic injuries. CT has the advantages as it may reveal other unsuspected intrathoracic injuries; a negative scan obviates the need for aortography, which carries a combined morbidity and mortality of 1.7% and is a costly investigation. However, the disadvantages are a positive scan merely delays the definitive aortogram and surgery. Helical CT has a sensitivity of 95% for detection of aortic injuries, but a specificity of 40%, rate requiring further investigation, and finally there are differences in defining the criteria for aortic injury [8].

12.6.3 Needle Cricothyroidotomy

A large-bore (14 gauge or larger) intravenous cannula may be used for needle cricothyroidotomy, in the absence of dedicated equipment.

Following appropriate skin preparation, a needle-mounted catheter on a syringe half-filled with water is advanced through the cricothyroid membrane in its midline directed caudally at 45°, whilst maintaining negative pressure on the plunger. Easy flow of air confirms entry into the airway, at which point the catheter should be advanced over the needle to its hilt.

Oxygenation may be achieved by attaching high-flow (15Lpm) oxygen to the catheter via a three-way tap open to air. Cyclical intermittent occlusion (1 s) and release (3 s) of the side limb of the three-way tap allows oxygenation and some degree of ventilation, as a temporising measure to a more definitive airway.

12.6.4 Percutaneous Cricothyroidotomy

A standard Seldinger technique may be adopted, using purpose-made commercially available kits.

Following cannulation of the airway as described for needle cricothyroidotomy above, the guidewire is threaded into place and the cannula removed. A small skin incision is performed and tract dilatation and airway catheter insertion performed either simultaneously or successively, depending on the equipment in use, prior to securing in place.

12.6.5 Surgical Cricothyroidotomy

Emergency surgical cricothyroidotomy may be performed using a scalpel, curved blunt dissection forceps (e.g. Kelley), gum-elastic bougie and a small (size 6) endotracheal or tracheostomy tube.

Following skin preparation and identification of landmarks, a 2 cm horizontal incision is made through the skin and soft tissues above the cricothyroid membrane. A horizontal stab incision is made into the cricothyroid membrane using the scalpel (whilst taking care not to injure the back wall of the airway). This is then dilated using blunt dissection forceps and a gum-elastic bougie inserted into the trachea. The appropriate-size tube is then positioned over the bougie and secured.

12.6.6 Tension Pneumothorax

Injury to the visceral pleura or upper airway can result in rapid accumulation of air in the pleural space and collapse of the lung. A flap laceration of the lung parenchyma may create a one-way valve, causing intrapleural pressure to rise and mediastinal structures to be compressed. The venous return to the heart is thus compromised. The classic symptoms and signs are chest pain, air hunger, respiratory distress, tachycardia, hypotension, tracheal deviation to the contralateral side, hyper-resonance on percussion, unilateral absence of breath sounds and neck vein distension.

The diagnosis of this condition is clinical, not radiological. Immediate needle thoracocentesis through the second intercostal space in the mid-clavicular line converts the tension pneumothorax into a simple pneumothorax, which subsequently should be treated with chest drain insertion. If tension pneumothorax occurs on both sides, unilateral signs may be absent. Bilateral needle thoracocentesis or thoracostomy followed by bilateral chest drain insertion is required.

12.6.7 Thoracostomy

Chest drainage [14] may be achieved safely in an emergent scenario, at either of the following sites.

The 'safe triangle' is defined anteriorly by the lateral border of pectoralis major (anterior axillary line), posteriorly by the mid-axillary line (classically by the anterior border of latissimus dorsi—that is, the posterior axillary line; however, this places the long thoracic nerve of Bell at risk during insertion) and inferiorly by the nipple line. Inadvertent low chest tube siting is common [15].

An anterior thoracostomy may be placed in the second or third intercostal spaces, at or just lateral to the mid-clavicular line. Care should be taken to avoid instrumenting superiorly at this site, to minimise the risk of subclavian vascular injury and to be mindful that medial insertion places the internal mammary vessels at risk.

Consider the positioning of the intercostal bundle just inferior to the ribs. Intercostal dissection and tube insertion should skim just above the lower rib, so as to minimise bleeding and pain complications.

Where possible, avoid insertion at sites of known rib fractures or external injury. Bedside image guidance in the form of ultrasound may guide the competent user to target other sites but should only be used in the stable patient.

Patients are classically positioned semi-recumbent at a 45-degree angle. The arm should be abducted and externally rotated (placing the hand above and behind the patient's head) to facilitate insertion into the safety triangle. In unstable patients, the supine position may be used, with abduction or extension of the arm facilitating lateral insertion.

12.6.8 Needle Thoracocentesis

A long, large-bore needle-mounted catheter is inserted into the pleural space either anteriorly or laterally in the safe sites described above [16] and the needle then removed to leave the soft catheter in situ. Initial success rates are low, with an even higher incidence of early failure due to catheter kinking or displacement [17].

The use of longer, dedicated pleural thoracocentesis needles may increase the success and longevity of this intervention [18]. Repeated instrumentations (placed progressively lateral to the mid-clavicular line) may be attempted to temporise, if necessary. Custom-made decompression needles offer the benefit of inbuilt one-way valves which aid rapid decompression (Fig. 12.2a) [19].

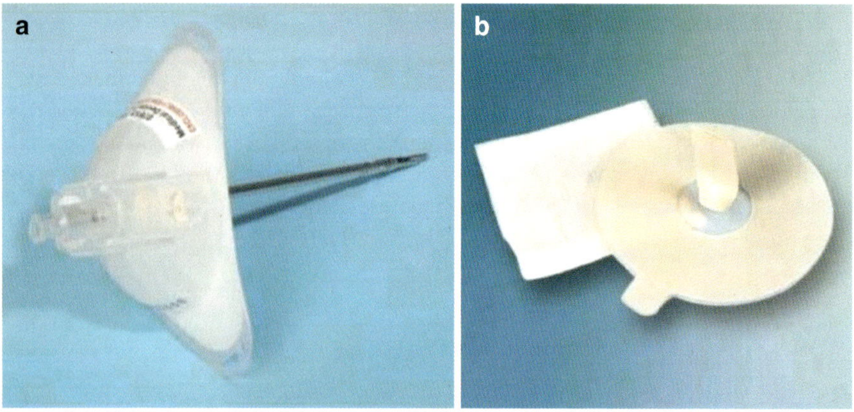

Fig. 12.2 (**a**) ThoraQuik needle decompression device. (**b**) Asherman Chest Seal

Nonetheless, needle thoracocentesis is a decompressive intervention and not a definitive pleural drainage system, which thus should be succeeded by tube thoracostomy [20].

12.6.9 Open Thoracostomy

An 'open' or 'finger' thoracostomy may be used to achieve decompression of the pleural space, quickly draining both blood and air. A scalpel and curved blunt dissection forceps are sufficient equipment for this purpose. Bilateral open thoracostomy may only be performed in patients receiving positive-pressure ventilation.

Following skin preparation with an antiseptic solution, generous infiltration of local anaesthetic (20 mL of 1% Lignocaine) through the tissues (particularly to the skin and parietal pleura) should precede insertion in the awake patient.

A generous (at least 3 cm), full-thickness incision is made through the skin and subcutaneous tissues, along the direction of the ribs. Blunt dissection (Roberts or Kelly) forceps are used to dissect a tract through the chest wall and intercostal musculature just at the upper border of the rib, with intermittent finger palpation to confirm positioning. Dissect one single tunnel perpendicular to the chest wall, avoiding long or multiple blind subcutaneous tracts that may complicate insertion. The closed dissection forceps should be used to puncture the pleura in a controlled fashion; opening the dissection forceps prior to extracting from the chest will dilate the pleural defect and tract through the chest wall.

A finger should be inserted into the pleural space and swept circumferentially along the inside of the chest wall, to confirm safe entry to the pleural space and sweep away any loosely adherent lung. Failure to digitally confirm safe entry and sufficient intrapleural space may demand re-attempting insertion at an alternate site.

Note that soft tissue may reappose to occlude the thoracostomy, requiring repeated digital or blunt dissection. Patient and equipment positioning may also occlude the thoracostomy site. Open thoracostomy may be considered an interim in the prehospital or trauma resuscitation setting but should be converted to a tube thoracostomy once appropriate.

12.6.10 Tube Thoracostomy

A large-bore—at least 28Fr—chest tube should be mounted on the dissecting forceps, just proximal to its tip, and inserted through the tract formed as described above [21].

Ensure that all chest tube fenestrations are located well within the pleural cavity, adjusting for variable subcutaneous tissue depth in different patients. The tube should generally be oriented apically when attempting to drain air and basally for fluid. Clamping of the tube until it is connected to a drainage system may reduce soiling, particularly when draining fluid.

Once positioned, the chest tube should be connected to an underwater seal and secured using a heavy, braided suture.

Tube placement should be confirmed by plain film imaging, once the clinical situation allows.

12.6.11 Open Pneumothorax

This results from an opening through the chest wall into the pleural cavity. If the opening exceeds two thirds of the diameter of the trachea, preferential air flow through the defect prevents generation of the negative intrapleural pressure required to expand the lung. The initial management consists of covering the defect to create a one-way valve to evacuate the air in the pleura. This can be done with an Asherman Chest Seal (Fig. 12.2b) or, if this is not available, a dressing plastered on three sides. As soon as possible, a chest drain should be placed, remote from the wound.

12.6.12 Massive Haemothorax

Massive haemothorax may occur with accumulation of 1500 mL of blood in the pleural cavity with resulting hypovolaemia and hypotension. Management consists of replacement of circulating volume and decompression of the chest with large chest drains (>28 FG). Immediate drainage of 1500 mL of blood may need urgent thoracotomy and definitive haemostasis [22]. If initial drainage is less than 1500 mL, there may still be a need for a thoracotomy if blood loss exceeds 200 mL/h over the next few hours. Pending this decision, the patient must be closely monitored in a high-dependency setting.

12.6.13 Cardiac Tamponade

Although cardiac tamponade is associated more with penetrating trauma, it is not uncommon to have it in blunt trauma. This can be caused by rib fractures causing pericardial or myocardial laceration and missile injuries in RTC caused by debris as well as myocardial rupture.

12.7 Tips and Tricks in Emergency Access

12.7.1 Thoracotomy and Thoracosternotomy

The patient should be sedated, paralysed and intubated prior to commencing the procedure. Double-lumen intubation or the use of a bronchial blocker may be used to achieve selective lung isolation; however, this is technically challenging and often time-consuming. A single-lumen tube with brief periods of apnoea may be undertaken to facilitate vision or intervention, if required. The left lung may additionally be isolated by selectively advancing a single-lumen tube down to the right main bronchus [23].

The patient should be supine, with the arms secured in a flexed position above the patient's head (where practical).

A scalpel, dissection scissors and rib spreader (e.g. Finochietto) and heavy trauma shears are sufficient for the purposes of accessing the chest.

Note the risk of profuse bleeding from chest wall and internal mammary vessels that are at risk of iatrogenic injury during emergency access to the thoracic cavity. This typically occurs with return of spontaneous circulation and should be actively sought and stemmed.

12.7.2 Anterior Thoracotomy

The anterior thoracotomy is preferred for access to the traumatised chest in clinical instability. A left-sided approach is adopted in all patients in cardiac arrest, to allow internal cardiac massage. Right-sided thoracotomy is indicated in patients with a spontaneous circulation and right-sided trauma.

Following appropriate (bilateral) skin preparation, a curved submammary incision through the skin, subcutaneous tissue and muscle (anterior border of latissimus dorsi) is performed extending from the sternal border to the mid-axillary line (Fig. 12.3a).

The chest is then entered bluntly using dissecting forceps (Roberts) in the fourth intercostal space (just above the fifth rib, avoiding injury to the intercostal bundle), with a finger then inserted to retract the lung away whilst transecting the intercostal

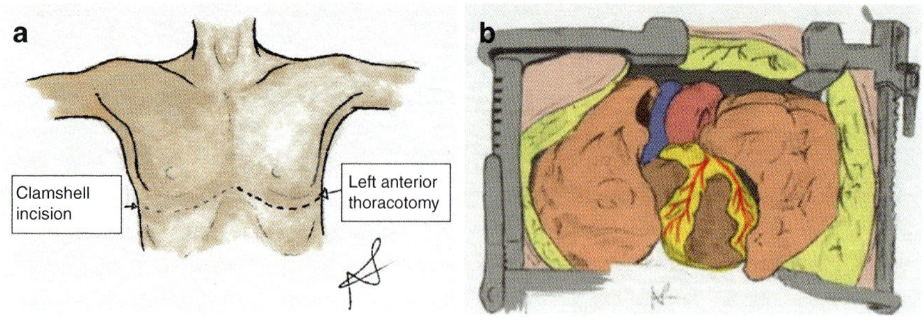

Fig. 12.3 (**a**) Anterolateral thoracotomy and clamshell incision. (**b**) Clamshell incision with exposed thoracic cavity

muscles along the length of the incision with scissors. A brief period of apnoea with ventilator disconnection allows the lung to collapse once the pleura is breached, reducing the risk of iatrogenic injury.

Improved access may be achieved by extending the incision across the contralateral sternal edge and horizontally splitting the sternum using heavy shears or a saw (e.g. Gigli) and/or by cutting the fifth rib posteriorly.

12.7.3 Thoracosternotomy

Where access to both sides of the chest is required, bilateral anterior thoracotomies may be performed and joined by a horizontal sternal division to give a 'clamshell' incision. The use of rib retractors bilaterally (or a single retractor placed at the sternum) will lift the upper chest, providing excellent access (Fig. 12.3b).

12.8 Tips and Tricks in Managing Injuries Associated with Blunt Trauma

12.8.1 Rib Fractures

The true incidence of rib fractures is not known, as 50% may not be apparent on a chest radiograph [24]. Patients rarely present with isolated rib fractures; the majority have associated intrathoracic injuries, and of particular significance are fractures of the first rib. These are uncommon injuries because of the first rib's rigid structure and relatively protected location. They are indicative of severe trauma and should prompt a search for associated visceral injury.

12.8.2 Flail Chest

Flail chest occurs where a portion of the chest wall is free floating due to multiple segmental rib fractures and occurs in about 5% of thoracic trauma patients. The ensuing pulmonary insufficiency results from three pathophysiological processes:

1. A negative intrapleural pressure cannot be maintained due to the paradoxical motion of the flail segment.
2. Pulmonary contusions sustained at the time of the injury cause haemorrhage and oedema of the lung underlying the flail.
3. Severe pain associated with the multiple fractured ribs results in hypoventilation.

The inadequacy of the resulting ventilation is indicated by arterial blood gas analysis. Treatment consists of appropriate analgesia to enable more effective chest wall movement, with ventilatory support if appropriate. Early fixation should be considered in these patients with respiratory compromise to prevent prolonged ventilation [25]. This can be done by using Stratos clasping device which stabilises the fracture and holds them together or Synthes plates and screws.

12.8.2.1 Rib Fixation

The access is approached through a lateral thoracotomy with individual surgeon preference varying between vertical axillary incision or lateral thoracotomy-like skin incision. The latissimus dorsi muscle fibres are divided to expose the serratus anterior. The serratus aponeurosis is divided to expose the ribs. The sites of fractures are identified. The periosteum is cleared to delineate the ribs; the ribs are stabilised with the stabilisers. The choice of the adjuncts varies between surgeons and is also dictated by the underlying ribs.

The Synthes system uses plates and screws; hence, healthy bones are a requirement as osteoporotic bones may disintegrate when the screws are fitted. Healthy bones need to be measured with the calipers to define the rib height. This allows selection of the correct size of screws. It is advisable to place three screws on each side of the fracture. It will be necessary to drill the holes prior to placing the self-locking screws. There are different plates which are in keeping with the size of the ribs; alternatively there are small plates as well. It is not necessary to fix every fracture, and usually fixing alternate ribs offers enough stability and relieves pain (Fig. 12.4a).

The Stratos system uses clasped adjuncts which wrap around the fractures to offer stability; care is taken to avoid the intercostal bundle whilst placing these adjuncts. If there are multiple fractures, there are long rods which allow interlinking the claspers (Fig. 12.4b).

12.8.3 Cardiac Tamponade

Although this is more common in penetrating trauma, blunt chest injury may also result in rupture of a cardiac chamber and subsequent tamponade. Injury to the heart or pericardial vessels causes blood to accumulate within the pericardial cavity. Increased intra-pericardial pressure acting on the low pressure atria and venae cavae reduces venous return, with consequent haemodynamic instability, manifesting

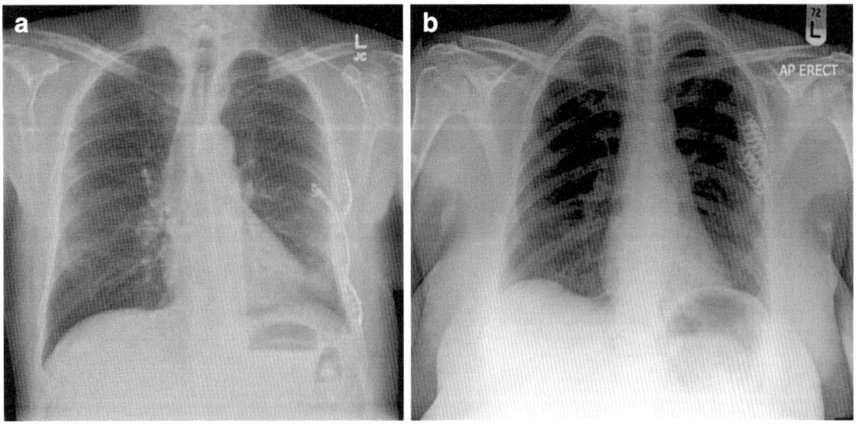

Fig. 12.4 (**a**) Rib fixation with plates and screw (Synthes). (**b**) Rib fixation with plates and screw (Stratos)

clinically as Beck's triad of increased jugular venous distension, hypotension and muffled heart sounds. Management consists of immediate surgical drainage and vascular repair. The condition may be temporarily relieved by the creation of a subxyphoid window, through which the pericardial cavity can be opened. Fluid resuscitation and needle pericardiocentesis have been shown to be of limited benefit [26].

12.8.4 Sternal Fractures

Sixty-six percent of traumatic sternal fractures is the result of an impact with a steering wheel. Wojcik and Morgan [27] report the incidence of associated cardiac contusion at 6%. Patients do not usually require inotropic support or develop dysrhythmias, and these injuries are managed conservatively. However, if the sternum is unstable, there are adjuncts which can be used to fix sternal fractures.

12.8.5 Pulmonary Injuries

Blunt trauma is more commonly associated with lung contusion, but if there are rib fractures caused by a blunt mechanism, pulmonary lacerations and pneumothoraces can ensue.

Blunt contusion of the lung can lead to sequestration of blood. In the absence of active bleeding, if the patient requires, volume contusion has to be born in mind as this can lead to volume loss. Another complication of blunt trauma is pulmonary haematoma. Although it is difficult to distinguish in the initial imaging, delayed films will demonstrate the haematoma as a more circumscribed area.

Most lacerations and air leaks may stop with chest drainage and conservative management. However if there is persistent air leak, surgical intervention may be warranted. Mostly surgical intervention in this cohort is performed as a planned procedure with the patient stable.

The choice of thoracoscopic or open approach is dictated by the stability of the patient to tolerate single-lung ventilation and surgeon's expertise.

12.8.6 Laceration

Lacerations are identified and are sutured with absorbable sutures. Alternatively, the laceration can be excluded and excised with a firing of stapler. The use of glues and adjuncts is best avoided as there is an increased risk of infection.

12.8.7 Tractotomy

A traversing injury has to be laid opened and explored (tractotomy), and major vessels and bronchi should be oversewn or repaired. This can be done by passing a pair of forceps and cutting it open or using a linear cutting surgical stapler, placing the anvil in the track and the staple cartilage on the lung surface. This lays the track open whilst sealing the edges.

12.8.8 Lung Resection

Repair of damage to major vessels in the hilum may require hilar control with clamps and sometimes may necessitate opening the pericardium. Sometimes the only option may be a lobectomy if there is destruction of the lobe with the missiles or glass pieces although the morbidity and mortality are very high.

12.8.9 Blunt Cardiac Trauma

The incidence of myocardial injury in victims of blunt chest trauma is 15–75%; however, a high index of suspicion is necessary, as myocardial injury often occurs in the absence of external signs. Blunt injury to the heart is almost always secondary to rapid deceleration in RTA when deceleration causes the heart to be crushed between the sternum and the spine. Primary crush accidents or a direct injury to the anterior chest wall will cause the same injuries.

Blunt cardiac injury causes disruption of the valvular apparatus, myocardial contusion or cardiac chamber rupture. ECG findings are variable, and measurement of the creatine kinase MB isoenzyme has been shown to be a sensitive marker of myocardial damage with a rise of greater than 6% of total CK-MB which is predictive of subsequent myocardial events. Elevated troponin I correlates with ECG changes and is indicative of myocardial damage. Echocardiography is very useful in assessing the contused myocardium.

12.8.10 Aortic Transection

Blunt rupture of the thoracic aorta is most commonly associated with rapid deceleration during RTC. This is caused by two mechanisms: (1) the *osseous pinch* effect where the deceleration or impact pushes the sternum backwards towards the vertebral column and the aorta is pinched between the two and (2) the *bell clanger effect* where the blood in the aorta pulls forwards like a bell clanger against the aorta which is fixed at the level of the isthmus. The majority of these patients die at the scene, and less than 25% survive to reach the hospital. The patient usually presents with a history of a blunt deceleration injury. Clinical presentation of the aortic injury is usually non-specific, with 20–50% of patients shocked and dyspnoeic. 30–50% of patients complain of interscapular or retrosternal pain. Reduced blood pressure in the arms compared to the legs is present in 7–40% of patients and is highly suggestive of acute aortic transaction. The strategies of management of aortic injuries are beyond the scope of this chapter; however, the principles are clamp and sew technique or repair under partial or complete cardiopulmonary bypass.

12.8.11 Diaphragmatic Injuries

Blunt trauma can cause diaphragmatic rupture due to sudden pressure changes; this is more common on the left side as the right is buttressed by the liver. Current CT scanners can identify diaphragmatic tears and ruptures (Fig. 12.1a, b). However the definitive diagnostic tool still remains a thoracoscopic examination as it allows clearance of the haemothorax, assessing the diaphragm as well as repairing it. The repair depends on the size of the rupture which can be closed primarily with non-absorbable sutures and if large buttressed with a mesh. A missed diaphragmatic injury may manifest later as herniation of abdominal contents more in the left than in the right. This may lead to intrathoracic obstruction or perforation with life-threatening consequences.

12.8.12 Tracheobronchial Injuries

The incidence of tracheobronchial injuries is between 0.85 and 2.8% in patients with blunt trauma, though many suffering major airway injury will die at the scene of the accident. Tracheal injuries can occur in deceleration RTA when the extended neck strikes the dashboard or steering wheel, crushing the trachea against the vertebral bodies. Tracheobronchial disruption is more common in the right side as the right main bronchus is unprotected unlike the left which is enclosed between the aorta and pulmonary artery and the weight of the right lung is more than the left.

12.8.13 Oesophageal Injury

Primary injury to the oesophagus is very rare in BTT due to its deep position within the mediastinum. However, it may occur as a secondary phenomenon caused by barotrauma. If there is blunt rupture of the oesophagus, primary repair with buttress done rapidly offers the best outcomes; however, if there is delay and soiling, diversion and chest drainage will stabilise the patient to enable transfer to a specialist centre.

12.9 Post-injury Care and Management

It is important to highlight the value of chest physiotherapy, analgesia and serial observation and imaging. Chest trauma victims can change their clinical stability very rapidly; hence, intense monitoring is mandatory. Pain management particularly if there are multiple ribs fractured or flail segments is provided with patient-controlled analgesia, intercostal blocks and epidural. A good regime of exercise, mobilisation and breathing exercise is vital in preventing pulmonary collapse and superadded infection especially in frail elderly patients. It is important to nurse elderly patients with input from elderly care physicians to address their comorbidity whilst treating with the thoracic trauma. Finally, they need a delayed imaging to rule out any delayed haemopneumothoraces both from a clinical and medicolegal perspective.

12.10 Delayed Presentations and Complications of Thoracic Trauma

Patients may re-present, or present late, with delayed complications resulting from blunt thoracic trauma. These commonly include retained, delayed or recurrent haemothorax, which may become secondarily infected resulting in pleural empyema in a quarter of patients [28] and occult diaphragmatic injury that may present with late dyspnoea as a result of paralysis or herniation of abdominal contents [29].

12.11 Role of Video-Assisted Thoracoscopic Surgery (VATS) in Thoracic Trauma

Minimally invasive surgery may be an appropriate initial approach in selected patients. It offers the advantage of better visualisation in hard-to-reach areas, whilst minimising the additional physiological insult associated with any surgical intervention. One should note both the diagnostic and therapeutic value of this approach [30].

Successful VATS without significant morbidity has been described in acute bleeding (with successful haemostasis), retained haemothorax and post-traumatic empyema (with adequate clearance and satisfactory lung expansion), diaphragmatic injuries (with definitive repair) and persistent air leak (with endoscopic control by means of repair and parenchymal resection) [31]. Rib fracture fixation may be performed by means of a VATS-assisted approach. Conversion thoracotomy is reported in circa 10–20% of cases [32, 33]. Early VATS intervention may also reduce lengths of hospital stay and associated costs in this patient group [34, 35].

Conventional VATS port positioning may be adopted, whilst being mindful of associated localised soft tissue and bony injury at potential access sites, as well as of the increased potential for visceral damage in the presence of altered anatomy.

Conclusion

Civilian blunt trauma is a common problem faced by most emergency units. The trauma network and good prehospital care have resulted in channelling these patients to appropriate units. Most thoracic traumas are best managed with resuscitation and chest drains; however, the analgesia, antibiotics and chest physiotherapy have invaluable role to play in the ultimate outcome. Resuscitative and emergency thoracotomies are still invaluable skill set for clinicians involved in the care of trauma patients as these procedures save lives. Appropriate referral to specialist centres and follow-up are essential to avoid delayed complications.

Acknowledgements Illustrated diagrams by Master Akhash V Rathinam.

References

1. Al-Koudmani I, Darwish B, Al-Kateb K, Taifour Y. Chest trauma experience over eleven-year period at al-mouassat university teaching hospital-Damascus: a retrospective review of 888 cases. J Cardiothorac Surg. 2012;7:35.
2. Sobrino J, Shafi S. Timing and causes of death after injuries. Proc (Bayl Univ Med Cent). 2013;26(2):120–3.
3. Bulger EM, Arneson MA, Mock CN, Jurkovich GJ. Rib fractures in the elderly. J Trauma. 2000;48(6):1040–7.
4. Gwinnutt CL, Driscoll PA. Advanced trauma life support. Eur. J. Anaesthesiol. 1996;13(2):95–101.
5. Fallouh H, Dattani-Patel R, Rathinam S. Blunt thoracic trauma. Surgery. 2017;35(5):262–8. Oxford International Edition.
6. Kram HB, Appel PL, Wohlmuth DA, Shoemaker WC. Diagnosis of traumatic thoracic aortic rupture: a 10-year retrospective analysis. Ann. Thorac. Surg. 1989;47(2):282–6.
7. Ordonez CA, et al. Computed tomography in hemodynamically unstable severely injured blunt and penetrating trauma patients. J. Trauma Acute Care Surg. 2016;80(4):593–7.
8. Steenburg SD, Ravenel JG, Ikonomidis JS, Schonholz C, Reeves S. Acute traumatic aortic injury: imaging evaluation and management. Radiology. 2008;248(3):748–62.
9. Kirkpatrick AW, et al. Hand-held thoracic sonography for detecting post-traumatic pneumothoraces: the Extended Focused Assessment with Sonography for Trauma (EFAST). J. Trauma. 2004;57(2):288–95.
10. Bruckner BA, et al. Critical evaluation of chest computed tomography scans for blunt descending thoracic aortic injury. Ann. Thorac. Surg. 2006;81(4):1339–46.
11. Ellis H. Applied anatomy of cricothyrotomy and tracheostomy. Br J Hosp Med (Lond). 2006;67(9):M168–9.
12. Langvad S, Hyldmo P, Nakstad A, Vist G, Sandberg M. Emergency cricothyrotomy—a systematic review. Scand J Trauma Resusc Emerg Med. 2013;21(1):43.
13. Schober P, Hegemann MC, Schwarte LA, Loer SA, Noetges P. Emergency cricothyrotomy—a comparative study of different techniques in human cadavers. Resuscitation. 2009;80(2):204–9.
14. Laws D, Neville E, Duffy J. BTS guidelines for the insertion of a chest drain. Thorax. 2003;58(Suppl 2):ii53–9.
15. Elsayed H, Roberts R, Emadi M, Whittle I, Shackcloth M. Chest drain insertion is not a harmless procedure—are we doing it safely? Interact. Cardiovasc. Thorac. Surg. 2010;11(6):745–8.
16. Inaba K, et al. Cadaveric comparison of the optimal site for needle decompression of tension pneumothorax by prehospital care providers. J. Trauma Acute Care Surg. 2015;79(6):1044–8.
17. Kaserer A, Stein P, Simmen H-P, Spahn DR, Neuhaus V. Failure rate of prehospital chest decompression after severe thoracic trauma. Am. J. Emerg. Med. 2017;35(3):469–74.
18. Clemency BM, Tanski CT, Rosenberg M, May PR, Consiglio JD, Lindstrom HA. Sufficient catheter length for pneumothorax needle decompression: a meta-analysis. Prehosp Disaster Med. 2015;30(3):249–53.
19. Rathinam S, Grobler S, Bleetman A, Kink T, Steyn R. Evolved design makes ThoraQuik safe and user friendly in the management of pneumothorax and pleural effusion. Emerg. Med. J. 2014;31(1):59–64.
20. Rottenstreich M, Fay S, Gendler S, Klein Y, Arkovitz M, Rottenstreich A. Needle thoracotomy in trauma. Mil. Med. 2015;180(12):1211–3.
21. Inaba K, et al. Does size matter? A prospective analysis of 28-32 versus 36-40 French chest tube size in trauma. J. Trauma Acute Care Surg. 2012;72(2):422–7.
22. Evans BJ, Hornick P. Penetrating injuries to the chest. Surgery. 2005;23(11):406–9.
23. Biere SS a Y, et al. Minimally invasive versus open oesophagectomy for patients with oesophageal cancer: a multicentre, open-label, randomised controlled trial. Lancet. 2012;379(9829):1887–92.
24. Carrero R, Wayne M. Chest trauma. Emerg. Med. Clin. North Am. 1989;7(2):389–418.

25. Marasco SF, et al. Prospective randomized controlled trial of operative rib fixation in traumatic flail chest. J. Am. Coll. Surg. 2013;216(5):924–32.
26. Smith MD, et al. Transesophageal echocardiography in the diagnosis of traumatic rupture of the aorta. N. Engl. J. Med. 1995;332(6):356–62.
27. Wojcik JB, Morgan AS. Sternal fractures—the natural history. Ann. Emerg. Med. 1988;17(9):912–4.
28. DuBose J, et al. Development of posttraumatic empyema in patients with retained hemothorax: results of a prospective, observational AAST study. J. Trauma Acute Care Surg. 2012;73(3):752–7.
29. Thiam O, et al. Traumatic diaphragmatic injuries: epidemiological, diagnostic and therapeutic aspects. Springerplus. 2016;5(1):1614.
30. Abolhoda A, Livingston DH, Donahoo JS, Allen K. Diagnostic and therapeutic video assisted thoracic surgery (VATS) following chest trauma. Eur. J. Cardiothorac. Surg. 1997;12(3):356–60.
31. Manlulu AV, Lee TW, Thung KH, Wong R, Yim APC. Current indications and results of VATS in the evaluation and management of hemodynamically stable thoracic injuries. Eur. J. Cardiothorac. Surg. 2004;25(6):1048–53.
32. Milanchi S, Makey I, McKenna R, Margulies DR. Video-assisted thoracoscopic surgery in the management of penetrating and blunt thoracic trauma. J. Minim. Access Surg. 2009;5(3):63–6.
33. Gabal A, Alghorori M. Role of emergency VATS in blunt chest trauma patients. J Cardiothorac Surg. 2013;8(Suppl 1):O73.
34. Chou Y-P, Lin H-L, Wu T-C. Video-assisted thoracoscopic surgery for retained hemothorax in blunt chest trauma. Curr Opin Pulm Med. 2015;21(4):393–8.
35. Smith JW, Franklin GA, Harbrecht BG, Richardson JD. Early VATS for blunt chest trauma: a management technique underutilized by acute care surgeons. J Trauma. 2011;71(1):102–7.

Penetrating Injuries

13

Eshan L. Senanayake and Timothy R. Graham

Abstract

The majority of penetrating injury results from stab injuries with a knife or gunshot wound injuries. Other penetrating injuries are less common; however the mechanism of injury is crucial in the diagnosis and subsequent exclusion of other thoracic injuries caused by penetrating trauma. Penetrating injuries to the thoracic cage are life-threatening and can result in all of the life-threatening thoracic trauma injuries: airway disruption, tension pneumothorax, open pneumothorax, massive haemothorax, flail chest and cardiac tamponade. Further potential life-threatening injuries such as oesophageal injury and aortic disruption are also possible with penetrating injuries to the thorax. These injuries should be dealt with in a systematic approach based on the principles of advanced trauma life support and should be managed in a definite centre of care, in the right environment, with the necessary expertise and equipment.

Keywords

Cardiac tamponade · Stab injury · Chest drain · Thoracic trauma · Haemothorax Pneumothorax · Aortic injury · Thoracotomy · Median sternotomy · Gunshot wound

13.1 Introduction

Penetrating trauma can be broadly differentiated into trauma following a stab wound (SW) or a gunshot wound (GSW) and can affect any portion of the thorax, anatomically classified by the chest wall, lungs, trachea and major bronchi, heart, great vessels or other major vascular structures, oesophagus or diaphragm. Based on the

E.L. Senanayake • T.R. Graham (✉)
Queen Elizabeth Hospital, University Hospital Birmingham NHS FT, Birmingham, UK
e-mail: tim.graham@uhb.nhs.uk

D. Parikh, P.B. Rajesh (eds.), *Tips and Tricks in Thoracic Surgery*,
https://doi.org/10.1007/978-1-4471-7355-7_13

principles of advanced trauma life support (ATLS) management, identification of the above injuries should be performed within the primary survey. Survival is based on rapid assessment, diagnosis and appropriate early surgical management. Penetrating injures to the thorax range from minor soft tissue lacerations to extensive GSW injuries, and similarly the site and size of penetrative entry do not necessarily reflect the extent of injury—a SW can traverse through multiple directions and not necessarily perpendicular to the point of entry, and a GSW entry site is often smaller than the exit wound. Similarly a high index of suspicion should be placed on junctional injuries, i.e. diaphragm, root of the neck and axilla, as these injuries cross potentially multiple anatomical structures.

Stab wounds are limited to the depth and direction of travel (track of penetration) and only transfer the manual kinetic energy to the surrounding tissues. In contrast, GSW transfers the kinetic energy of the travelling bullet (kinetic energy = ½ mass × velocity^2) and the radial injury to the surrounding tissue. In general hand gun wounds have low-energy transfer, and high-velocity rifles have high-energy transfer injuries.

Other forms of penetrating injury including blast injury are uncommon but can cause similar devastating injuries, and hence the mechanism of injury is important in assessing the extent of tissue damage caused.

13.2 Radiological Imaging

Imaging the thorax after trauma is dependent on the mechanism and extent of injury. Often the patient will be a polytraumatic patient particularly following blunt trauma, which can also be associated with penetrating trauma to the thorax. Therefore a trauma series of radiological imaging, which includes the thorax, is appropriate. However if isolated penetrating trauma to the thorax is present, then a simple chest radiograph can be invaluable followed by a more extensive evaluation with a CT of the thorax. Further extensive imaging is based on these initial findings. Stability of the patient and index of suspicion regarding extent of injury are required when deciding if a CT is required prior to surgical intervention.

13.3 Resuscitative Thoracotomy

A resuscitative thoracotomy is one where a thoracotomy is performed immediately, as an integral part of the initial resuscitation. This can be performed at the scene of the injury, in the emergency department or operating room. A resuscitative thoracotomy is performed with the aim of achieving one or more of the following:

- Release of cardiac tamponade
- Local control of intrathoracic vascular haemorrhage
- Local control of cardiac haemorrhage
- Local control of massive airway bleeding
- Allow open cardiac massage
- Control of massive air embolism
- Occlusion of the descending thoracic aorta (cross clamping)

An emergency or urgent thoracotomy is performed under more controlled circumstances, dictated by the clinical stability of the patient, and is not part of the initial resuscitation process but would be performed early after the initial resuscitation, if indicated. The patient should maintain clinical and physiological stability but would still fit the indications for an emergency or urgent thoracotomy. This procedure may be performed in the emergency department. However if the patient remains clinically stable enough to be transferred to the operating room, the procedure could be performed more effectively with better equipment and a more suitable environment.

Survival following a thoracotomy for a stab wound is higher than that seen following a gunshot wound, and this has remained consistent over the last 20 years. Approximately 18–25% survived a resuscitative thoracotomy in the emergency department following a stab wound, and 4.7–7.3% survived following a gunshot wound [1–3]. Similarly overall survival post penetrating trauma is higher following a SW compared to GSW injuries, and survival following an isolated stab wound to the heart is associated with higher overall survival rates.

13.3.1 Indications for a Resuscitative Thoracotomy

Indications (and contraindications) for a resuscitative thoracotomy stem from several retrospective data from case series and case reports and are widely debated [4]. Therefore it is difficult to reach clear conclusions from these studies.

Absolute Indications

- Cardiac arrest following an isolated penetrating thoracic injury, with previously witnessed cardiac output (pulse, blood pressure, consciousness) requiring <15 min pre-hospital CPR
- Unresponsive hypotension (<70 mmHg despite vigorous fluid resuscitation) following penetrating thoracic injury

Recommended Indications

- Rapid exsanguination from the chest drains (>1500 mL) following blunt or penetrating thoracic injury
- Unresponsive hypotension (<70 mmHg despite vigorous fluid resuscitation) following blunt thoracic injury

Relative Indications

- Penetrating thoracic injury with traumatic arrest without witnessed cardiac output
- Penetrating non-thoracic injury with traumatic arrest with previously witnessed cardiac output
- Blunt thoracic injury with traumatic arrest with previously witnessed cardiac output requiring <5 min pre-hospital CPR

13.3.2 Contraindications for a Resuscitative Thoracotomy

Absolute

- Any patient with a cardiac output and hypotension, responding to fluid resuscitation
- Blunt trauma without witnessed cardiac output (>5 min of pre-hospital CPR)
- Penetrating abdominal trauma without cardiac output
- Absence of signs of life at the scene and on arrival (>15 min of pre-hospital CPR)
- Improperly trained team and expertise
- Severe head injury
- Severe multisystem injury
- Insufficient equipment

Relative

- Pre-existing patient factors, i.e. extreme of age, quality of life, pre-existing disease

13.4 Surgical Access for Penetrating Trauma

13.4.1 Resuscitative or Emergency Thoracotomy

Emergency anterolateral thoracotomy is performed via the fourth or fifth intercostal space with the patient prone. The incision can be extended across the sternum and to the contralateral side, to convert to a bilateral anterior thoracotomy or extended posteriorly. A scalpel is used to cut through the pectoralis muscle groups and curved Mayo scissors to cut through the intercostal muscles. Alternatively tough cut (trauma) scissors can be used. The sternum can be transected using a Gigli saw or tough cut scissors. The internal mammary arteries are transected and subsequently ligated. A large self-retaining rib retractor is used to provide access, and two on either side can be used during a bilateral anterior thoracotomy to provide maximum exposure. The pericardium is opened widely cranio-caudally staying anterior to the phrenic nerve. Although a limited anterolateral thoracotomy provides relief of tamponade, further access to the mediastinum and hilum is restricted. Hence bilateral anterior thoracotomy is preferred in the trauma setting.

Once the pericardium is opened, blood and clot can be evacuated (relief of tamponade) and the heart visualised. If required internal cardiac message can be performed using a single-handed or double-handed technique. Care should be taken not to cause iatrogenic injury to the right ventricle, during single-handed cardiac message.

The descending thoracic aorta can be clamped by manual compression by hand or placement of a large swab at the end of Rampleys forceps (or equivalent) to aid manual non-traumatic compression. Ideal dissection of the parietal pleura off the descending thoracic aorta and blunt dissection of the aorta to gain complete control will be difficult given the time pressure and emergency circumstances.

13.4.2 Access for Urgent Entry to the Thorax

In the more urgent setting, surgical access to the thorax is dictated by the type of injury and the most optimum access required for surgical repair and is usually performed in the operating theatre. Median sternotomy remains the most suitable form of access to the mediastinum, heart and great vessels and allows access for the use of other adjuncts such as cardiopulmonary bypass; however the need of a power saw and potential lack of expertise remain a limiting factor. Isolated lung injury can be accessed via an anterolateral or posterolateral approach based on the location of the injury. Video-assisted thoracoscopic surgery (VATS) can also be helpful during repair of limited lung parenchymal injury, evaluation of the extent of thoracic injury or management of a simple haemothorax.

13.4.3 Cardiac Injury

Cardiac injury is a significant challenge to manage [5] and is commonly associated with cardiac tamponade which remains a clinical diagnosis. Cardiac tamponade following a stab wound to the heart generally seals the entry site and thus allows finite time for definite management. However the degree of cardiac tamponade will dictate the metabolic and physiological picture of the patient and survivability. Those who survive to the operative room have a lower mortality compared to those that require resuscitative or emergency thoracotomy [6]. Commonly, it is the right ventricle that is injured and less frequently the left ventricle [7], and multichamber injuries are less common. Echocardiographic assessment can help make the diagnosis [8]. CT thorax can be helpful in identifying mediastinal shrapnel and foreign bodies.

Management of cardiac injury is surgical repair of the cardiac laceration. Bleeding is initially controlled using gentle manual compression. Alternatively a Foley catheter can be passed through the laceration and the balloon gently inflated followed by gentle traction to stop the bleeding. Laceration to the ventricle wall is repaired using a 2-0 or 3-0 Prolene or Ethibond full-thickness mattress suture technique across the laceration. Teflon or pericardial pledgets can be used to prevent cutting through the muscle. Similarly atrial laceration can be repaired using a 4-0 Prolene with or without pledgets, by placement of a mattress suture or purse string around the defect.

Care should be taken with lacerations near a coronary vessel—a horizontal mattress suture that runs underneath the coronary artery can be used to control bleeding. If there is laceration of the coronary artery, initially proximal and distal control should be performed by manual compression or placing sloops around the coronary artery to restrict flow and direct repair, or preferably coronary artery bypass grafting using long saphenous vein for conduit should be performed. Intra-coronary shunts may be used as a temporising measure.

Intraoperative assessment with transoesophageal echocardiography (TOE) can confirm and/or exclude other valvular injuries and assess regional wall motion abnormalities and should be used routinely. If a perfusionist is available, cell salvage can be used to conserve blood loss. Non-significant valvular or septal injuries can be repaired electively but would be dependent on the haemodynamic status of the patient and the presence of other life-threatening injuries, as cardiopulmonary bypass (CPB) is mandatory for repair of these latter injuries.

13.4.4 Great Vessel Injury

Intra-pericardial great vessel injury is rare but occurs as a result of significant mediastinal injury caused by a long track of penetration. The majority of great vessel injury is caused by penetrating trauma [9]. These can be difficult to repair. The most suitable surgical access is via a median sternotomy if mediastinal vascular injury is suspected; this allows extension into the root of the neck if required. Descending thoracic injury is best approached via a thoracotomy. As radiological imaging can be unreliable in the trauma setting, adjuncts such as cardiopulmonary bypass and TOE should be available to help deal with any eventuality [10]. As time is of the essence with penetrating trauma to the great vessels, radiological imaging may not be possible, and emergency/urgent surgery would be often required.

Initial surgical management is vascular control proximal and distal to the site of injury. Ensure both anterior and posterior walls of any vessel are inspected thoroughly as a posterior tear (from a through-and-through injury) can only become evident (in the absence of good preoperative imaging) when the anterior tear is extended and inspected from within the vessel or when cardiopulmonary bypass (if used) is discontinued and you are faced with extensive bleeding. Hypothermic circulatory arrest can be used to aid thorough inspection of the aorta and aid surgical repair [10, 11]. Alternatively cardioplegic arrest can be employed to provide diastolic arrest and a bloodless field. If the pulmonary artery is difficult to access, transecting the aorta can provide improved surgical access to the pulmonary arteries. The above techniques require the use of cardiopulmonary bypass (CPB).

The descending thoracic aorta injuries can be repaired by cross clamping the aorta and placing an interposition graft being mindful of the total ischaemic time (lack of lower limbs, visceral organs and spinal cord perfusion). In circumstances that require extensive ascending aorta or aortic arch repair, with the use of an interposition graft, the use of selective antegrade cerebral perfusion to maintain continuous cerebral perfusion during the repair is warranted. Such extensive aortic repairs will require thorough operative planning that includes site of cannulation for CPB, modes of CPB, myocardial protection, cerebral perfusion, visceral perfusion, spinal cord perfusion, etc. and hence best performed by a surgeon with the relevant expertise in aortic surgery.

Simple lacerations to the great vessels can be managed using standard vascular techniques of direct surgical repair. Isolated vascular injuries can be oversewn with 3-0 or 4-0 Prolene. A side-biting vascular clamp can be helpful, but good proximal and distal control of the vessel is important. Repair of injuries to the SVC or IVC can be limited by surgical access, as manipulating the heart can cause haemodynamic instability. In these circumstances, again cardiopulmonary bypass can be helpful to achieve stability. Ligation of the SVC and IVC should only be considered if a further shunting procedure is possible. In contrast the innominate vein can be ligated if required.

Vascular junctional injuries are difficult to control, i.e. root of the neck and clavicle. Here again, control with gentle traction using a Foley catheter can be useful until full exposure of the site of injury is possible. Exposure can either be via a median sternotomy extended into the neck or a 'trap-door' incision (upper sternotomy and with fourth intercostal space anterior thoracotomy) or a clavicular/subclavicular incision. Approach should be decided based upon the surgeons' familiarity and degree of injury. These vascular injures can be repaired primarily or by placement of an interposition or bypass graft [12].

Similarly injuries to the vascular structures within the hilum are difficult to control, and access through a posterolateral thoracotomy or bilateral anterior thoracotomy is helpful. The pulmonary artery and veins can be controlled by placement of rubber sloops and snugging down to reduce blood flow. Primary repair should initially be attempted, and lung resection and pneumonectomy should be a last resort.

13.4.5 Chest Wall Injury

Penetrating injury to the chest wall alone can be managed with minimal surgical intervention, i.e. interrupted closure (allow drainage if the site gets infected) of the soft tissue with monofilament sutures (reduce infection). Associated pneumothorax or haemothorax can be managed with intercostal chest drain insertion. Haemothorax may result from damage to the intercostal or internal mammary vessels; ongoing bleeding will need ligation or electrocautery.

13.4.6 Airway Injuries

Penetrating injury to the trachea or bronchus is rare (1–2% of thoracic injuries) and devastating [13]. Tracheal injuries commonly occur from a stab injury to the neck. Injuries in the laryngotracheal region may require a surgical airway if endotracheal intubation proves difficult (cricothyroidectomy or tracheostomy). Gunshot wounds are the commonest cause of central airway injuries. Associated pulmonary injuries should be immediately treated with intercostal chest drain insertion; massive air leak should raise the suspicion of a major bronchial injury.

Initial management should involve successful and secure intubation followed by bronchoscopy for thorough evaluation of the injury and the entire bronchial tree.

Proximal tracheal injuries are managed with intubation distal to the injury. Injury to the main bronchi can be managed with double-lumen intubation to prevent contamination of the good lung from blood and debris or with bronchial blockers or a Fogarty catheter to occlude the injured bronchus.

Definitive treatment is by resection and repair of the injured segment, and hence surgical access is dependent on the site of injury, i.e. cervical, upper sternotomy or posterolateral thoracotomy. During repair of a bronchial injury, control of the hilum is required and will aid in managing unsuspected vascular injury. Placing sloops around the pulmonary arteries and veins will allow rapid control if required. Repair of the airway should follow standard principles of a sleeve resection, i.e. tension-free without compromising blood supply. Larger airway defects may require an appropriate lung resection, i.e. lobectomy or sleeve resection with pneumonectomy being the last resort due to poor outcomes associated with pneumonectomy post trauma.

13.4.7 Lung Parenchymal Injury

As with all penetrating trauma, injury to the lung tissue can be simple and may not need surgical intervention, or it can be severe particularly following a deep penetrating injury or GSW. In a stable patient, investigation with a chest radiograph is often adequate, and any associated pneumothorax or haemothorax, which is common, can be managed with simple intercostal chest drainage and drain management alone. Subsequent management is based on chest tube drainage, presence of an air leak and lung re-expansion. The majority of lung parenchymal injuries even following GSW injuries can be managed in this conservative manner without the need for a thoracotomy [14].

Placement of a large bore 28Fh drain is advisable in all trauma patients who have even a small pneumothorax or pleural collection as there is potential for this to get worse. In those with an initial normal chest radiograph, serial evaluation is important and dictated by the clinical status of the patient and nature of injury [15].

If a patient requires a thoracotomy, i.e. for persistent large air leak or ongoing bleeding (>1.5 L of total blood loss), a posterolateral thoracotomy is preferred to allow adequate access to the hilum on single-lung ventilation. Usual control of the vessels in the hilum is required. A nonanatomic lung resection will allow more lung parenchyma to be spared if there is healthy lung tissue, after a generous margin is achieved. Resection can be performed using standard stapling devices. An anatomic lung resection may be required if there is extensive tissue loss/injury. A tractotomy can be performed with deep injuries to the lung parenchyma to aid haemostasis. Stress before a pneumonectomy is to be avoided as the morbidity increases. The bronchial stump will require extra coverage due to the potential infected space and to avoid a bronchopleural fistula.

13.4.8 Injury to the Diaphragm

These are difficult to diagnose and a high index of suspicion should prevail. Simple laceration to the diaphragm may not be initially evident, and the patient may re-present with herniation of the abdominal contents with potential for bowel incarceration. VATS or laparoscopy can be helpful in assessing the diaphragm if a diaphragmatic injury is suspected, negating the need for an invasive laparotomy [16]. In skilled hands, repair of the diaphragm using VATS would reduce the overall morbidity of performing a thoracotomy or laparotomy if there is no intra-abdominal injury suspected. Alternatively the diaphragm can be repaired via a laparotomy using an interrupted repair technique.

13.4.9 Oesophageal Injury

Penetrating injury to the oesophagus is rare (associated with major trauma, i.e. GSW) and easy to miss unless there is a high index of suspicion. Injury to the cervical oesophagus is more common. Oesophageal injury is associated with high morbidity given the risk of mediastinal contamination and high risk of associated mediastinal injury. Ideally a Gastrografin swallow or oral contrast with CT will help the diagnosis, but this is dependent on the stability of the patient. Flexible bronchoscopy (to exclude airway injury) and oesophagoscopy also can help with diagnosis [17]. Thoracotomy should be performed on the side of the associated major lung injury.

The oesophagus should be repaired using primary closure after debriding back to healthy tissue. A two-layered closure is required with a watertight closure of the mucosal layer, followed by the muscular second layer. The repair should be covered with an intercostal muscle flap and the area well drained with chest drains. A nasogastric or nasojejunal feeding tube should be placed at the time of the operation to enable feeding.

13.5 Conclusions

Penetrating injury to the thorax can cause a varied degree of injury (simple to severe) to any structure within the thorax and to those outside the thorax, at junctional sites. A high index of suspicion should prevail with regard to the extent of injury caused. Expeditious diagnosis and management is important to limit mortality and morbidity. A low threshold for operative intervention should be maintained for patients with penetrating injury to the mediastinal region.

13.6 Complications

Acute respiratory distress syndrome (ARDS) is common after thoracic trauma, and mortality associated with ARDS is high. ARDS is often associated with pneumonia and pulmonary contusions. Management is supportive in nature with mechanical ventilation. Rarely extracorporeal membrane oxygenation is required to support these patients.

Pneumonia is a common infective complication following thoracic trauma, and management is along the standard principles of intensive care therapy. Similarly an infected pleural space is common and should be managed similar to a para-pneumonic infection; however post-traumatic empyemas may have a combination of Gram-positive and Gram-negative organisms.

Complications with bronchopleural fistulae are difficult to manage. Large air leaks can impact on ventilation requirements and may need operative intervention. In these cases the parenchymal tissue can be extremely fragile and friable. The parenchymal injury should be exposed and major bronchioles oversewn followed by layered closure of the lung parenchyma and finally the visceral pleura. Layered closure is important to prevent a late lung abscess.

Arteriovenous fistulas can present as late complications following penetrating injury to the great vessels and require surgical repair. CT and angiography are required for operative planning. Prosthetic graft placement may be required for the great vessels at surgery.

References

1. Vij D, Simoni E, Smith RF, Obeid FN, Horst HM, Tomlanovich MC, et al. Resuscitative thoracotomy for patients with traumatic injury. Surgery. 1983;94(4):554–61.
2. Ivatury RR, Kazigo J, Rohman M, Gaudino J, Simon R, Stahl WM. "Directed" emergency room thoracotomy: a prognostic prerequisite for survival. J Trauma. 1991;31(8):1076–81; discussion 1081–2.
3. Durham LA 3rd, Richardson RJ, Wall MJ Jr, Pepe PE, Mattox KL. Emergency center thoracotomy: impact of prehospital resuscitation. J Trauma. 1992;32(6):775–9.
4. Mejia JC, Stewart RM, Cohn SM. Emergency department thoracotomy. Semin Thorac Cardiovasc Surg. 2008;20(1):13–8. Epub 2008/04/19.
5. Embrey R. Cardiac trauma. Thorac Surg Clin. 2007;17(1):87–93, vii. Epub 2007/07/27.
6. Asensio JA, Berne JD, Demetriades D, Chan L, Murray J, Falabella A, et al. One hundred five penetrating cardiac injuries: a 2-year prospective evaluation. J Trauma. 1998;44(6):1073–82. Epub 1998/06/24.
7. Navid F, Gleason TG. Great vessel and cardiac trauma: diagnostic and management strategies. Semin Thorac Cardiovasc Surg. 2008;20(1):31–8. Epub 2008/04/19.
8. Aaland MO, Bryan FC 3rd, Sherman R. Two-dimensional echocardiogram in hemodynamically stable victims of penetrating precordial trauma. Am Surg. 1994;60(6):412–5. Epub 1994/06/01.
9. Brinkman WT, Szeto WY, Bavaria JE. Overview of great vessel trauma. Thorac Surg Clin. 2007;17(1):95–108. Epub 2007/07/27.
10. Senanayake EL, Jeyatheesan J, Rogers V, Wilson IC, Graham TR. Stab to the chest causing severe great vessel injury. Ann Thorac Surg. 2012;94(5):1716–8. Epub 2012/10/27.
11. Fulton JO, Brink JG. Complex thoracic vascular injury repair using deep hypothermia and circulatory arrest. Ann Thorac Surg. 1997;63(2):557–9. Epub 1997/02/01.
12. Demetriades D. Penetrating injuries to the thoracic great vessels. J Card Surg. 1997;12(2 Suppl):173–9; discussion 179–80. Epub 1997/03/01.
13. Karmy-Jones R, Wood DE. Traumatic injury to the trachea and bronchus. Thorac Surg Clin. 2007;17(1):35–46. Epub 2007/07/27.
14. Inci I, Ozcelik C, Tacyildiz I, Nizam O, Eren N, Ozgen G. Penetrating chest injuries: unusually high incidence of high-velocity gunshot wounds in civilian practice. World J Surg. 1998;22(5):438–42. Epub 1998/05/02.
15. Meyer DM. Hemothorax related to trauma. Thorac Surg Clin. 2007;17(1):47–55. Epub 2007/07/27.
16. Cetindag IB, Neideen T, Hazelrigg SR. Video-assisted thoracic surgical applications in thoracic trauma. Thorac Surg Clin. 2007;17(1):73–9. Epub 2007/07/27.
17. Flowers JL, Graham SM, Ugarte MA, Sartor WM, Rodriquez A, Gens DR, et al. Flexible endoscopy for the diagnosis of esophageal trauma. J Trauma. 1996;40(2):261–5; discussion 265–6. Epub 1996/02/01.

Part IV

Thoracic Wall

for the chest wall tumours, and majority of them are resectable, if localized to the chest wall. A collaborative effort between Surgeon, Radiologist and oncologist is required to have optimal outcome in the management of these tumours.

14.2 Pathology

The primary chest wall tumours are classified according to their malignant potential and tissue of origin—bone or soft tissue (Table 14.1).

14.3 Diagnosis

These chest wall tumours are often slow growing and are misinterpreted. Patients give history of a lump or chest discomfort and are often treated with analgesics and reassurance for a period of time. The soft tissue tumours are usually painless, whereas bony tumours are painful as result of periosteal damage and expansion. Symptoms due to compression of adjacent structures or presence of pleural effusion can bring to light underlying chest wall tumour, growing into the chest cavity (Fig. 14.1).

The CT and MRI scan are critical imaging modalities in diagnosing, staging and planning treatment. The CT scan assesses the extent of bone and soft tissue involvement, probable diagnosis, extension into the adjacent areas and distant metastasis. The MRI further delineates relationship of the tumour with neurovascular structures.

Even though the imaging characteristics can assist in establishing the diagnosis, tissue biopsy is essential to obtain definitive diagnosis and plan further treatment. The tissue can either be obtained with core needle, incisional or excisional biopsy.

Table 14.1 Classification of chest wall tumours

Tissue	Benign	Malignant
Bone	Osteoblastoma Osteoid osteoma	Ewing's sarcoma Osteosarcoma
Cartilage	Enchondroma Osteochondroma	Chondrosarcoma
Fibrous tissue	Fibrous dysplasia	
Bone marrow	Eosinophilic granuloma	Solitary plasmacytoma
Osteoclast	Aneurysmal bone cyst Giant cell tumour	
Adipose tissue	Lipoma	Liposarcoma
Fibrous tissue	Fibroma	Fibrosarcoma
Muscle	Leiomyoma Rhabdomyoma	Leiomyosarcoma Rhabdomyosarcoma
Nerve	Neurofibroma Schwannoma	Neurofibrosarcoma Neuroblastoma
Vascular	Haemangioma	Haemangiosarcoma

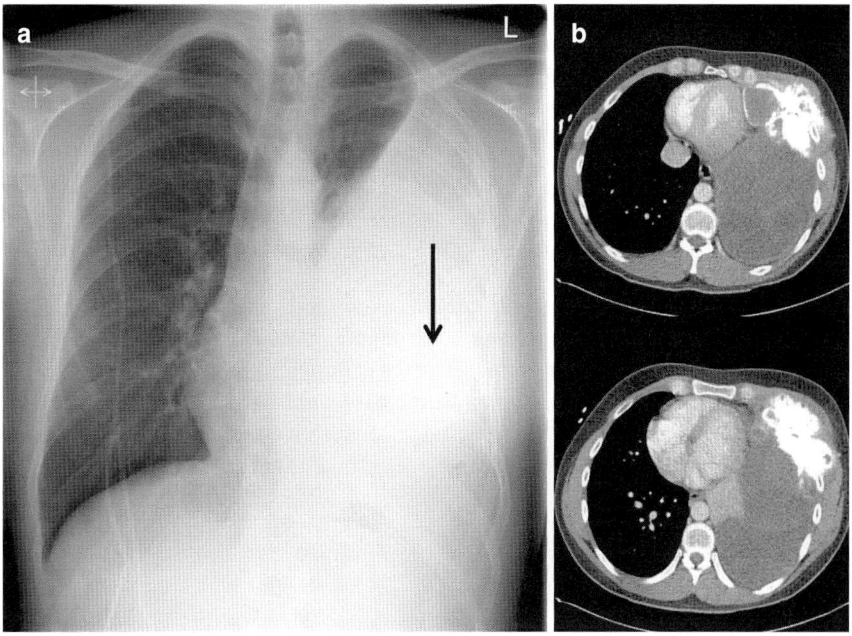

Fig. 14.1 (**a**) Chest X-ray demonstrating large pleural effusion. Arrow pointing to underlying chest wall mass. (**b**) CT scan confirming findings of the chest X-ray

It is important to obtain sufficient tissue, avoid spillage and avoid disrupting tissue planes, and the incision for biopsy should be planned in such a way that it can be incorporated into definitive surgical resection at the later stage.

14.4 Surgical Management of Chest Wall Tumours

The surgical resection of chest wall tumours is complex and challenging. The malignant tumours of chest wall include primary or secondary tumours. Direct invasion of the chest wall by lung or breast cancer represent common indication for chest wall resection [2]. The patients with primary malignant chest wall tumours need to be discussed in a multidisciplinary team meeting specializing in the treatment of these malignancies. Majority of chest wall tumours require surgical resection either alone or as a part of multimodality treatment. The Ewing's sarcoma in particular is treated with well-established protocol consisting of chemotherapy followed by surgery and radiotherapy [3]. The osteosarcomas and spindle cell sarcomas often receive chemotherapy in addition to surgical resection. Role of chemotherapy in soft tissue sarcomas remains unproven, and radiotherapy is not recommended, unless the tumour is large and high grade, and resection margins are close [4]. The radiotherapy however doesn't compensate for poor surgery resulting in positive resection margins.

14.5 Principles of Surgical Resection

14.5.1 Curative Resection

The aim of surgery for chest wall tumours should be curative, ensuring wide en bloc excision with tumour-free resection margins. The adequacy of resection margin depends on malignant potential of the tumour, location and overall fitness of the patient. The usual recommendation is either 4 cm clear circumferential margin or one healthy rib and intercostal space on either side of the tumour. However, it may not always be feasible to have 4 cm margins all around, particularly for the tumours closer to vertebrae, thoracic outlet or those abutting the mediastinum. In these situations, the surgery still must ensure microscopic tumour-free margins. In low-grade tumours, particularly Grade I chondrosarcomas, 2 cm clear margin may be sufficient for cure. The surgeon must never compromise the extirpative surgery because of concern with size of the defect being created and its subsequent closure.

Rarely, chest wall resection may be required for palliative purposes to relieve intractable pain or remove ulcerated, fungated foul-smelling mass, thus improving the quality of life of the patient. It may give the opportunity of local control in conjunction with chemo- and radiotherapy [2].

14.5.2 Operability

Once the recommendation to resect the tumour is made, the patient needs to be reviewed for assessment with regard to fitness for major thoracic surgical procedure. The general well-being of patient is noted, the comorbidities are explored and subjective and objective assessment of cardiorespiratory fitness is carried out. It is important for the patient to quit smoking and in borderline cases to be enrolled in pulmonary rehabilitation programme.

14.5.3 Planning Resection

It is ideal for the surgeon to review the images of the patient with the radiologist, to obtain clear idea about the location and extent of the tumour, involved adjacent structures needing resection and in particular relation with the thoracic outlet, vertebrae, mediastinum, diaphragm and abdominal organs. The plastic surgeon should also be involved in the planning phase to decide the soft tissue and skin flaps that will require harvesting, review their quality and vascularity with the assistance of the radiologist. It is imperative to have a clear preoperative information of extent of resection, as the frozen section examination is not possible for bony tumours. The extent of chest wall to be removed and its impact on the patient should be anticipated preoperatively, and surgery offered, only if it is certain that tumour is resectable and patient will tolerate the operative procedure. An attempt to remove tumour with positive tumour margins does not provide any prognostic benefit to the patient.

14.5.4 Entry into the Chest

It is important that the tumour mass is removed en bloc with other involved structures, without disrupting it. For that reason, during the review of the images, the safe entry point into the chest away cavity is identified. A small intercostal opening can be made at a distance from the tumour and finger exploration carried out, which can guide on further extension of the incision.

14.5.5 Chest Wall Reconstruction

The oncologic principle of undertaking en bloc resection with wide resection margins will result in defect in the chest wall, which needs to be reconstructed for the following reasons.

(a) Maintain structural integrity to protect underlying organs, prevent herniation of the lung and maintain adequate intrathoracic volume. In special circumstances, reconstruction is performed to maintain stability of spine, prevent impaction of the scapula and repair of the diaphragm.
(b) Maintain functional integrity of chest wall to prevent paradoxical movement, minimize pain and preserve respiratory mechanics for adequate ventilation.
(c) Achieve good cosmetic outcome.

14.5.6 Planning the Operation

It is important to anticipate and arrange for assistance from other specialities like spinal or vascular surgery. The operating room team needs to be briefed about the operative procedure in detail, including requirements of various surgeons, intraoperative change in the position of the patient and possibility of longer operating time. The pain control strategy, need for single-lung ventilation and positioning of patient needs to be elaborated. The surgical incisions are planned to include previous sites of biopsy and facilitate harvest of the muscle flaps.

14.5.7 When to Reconstruct

The reconstruction of the chest wall is controversial in terms of the indication and material used for the purpose. The large full-thickness defects in the chest wall leave the segment vulnerable to paradoxical motion, thus adversely affecting respiration. The evidence emerging with regard to fixation of flail segments in chest trauma improving ventilation and decreasing pulmonary complications further supports the need to reconstruct chest wall defects after surgery [5]. The decision to reconstruct should be based not only on the size of the defect but also its location. Generally, lesions less than 5 cm in size in any location and those up to 10 cm posteriorly do not need reconstruction for functional reasons [6]. However, these defects may need to be repaired with prosthetic material to protect organs, prevent lung herniation and for aesthetic purposes. The posterior defects in proximity to tip of the scapula may also require reconstruction to prevent its entrapment in the defect during certain movements.

14.5.8 What Prosthetic Material to Reconstruct?

The ideal characteristics of prosthetic material for chest wall reconstruction include rigidity to prevent paradoxical motion, inertness to allow ingrowth of fibrous tissue and decrease likelihood of infection, malleability to fashion it into appropriate shape and radiolucency to allow radiographic follow-up of the underlying problem [7]. The material used for reconstruction could be rigid or nonrigid in nature. The nonrigid material like meshes and patches are easy to manipulate, handle and suture to the edges of the defect. These include Vicryl, Prolene, or Marlex mesh, PTFE (polytetrafluoroethylene—Gore_tex) or biological patches. The Vicryl and biological meshes can be used in patients at risk of getting infection. The interstices of knitted meshes allow tissue to grow through, are permeable to fluids and hence prevent occurrence of seroma [8]. The rigid materials are various osteosynthesis systems consisting of titanium implantable material (Stratos Germany and Synthes Switzerland) and more commonly used mesh-methyl methacrylate cement composite graft (Fig. 14.2).

The choice of the prosthetic material is based on surgeon's preference, and all of them work reasonably well [9]. The larger defects and those in anterior or anterolateral location, involving costal margin and requiring diaphragm reconstruction, are better reconstructed with rigid prosthesis. While comparing chest wall resection and reconstruction using rigid and nonrigid prosthesis, use of latter was associated with decreased frequency of respiratory complications and improved outcomes [10].

The use of polypropylene mesh-methyl methacrylate composite graft was first described in 1981 and has been used widely with good results [6, 11, 12].

A thin layer of methyl methacrylate is created by filling it in a pocket constructed in double-layered polypropylene mesh, corresponding to the size and shape of the defect in the chest wall. The prosthesis can be gently contoured to the curve of the chest wall.

The size of the pocket created in the mesh is constructed few mm smaller than the dimensions of the chest wall defect to prevent rubbing of prosthetic plate with surrounding bony structures and the resultant pain. About 2–3 cm of double-layered mesh is left around the pocket to be used for suturing the graft to the chest wall. The pleural cavity is washed out; a chest drain is placed and secured. The composite graft is then secured to the edges of the chest wall defect using interrupted strong nonabsorbable sutures (Ethibond no 3). The two layers of the mesh are placed on either side of the edges of the defect, as the sutures are tied securely (Fig. 14.3).

Alternately, the titanium bars of osteosynthesis system can be used to bridge the defects by replacing the resected ribs individually (Fig. 14.4). There is theoretical advantage of more physiologic rib movements with use of titanium bars. However, they are prone to infection, displacement and rupture, requiring reoperation for their removal (Fig. 14.5).

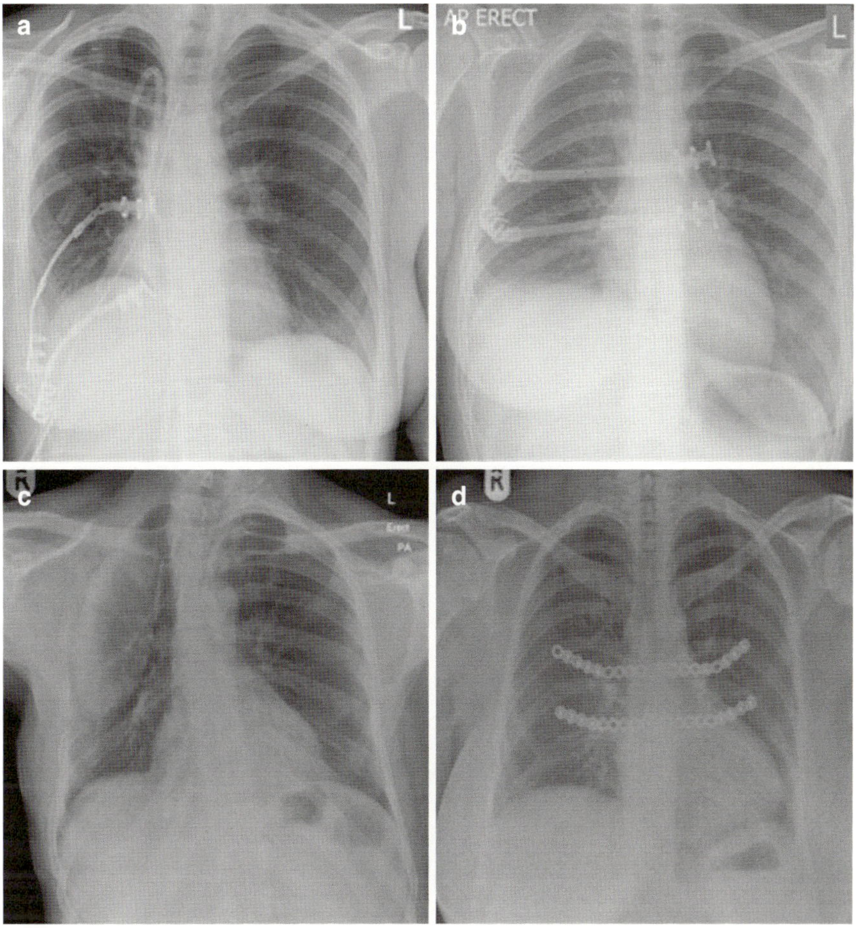

Fig. 14.2 (**a**, **b**) Stratos osteosynthesis system. (**c**) Methyl methacrylate-Marlex composite graft. (**d**) Synthes titanium bars used for rigid reconstruction

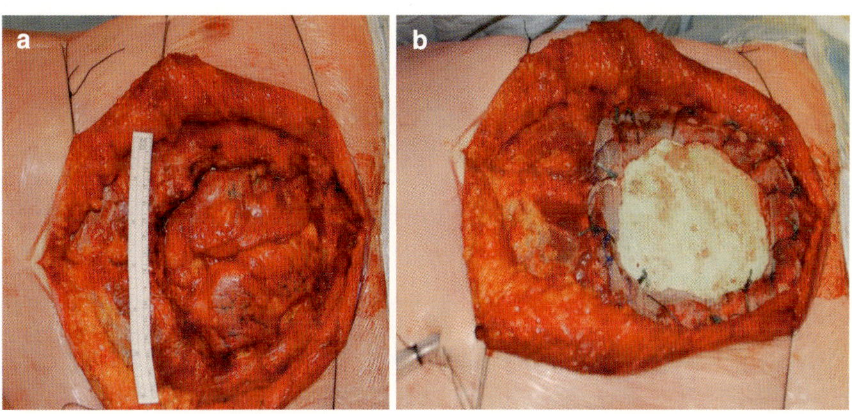

Fig. 14.3 (**a**) Chest wall defect after sternectomy (**b**) reconstruction using methyl methacrylate-Marlex mesh composite graft sutured to the edges, with layers of Marlex placed on either side of the edges

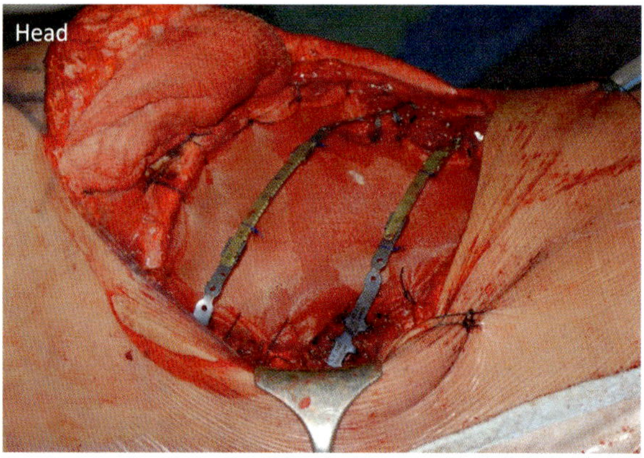

Fig. 14.4 The Stratos osteosynthesis system used to reconstruct lateral chest wall defect. A synthetic mesh has been sutured to the edges to allow platform to place muscle flaps to cover the prosthesis

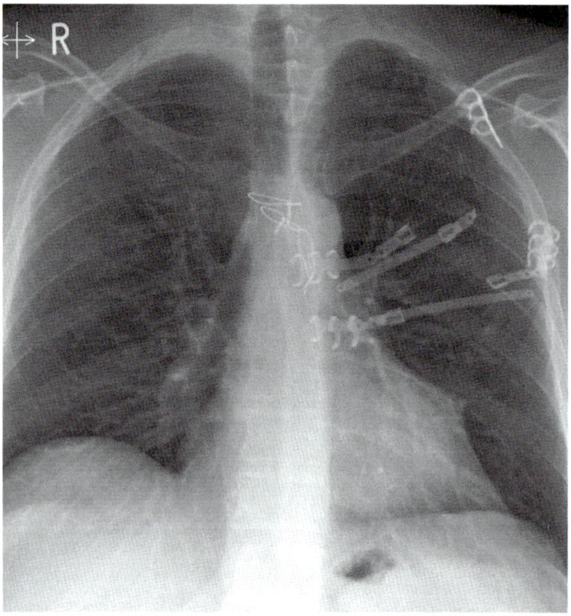

Fig. 14.5 Fractured titanium bars few months postoperatively

Once the chest wall stability has been established, well-vascularized soft tissue is harvested to cover the prosthetic material. Over the past few years, the use of muscle and musculocutaneous flaps has become mainstay in chest wall reconstruction [2, 9, 13]. The vascularized tissue obliterates the dead space and decreases the risk of infection of the prosthetic material used for reconstruction. In addition, it improves the cosmetic outcome of the reconstruction, improves convalescence and allows for timely adjuvant treatment, if required. The option of using soft tissue in the preoperative planning phase gives confidence to the surgeon to undertake radical resection of the tumour without undue concern about the size of the defect created.

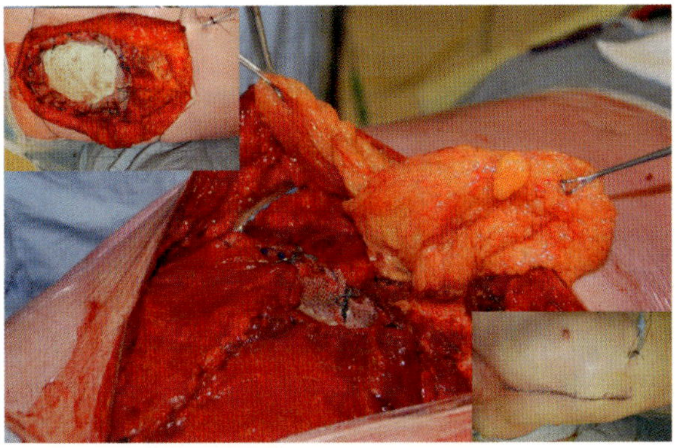

Fig. 14.6 The prosthesis (inset top left corner) covered with bilateral pectoral muscles and omentum. Final outcome (inset bottom right corner)

The thoracic trunk is well suited for vascularized coverage using many local muscles as pedicle grafts including latissimus dorsi, pectoralis major, serratus anterior, rectus abdominis and greater omentum (Fig. 14.6). Occasionally, if pedicled muscle flap is unavailable, then free tissue transfer flap can be utilized.

14.6 Special Situations

14.6.1 Diaphragm

The diaphragm may be detached from the chest wall in the process of removal of the lower ribs, or significant part of it may be resected en bloc with the tumour. If lower three to four ribs are only resected, the edge of the diaphragm can be attached directly to the higher ribs, without significantly compromising the volume of the pleural cavity. However, if more than four ribs or larger part of the diaphragm has been removed, then it will require reconstruction—to maintain adequate volume of the pleural cavity, isolate abdominal cavity and preferably preserve its function. A thick PTFE patch is ideal to replace the resected diaphragm. This is sutured to the edge of the residual diaphragm medially and secured to the methyl methacrylate-Marlex composite graft or titanium bar used for reconstruction of the chest wall defect laterally (Fig. 14.7).

14.6.2 Impaction of Scapula

Even a smaller chest wall defect created in relation to the tip of scapula will require intervention to avoid its entrapment and resultant discomfort. This could be prevented by either covering the defect with prosthetic material or excising the tip of the scapula.

7. LeRoux BT, Shama D. Resection of tumors of the chest wall. Curr Probl Surg. 1983;20:345–86.
8. Thomas PA, Brouchet L. Prosthetic reconstruction of the chest wall. Thorac Surg Clin. 2010;20:551–8.
9. McCormack PM. Use of prosthetic materials in chest-wall reconstruction. Assets and liabilities. Surg Clin North Am. 1989;69(5):965–76.
10. Weyant MJ, Bains MS, Venkatraman E, Downey RJ, Park BJ, Flores RM, et al. Results of chest wall resection and reconstruction with and without rigid prosthesis. Ann Thorac Surg. 2006;81:279–85.
11. McCormack P, Bains MS, Beattie EJ, Martini N. New trends in skeletal reconstruction after resection of chest wall tumors. Ann Thorac Surg. 1981;31(1):45–52.
12. Lardinois D, Müller M, Furrer M, Banic A, Gugger M, Krueger T, et al. Functional assessment of chest wall integrity after methylmethacrylate reconstruction. Ann Thorac Surg. 2000;69(3):919–23.
13. Cohen M, Ramasastry SS. Reconstruction of complex chest wall defects. Am J Surg. 1996;172(1):35–40.

Pleural Pathologies and Malignant Effusion

15

Gregor J. Kocher and Ralph A. Schmid

Abstract

This chapter focuses on the diagnosis and treatment of pleural disorders such as pleural effusion, pneumothorax, and pleural tumors. While in the management of benign pleural effusions, effective treatment of the underlying disease is crucial, drainage and pleurodesis are the mainstay of treatment for patients with recurrent malignant effusion. Pneumothorax, either primary or secondary, is another common pleural pathology, which often requires surgical treatment in the form of air-leak closure and pleurodesis, commonly performed by video-assisted thoracoscopic surgery (VATS). Solid tumors of the pleura are rather rare findings. Whereas pleural fibroma usually shows a benign course of disease, malignant pleural mesothelioma (MPM) is one of the most aggressive and most difficult to treat tumors of the human body. Only few cancers have caused so much controversy as MPM. For now, trimodality treatment concepts including chemotherapy, followed by extirpative surgery (e.g., extrapleural pneumonectomy or lung-sparing pleurectomy/decortication) and postoperative high-dose radiation therapy, seem to be the most promising strategy.

Keywords

Pleural effusion · Pneumothorax · Pleurodesis · Pleural fibroma · Malignant pleural mesothelioma · Pleurectomy decortication · Extrapleural pneumonectomy

G.J. Kocher, M.D. (✉) • R.A. Schmid, M.D.
Division of Thoracic Surgery, University Hospital Bern, Bern, Switzerland
e-mail: gregor.kocher@insel.ch; ralph.schmid@insel.ch

D. Parikh, P.B. Rajesh (eds.), *Tips and Tricks in Thoracic Surgery*,
https://doi.org/10.1007/978-1-4471-7355-7_15

15.1 Background

The pleural space is basically located between the visceral and parietal pleura and contains normally between 3 and 5 mL of fluid on each side. Common pleural pathologies include effusions, pneumothorax, and pleural tumors. In recent years videothoracoscopy has become one of the most frequent procedures, not only for the diagnosis but also for the treatment of most pleural pathologies.

15.2 Pleural Effusion

While the most common causes of transudative effusions are congestive heart failure and hypoalbuminemic states (e.g., malnutrition, cirrhosis), exudative effusions are mostly due to malignancy, infection (e.g., pneumonia), and pulmonary embolism. In patients aged over 60 years, more than 50% of exudative effusions are caused by malignancy, with breast cancer, bronchial carcinoma, ovarian carcinoma, and malignant lymphoma being the leading causes.

Thoracentesis usually allows differentiation between transudative and exudative effusions [1], and cytology is used to confirm suspected malignancy.

15.2.1 Benign Effusion

Primary treatment of nonmalignant pleural effusions should be directed at the underlying disease in all patients. Often repeated thoracentesis or the placement of a chest tube may be required to relieve symptoms until the underlying disease is well controlled. In case of recurrent or persistent symptomatic pleural effusion despite therapy of the underlying cause, additional surgical therapy has to be considered. Thoracoscopic talc pleurodesis and/or the placement of an indwelling pleural catheter (see also "malignant effusion") are the therapeutic options of choice. Early treatment of the underlying disease and adequate drainage of the pleural effusion are important to prevent the formation of dense layers of fibrin on the visceral pleura, which result in trapped lung. In patients with a trapped lung, pleurectomy and lung decortication may be more suitable.

15.2.2 Malignant Effusion

Asymptomatic patients with malignant pleural effusions usually do not require treatment.

Whereas in patients with a short life expectancy (<3 months) and slowly accumulating effusions, repeat outpatient thoracentesis is recommended, an indwelling pleural catheter (IPC) should be placed if a pleural effusion re-accumulates rapidly. The main advantage of an IPC is that it can even be placed under local anesthesia (e.g., in patients with severe comorbidities) and that its placement is associated with a shorter mean length of hospital stay and interval to the initiation of a systemic therapy compared to talcum pleurodesis. In patients with good performance status, chemical pleurodesis with talc in terms of a thoracoscopic poudrage is recommended [2], since it is usually a single definitive procedure without the inconvenience of an indwelling catheter that requires intermittent drainage. The combination of thoracoscopic talc pleurodesis with the intraoperative placement of an indwelling pleural catheter should be considered in patients with a high risk for recurrence (e.g., large effusion (>1000 mL), incomplete lung re-expansion). In those patients the IPC can be removed as soon as pleurodesis is complete (radiologic obliteration of pleural space with cessation of fluid drainage).

15.2.3 Tips and Tricks for Operative Management

The evacuation of large effusions by insertion of a chest tube and initialization of respiratory physiotherapy 2–3 days prior to surgery often allows better intraoperative lung re-expansion. Thoracoscopic talc poudrage (standard dose of 5 g calibrated talc) with or without the insertion of an indwelling pleural catheter can easily be performed through two ports in the seventh intercostal space, which are used for chest tube placement (or chest tube and IPC) in the end of the procedure. All loculations, including those in the fissures, should be broken down in order to allow mobilization and re-expansion of the whole lung. During the instillation of the talc powder through one of the ports, the lung can be retracted with a lung grasper in order to allow exposition of the whole parietal and visceral pleura for complete pleurodesis. Especially in the paravertebral space, where recurrence appears most frequently, proper distribution of the talcum powder is important. With the placement of two chest drains (apico-ventral and postero-basal), or one chest drain (anterior apical) and one IPC (postero-basal), respectively, the formation of recurrent encapsulated effusions may be prevented.

15.2.4 Alternative Ways of Operative Management

In certain malignancies (e.g., lymphoma, small cell lung cancer) evacuation of the pleural effusion by simple thoracentesis or chest tube placement should be preferred in order to allow rapid initiation of chemotherapy and/or radiotherapy, which may control the underlying disease and with that the recurrence of effusion.

Pleurectomy including decortication can be an option in patients with chronic pleural empyema and recurrent effusions due to trapped lung. The role of pleurectomy/decortication in malignant pleural mesothelioma will be discussed in a separate section.

The use of pleuroperitoneal shunts is not advisable anymore in most cases, since shunt occlusion is a common complication and the placement is more invasive than the implantation of an IPC, which is at least as effective. The only exception are patients in a hypoalbuminemic state who suffer from hepatic effusion, where a pleuroperitoneal shunt should be considered, since massive fluid loss including further depletion of proteins and electrolytes may be prevented.

15.2.5 Tips and Tricks to Avoid and Deal with Intraoperative Complications

Bleeding can generally be controlled with coagulation diathermy or argon beam coagulation.

Air leak can occur intraoperatively by accident or with the breakdown of adhesions. Therefore adhesions should only be separated carefully because pleurodesis will not be successful if persistent air leak with lung collapse is present. Small air leaks do often not require any treatment if the lung is well expanded. If bigger air leaks are present, the use of sealants (e.g., TachoSil®, PleuraSeal®, Progel®) may be considered. In case of deeper lacerations, the use of an endostapler in order to resect the affected part of the lung may be worthwhile.

15.2.6 Postoperative Management and Postoperative Complications

Re-expansion pulmonary edema is a rare complication that may occur after rapid evacuation of large pleural effusions (>1.5 L) or evacuation of pneumothorax in patients with lung collapse of >72 h duration. The condition may be prevented/attenuated by only allowing slow lung re-expansion (i.e., small drainage without suction, intermittent clamping of drainage after 1000 mL). Depending on the severity of the condition, a stepwise approach with supplemental oxygen, diuretics, non-invasive ventilation, or even invasive ventilation may be necessary.

ARDS has become an exceptionally rare complication after talc pleurodesis with the introduction of large size talc particles (calibrated talc) and adequate dosage of the talcum powder (standard dose: 5 g) [3].

Recurrence can either occur in terms of a localized encapsulated effusion or as a recurrent large effusion. Whereas localized effusions may best be treated by ultrasound- or CT-guided drainage, larger effusions may require re-intervention with a combination of talcum poudrage and IPC placement.

15.2.7 Conclusions

Treatment of benign pleural effusions is generally directed at the underlying disease. Patients with malignant effusions often profit from surgical drainage and pleurodesis in order to prevent recurrent effusions. Depending on the dynamics of the effusion, as well as the patients' condition and life expectancy, different treatment options may apply. Indwelling pleural catheters, thoracoscopic talc poudrage, and a combination of both are possible treatment options, which have to be tailored to the patients' situation.

15.3 Pneumothorax

Patients with primary pneumothorax are usually <30 years old, healthy young males, without any known underlying pulmonary disease and often present with chest pain as their main symptom. Secondary pneumothorax on the other hand often occurs in male patients over 45 years, with documented, preexisting pulmonary disease, and therefore shortness of breath is a common symptom when pneumothorax occurs.

15.3.1 Primary (PSP)

Primary risk for recurrence is 10% after the first and >50% after the second episode.

In PSP, surgery is therefore indicated in case of recurrence or if primary pneumothorax is complicated by tension, prolonged air leak (>48 h) with incomplete lung re-expansion, or hemothorax. Furthermore certain patients with a profession or lifestyle at risk, such as divers, flying personnel, pilots, or those living in a remote area for a longer time, may be candidates for surgery after the first episode. In small PSP (i.e., size <20% or <3 cm apex-cupula distance) in case of first episode, observation with optional oxygen supplementation and radiographic control after 12–24 h is usually sufficient. In larger first episode PSP, simple needle aspiration may be considered. If aspiration fails to re-expand the lung, the insertion of a small-bore chest drain is indicated.

15.3.2 Secondary (SSP)

Primary risk for recurrence is 50% after the first and >80% after the second episode.

Surgery is generally indicated in all patients with SSP due to the high risk of recurrence and the relatively high potential of a life-threatening event in case of recurrent pneumothorax, since those patients already suffer from respiratory limitation caused by their underlying disease.

15.3.3 Tips and Tricks for Operative Management

Cornerstones of the surgical treatment are resection of blebs/bullae on one hand and pleurodesis (e.g., mechanical or chemical) on the other hand. Usually two ports in the same intercostal space (sixth or seventh) are sufficient to perform the procedure (Fig. 15.1).

Resection of blebs/closure of the air leak: After inspection of the lung, visualized blebs, which are often located at the apex of the lung, are resected by means of an endostapler. If an air leak is present, its exact location can be visualized by submersion of the partially inflated lung in saline. Staple lines must be placed in the region of healthy lung tissue in order to prevent tearing of fragile lung tissue, resulting in

15.3.7 Variations and Complex Presentations

Catamenial pneumothorax usually occurs on the right side within 48–72 h of the onset of menstruation in women aged between 30 and 40 years. Treatment is similar to that of PSP, although during VATS the surgeon has to look for endometriosis (pleural, diaphragmatic) as well as for holes in the diaphragm, which might require partial resection of the hemi diaphragm. In case of recurrence after the first operation, thoracoscopic talc poudrage is advisable, often in combination with a hormonal therapy (gonadotropin-releasing hormone analogue), which is administered in the immediate postoperative period for up to 6–12 months [5].

In patients with *lymphangioleiomyomatosis* as well as in patients suffering from *cystic fibrosis*, the eventual need for lung transplantation in the later course of the disease has to be kept in mind; therefore, mechanical pleurodesis (preferably abrasion) is the method of choice.

In patients with *acquired immunodeficiency syndrome (AIDS)*, the high incidence of pneumothoraces is often due to pneumocystis carinii organisms which cause repeated inflammation and the formation of blebs/bullae at both lung apices. Treatment consists again of resection of the apex combined with mechanical pleurodesis.

15.3.8 Conclusions

While the first episode of PSP can easily be treated conservatively in the absence of complicated pneumothorax, thoracoscopic resection of affected lung tissue combined with the induction of pleural symphysis by mechanical or chemical pleurodesis is the treatment of choice for recurrent and/or complicated PSP as well as for SSP.

15.4 Pleural Fibroma

Solitary fibrous tumors of the pleura are rare primary tumors that arise from mesenchymal cells in the areolar tissue subjacent to the mesothelial-lined pleura and usually show a benign clinical course. More than half of the patients are asymptomatic, while others may present with cough, shortness of breath, and/or chest pain. While 80% of these tumors arise from the visceral pleura and can be treated with simple wedge resection, the remaining 20% arise from the parietal pleura (Fig. 15.2) and sometimes require wider en bloc chest wall resection in order to prevent recurrence. Although histology is benign in 78–88% of cases, a careful follow-up is needed because of the relatively high risk of recurrence, especially if the tumor is sessile and/or malignant. In case of local recurrence, re-resection is recommended [6].

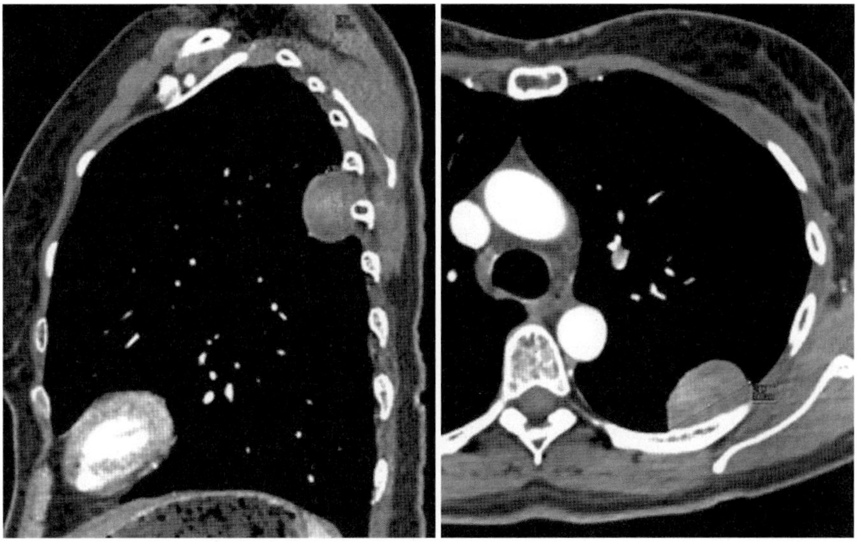

Fig. 15.2 CT scan showing sessile type of a solitary pleural fibroma (tumor marked with star)

15.4.1 Tips and Tricks for Operative Management

Since recurrence is clearly associated with histology and morphology of pleural fibroma, tumors with a high recurrence rate, i.e., those which are sessile, arising from the parietal pleura and/or showing malignant histology, a wider excision margin is strongly advisable. During surgery, care has to be taken not to spill any tumor tissue (i.e., no opening of the tumor capsule, tumor removal with endobag during VATS), in order to prevent local or portside recurrence. For the same reason, needle biopsies should be avoided in the preoperative course if CT scan already is suspicious enough for the diagnosis.

15.4.2 Alternative Ways of Management

Since these tumors show a potentially malignant transformative biological behavior, conservative treatment in terms of "wait and see" may only be considered in elderly patients with poor performance status and small tumors or in the presence of severe comorbidities that preclude surgery.

15.4.3 Postoperative Management

At the time, there is no adequate data to support the usage of radiotherapy and chemotherapy in the treatment of pleural fibroma apart from study protocols.

15.4.4 Conclusions

Solitary fibrous tumors of the pleura are rare tumors, which usually show a benign clinical course. Complete surgical resection is the mainstay of treatment. Recurrence is mainly seen in patients with malignant histology or those with a sessile tumor arising from the parietal pleura; thus, wider resection margins are recommended in these patients.

15.5 Malignant Pleural Mesothelioma (MPM)

MPM is an aggressive form of malignancy with a poor overall prognosis of less than 12 months from the time of diagnosis. Currently, selected patients with resectable disease and favorable prognostic factors (i.e., epithelial histologic type, excluded N2 or metastatic disease, good performance status with the ability to complete a trimodality treatment) are treated in a multimodal therapeutic approach involving chemotherapy, followed by surgical resection and adjuvant radiotherapy. Surgery in a "curative intent" aims at a best possible macroscopic complete resection, whereas it has to be noted that complete resection of this neoplasm with histologically negative margins is rarely achieved. The most complete cytoreductive procedure is extra pleural pneumonectomy (EPP), which involves en bloc resection of the visceral and parietal pleurae, lung, ipsilateral hemi diaphragm, and pericardium (Fig. 15.3).

Another option that is intended to cytoreduce the actual tumor burden is extended pleurectomy/decortication (P/D) with resection of the tumor including parietal and visceral pleurectomy with resection of the diaphragm and pericardium as required.

The optimal form of treatment remains highly controversial within the thoracic community: Recent studies show significantly lower 30-day mortality rates and a trend toward better overall survival for P/D compared to EPP [7]; in contrast to that, the MARS trial [8] fundamentally questioned the role of surgery in the treatment of MPM at all.

15.5.1 Tips and Tricks for Operative Management

For both, EPP and P/D, surgical resection may be facilitated if pleurodesis (e.g., talc poudrage) has already been carried out, since the pleural sheets and the tumor mass are sticking together, allowing easier en bloc resection. If thoracoscopic biopsy has been carried out as a previous procedure, the excision of the trocar sites is strongly advisable, even after local radiotherapy, in order to prevent tumor recurrence at the trocar sites.

The chest cavity is best accessed with the patient in a semi-lateral decubitus position, performing a muscle-sparing anterolateral thoracotomy through the fifth intercostal space, which also allows harvesting of the latissimus dorsi muscle for later coverage of the bronchial stump. First the chest cavity is entered in an extra pleural fashion with mobilization of the whole lung except for the diaphragmatic and pericardial part. Opening of the pleural space should be carefully avoided in order to

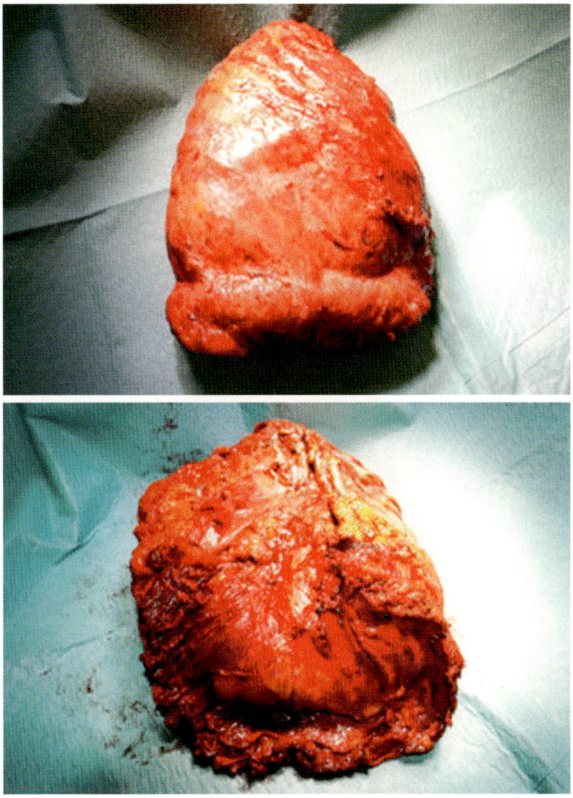

Fig. 15.3 En bloc specimen after right EPP with complete resection of the parietal pleura (above), right pericardium and diaphragm (below)

prevent spillage of the tumor. Whereas in EPP the pericardium is now opened, followed by division of the great vessels and bronchus, in P/D the pericardium is usually only resected if necessary to clear the tumor. Resection of the diaphragm is then performed while avoiding to enter the peritoneal cavity, if possible, in order to minimize abdominal tumor contamination. For this step a second, lower thoracotomy in the eighth intercostal space may be very helpful for complete resection and reconstruction of the diaphragm. A synthetic mesh serves as a replacement for the diaphragm, which should be fixated properly (optimally around the ribs) in order to prevent patch disruption or dislocation with herniation or even incarceration of abdominal organs. Furthermore the mesh should be placed in a normal ("physiologic") diaphragmatic position to prevent radiation injury of abdominal organs. Reconstruction of the pericardium can be performed with either synthetic meshes or preferably biologic material (e.g., decellularized bovine or porcine pericardium), but meticulous care has to be taken to prevent constriction of the heart and to allow sufficient pericardial drainage (i.e., use of permeable and/or fenestrated material) (Fig. 15.4).

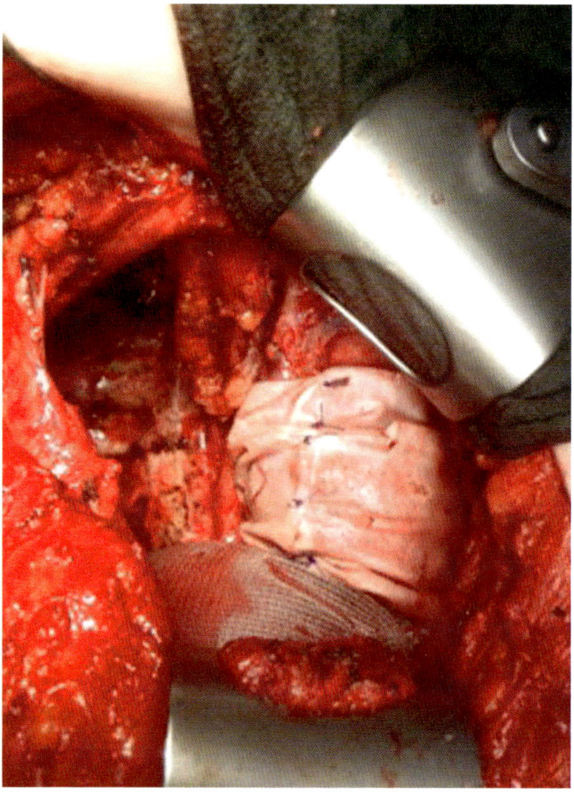

Fig. 15.4 Postoperative result after right EPP with reconstruction of the diaphragm (D – synthetic mesh), pericardium (P – porcine pericardium, fenestrated). The bronchial stump is covered with a latissimus dorsi muscle flap (M). *E* oesophagus, *SVC* superior vena cava (the phrenic nerve is clipped and divided)

15.5.2 Alternative Ways of Operative Management

Both surgical techniques (EPP and P/D) can of course also be performed through a posterolateral thoracotomy in the sixth intercostal space. Since the posterior rib spaces are narrower, resection of the sixth rib often allows better exposure of most structures. When choosing a posterior approach, the serratus anterior muscle can be used for coverage of the bronchial stump in EPP.

As discussed before, EPP allows more complete cytoreduction, with the prize of a higher 30-day mortality rate compared to P/D [7]. Common disadvantages of P/D on the other hand are postoperative air leak, empyema, hemorrhage, and incomplete macroscopic tumor removal in most cases. Furthermore, since the lung is left in place, postoperative radiotherapy is limited because of the risk of radiation pneumonitis.

Since there is existing data that tumor resection may not at all prolong survival in MPM [8], talc poudrage can be carried out as an alternative palliative surgical option, in patients who are unfit for tumor resection, aiming at the prevention of recurrent malignant effusions. As for all patients who suffer from MPM and undergo any form of thoracoscopy, also these patients should receive postoperative radiation of the trocar entry sites in order to prevent tumor ingrowth. Furthermore if palliative pleurodesis is performed, a combination with chemotherapy may be considered [8].

Selected patients with only localized tumor, as a rare subgroup of mesothelioma, may benefit from limited resection in terms of resection of visible tumor only (e.g., tumorectomy including pleurectomy). Preferably also these patients should receive postoperative radiation therapy in order to prevent recurrence. Radiation therapy may also be an option in inoperable patients who present with symptoms due to tumor infiltration of the chest wall.

15.5.3 Tips and Tricks to Avoid and Deal with Intraoperative Complications

General considerations: Since intraoperative identification of the oesophagus can sometimes be difficult due to tumor adhesions and/or dense adhesions after pleurodesis, a large bore orogastric tube should be in place during any surgical procedure.

As for EPP, also in P/D special attention has to be paid when performing decortication near the subclavian vessels and azygos/hemiazygos vein in order to prevent injury of these delicate structures. In order to prevent injury to the recurrent laryngeal nerve on the left side, the vagus nerve can be sought at its entry into the chest cavity and followed distally around the aortic arch.

EPP: Since multimodality concepts usually include neoadjuvant chemotherapy as well as adjuvant high-dose radiotherapy of the hemithorax with a corresponding risk for potentially fatal bronchopleural fistula (BPF), a well vascularized tissue flap should be used for coverage of the bronchial stump for prevention of BPF in these patients with already limited prognosis. We prefer the use of a latissimus dorsi muscle flap, but also serratus muscle or intercostal muscle flaps are suitable for stump protection.

P/D: Air leak can be a major problem after P/D. Superficial lung lesions occurring after removal of the visceral pleura usually do not require treatment. Deeper tears of the lung parenchyma should be sutured with a running monofilament synthetic absorbable suture (e.g., polydioxanone), and sometimes the use of lung sealants (e.g., TachoSil®, PleuraSeal®, Progel®) can be helpful.

15.5.4 Postoperative Management and Postoperative Complications

In EPP a chest drain connected to an underwate r seal without suction can serve as a monitor for postoperative bleeding in the first 12–24 h after surgery. Because of the risk of infection of the postpneumonectomy space, the drainage should be removed after a maximum of 24 h after the procedure. In P/D chest tube(s) can be removed as soon as there is no air leak, and the amount of drainage is less than

Thoracic Outlet Syndrome

16

Mark X. Gannon

Abstract

The thoracic outlet syndrome [TOS] is most easily conceived as three conditions in which the elements of the neurovascular bundle, compressed at the thoracic outlet, produce a venous, an arterial and a neurogenic form of TOS. In the absence of hard diagnostic criteria and with the relative frequency of neurogenic TOS [NTOS], clinical skills remain important in the diagnosis and treatment of NTOS. The elevated arm stress test [EAST] is helpful as is the finding of brachial plexus tenderness behind the scalenus anterior muscle, and improved diagnostic accuracy can be gained from using a chemo denervation test with local anaesthetic or botox to identify and select patients with NTOS.

Arterial TOS [ATOS] and venous TOS [VTOS] are more easily diagnosed. Subclavian artery aneurysm, stenosis and occlusion may present in a non urgent way, and the ischaemia and any associated neurological symptoms are treated on their merits. The majority of ATOS presents acutely with embolism and is usually managed in a staged way with embolectomy, decompression and bypass.

VTOS most usually presents with subclavian artery vein thrombosis and needs to be distinguished from other secondary causes of axillosubclavian venous thrombosis. Thrombolysis and positional venography allows patients to be identified who are most likely to benefit from decompression, venolysis and venoplasty.

Keywords

Thoracic outlet syndrome · Neurogenic · Vascular · Venous

M.X. Gannon
Department of Vascular Surgery, Birmingham Heartlands Hospital, Birmingham, UK
e-mail: mark.gannon@heartofengland.nhs.uk

D. Parikh, P.B. Rajesh (eds.), *Tips and Tricks in Thoracic Surgery*,
https://doi.org/10.1007/978-1-4471-7355-7_16

Thoracic outlet syndrome [TOS] is a collection of conditions caused by compression of the neurovascular structures to the upper limb as they cross the first rib. The names of the three conditions are determined by which of the neurovascular structures under compression is leading to the principal presenting symptom complex. Where the symptoms are principally pain + sensorimotor symptom, it is called neurogenic thoracic outlet syndrome [NTOS]; where they are principally associated with ischaemia or aneurysm, it is known as arterial thoracic outlet syndrome [ATOS]; and where the symptoms are caused by compression or thrombosis of the subclavian vein, it is called venous thoracic outlet syndrome [VTOS]. The three conditions are distinct but they are not mutually exclusive. The subclavian artery and the brachial plexus en route to the upper limb cross the first rib by passing through the scalene triangle between scalenus anterior and medius. This space may be narrowed and lead to compression because of bony or fibromuscular variations in anatomy often aggravated by tightening and fibrosis of the scalene muscles as a result of trauma or overuse. Compression of the subclavian vein takes place in the costoclavicular space where the anatomy is usually normal, but the venous compression is associated with muscle hypertrophy or overuse.

16.1 Neurogenic Thoracic Outlet Syndrome [NTOS]

NTOS is by far the commonest accounting for more than 90% of patient presentations [1]. It may be associated with recognisable skeletal abnormalities such as a cervical rib or prefixation of the first rib on the second, but most commonly there is no bony abnormality. The diagnosis is considered to be difficult to make because there is no clear objective diagnostic investigation which will reliably point to its presence. It is important therefore to take a detailed medical history and perform careful clinical examination. Common presenting symptoms include pain in the upper limb, in the neck, sometimes with occipital headache, tingling and paraesthesia in the upper limb, variable and intermittent changes in colour and weakness in various forms. The history should be distinguished from pain syndromes originating from the cervical spine, the shoulder and rotator cuff and sensory and motor dysfunction caused by compression of the major upper limb peripheral nerves. Most of these conditions have reliable reproducible patterns of pain, weakness or sensory change, whereas the patient with TOS will not fit easily into any one of these categories.

Significant proportions of patients presenting with NTOS have a history of hyper extension injury often associated with a traffic accident. In some there are posturally related occupational factors and in others consequences from hobbies and sporting activities. These aetiological factors, particularly the trauma, result in fibrosis and scarring of the scalene muscles, and the tightening and shortening is thought to be a contributory factor in the development of the symptoms [2].

Careful physical examination is necessary so that the clinician can rule out the principal alternate diagnosis. The typical features of spinal, shoulder and upper limb neurological compression syndromes and some understanding of regional complex pain syndrome need to be understood. There are some specific features that are helpful in making the diagnosis of NTOS; in particular the EAST [elevated arm stress test] as described by Roos [3] is helpful in that its use precipitates the symptoms in NTOS and one may simultaneously notice symptoms of arterial compression which may act as a proxy. Adson's test on the other hand is not a reliable test because of the frequency of false-positive results [4]. Tenderness on pressure and palpation over the scalene muscles in front of the brachial plexus is a helpful physical sign which is not usually present in the other conditions being considered [2].

Special investigations also serve to show what the presenting condition is not. Normal x-rays, CT scans, MRIs and conduction studies are often used to rule out other potential diagnoses. Plain x-rays and reconstructed spiral CT scans are very good at demonstrating osseous abnormalities. CT angiography is a reliable way of looking at the arterial flow across the thoracic inlet (Fig. 16.1). Nerve conduction studies have not been of great help in making a proactive diagnosis of TOS though recent studies looking at prolonged latency of the medial antebrachial cutaneous nerves are being examined as a potential diagnostic test [5].

A manoeuvre which does increase confidence in the diagnosis of NTOS and predicts the success of surgical decompression is chemical blockade of the scalenus anterior muscle. This can be done with local anaesthetic agents [6] which provide a rapid onset but short-lived blockade of the scalenus anterior function, or a more prolonged chemical denervation can be achieved by injecting the scalenus anterior muscle with botulinum toxin using ultrasound or CT guidance [7, 8] (Fig. 16.2). In both circumstances relief of symptoms following the block provides confidence that the symptoms are associated with compression in the scalene triangle. In individuals who are high risk for anaesthesia in surgery, chemodenervation with botulinum toxin can also provide an alternate therapeutic option. It is not unusual to find that after botox treatment, the relief of symptoms can often persist quite a lot longer than one would be able to explain from the effects of the toxin.

There are some features in the patient history which are associated with poorer surgical outcomes in NTOS. Patients with depression and high levels of self-reported pain, the unmarried and those of lower educational attainment tend to do less well [9]. In those patients with an ongoing compensation claim and with manual jobs, the outcomes are mixed.

16.2 Conservative Measures

The first line of treatment in patients diagnosed with NTOS is to pursue a course of physiotherapy, the purpose of which is to strengthen, stretch and mobilise the muscles of the shoulder girdle. Scapula mobilisation, shoulder mobilisation, stretching of the scalene muscles, mobilisation of the clavicle and first rib and physical means of managing muscular trigger points for the pain are all used to create circumstances in which the symptoms can improve. Modification of the working environment through a workplace assessment and modification of sports and pastimes can also be introduced where they are felt to be part of the precipitating problem [10, 11].

The long-term natural history of NTOS is not clearly documented, but the observation that it seldom occurs in older people suggests that work activity and postural matters may contribute. This is not to say that some people are not so disabled by the symptoms of NTOS that they would not sooner undergo surgical decompression if a course of physiotherapy is not successful [12].

Surgical decompression of NTOS can be achieved either by scalenectomy or by resection of the first rib by a supraclavicular or trans-axillary route. The experience of the individual surgeon may dictate a preference for one procedure over another, but outcomes in large series of patients operated on for NTOS show that good results can be achieved by a thorough scalenectomy to which only modest additional benefit is added by excision of the first rib [2]. Trans-axillary excision of the first rib produces outcomes similar to scalenectomy, but the approach is more limited in that it does not allow a thorough decompression of the plexus and provides no flexibility for access to the vascular structures if required. First rib excision by the trans-axillary route decompresses the scalene triangle by removing its base but does not address the developmental and acquired abnormalities of the scalenus muscles which are thought to be the cause of NTOS.

16.3 Arterial Thoracic Outlet Syndrome [ATOS]

ATOS is a condition that should be brought to mind when patients present with acute or chronic upper limb ischaemia as although it only accounts for 1–3% of all TOS it is not a rare condition in clinical practice. The subclavian artery is compressed in the scalene triangle. There are significantly more patients with cervical rib and first rib abnormalities among ATOS than there are in the other forms of TOS. The presentation may be non urgent or urgent. The subclavian artery compressed in the scalene triangle may lead to effort symptoms [sometimes called claudication] when the patient is active with their arms particularly in an elevated position as a result of the artery simply being compressed in the stress position. Or, there may be similar effort-related symptoms in all positions when stricture begins to develop in the subclavian artery, or a patient may have persistent symptoms if there is subclavian artery occlusion. Another non urgent presentation is with a pulsatile swelling in the supraclavicular fossa caused by subclavian artery aneurysm. This is a form of post-stenotic dilatation where the turbulent flow beyond the constrained artery in the scalene triangle produces turbulence that damages the artery wall and predisposes to aneurysm.

The urgent presentations of ATOS are almost all due to embolisation which may take place from a narrowed subclavian artery or from the laminated thrombus in a subclavian artery aneurysm. They may lead to macro or micro embolisation into the upper limb [13]. Micro embolisation may manifest with splinter haemorrhages or small areas of skin infarction in TOS, or it may present as Raynaud's phenomena though in many cases of patients with Raynaud's there is no evidence of occlusive or embolic disease and it may be understood as an autonomic component of NTOS. Acute limb ischaemia will accompany macro embolic events where thrombus from the disease subclavian artery embolises and occludes the upper limb circulation, frequently at points of arterial bifurcation in the axillary or brachial artery and sometimes presenting with more distal ischaemia from emboli which have broken up and occluded the smaller arteries in the forearm and hand. Elective surgical correction of the arterial abnormalities of ATOS is done in accordance with the clinical picture which presents. Stable effort-related symptoms in a non dominant arm with a complete occlusion of the subclavian artery may be managed conservatively, or more symptoms in the dominant arm of an active person may be managed with decompression and bypass. Ongoing and worsening symptoms from compression and stenosis as well as the finding of subclavian artery aneurysm will usually be managed by decompression and bypass. Surgical decompression is usually performed through the anterior supraclavicular approach, and scalenectomy is a required part of adequate exposure of the subclavian artery for interposition grafting with either the long saphenous vein or prosthetic interposition graft [13].

The acute presentations of ATOS may require a staged approach, the initial stage requiring embolectomy and the restoration of adequate arterial flow followed by anticoagulation with later planned decompression and bypass or interposition grafting.

For those patients with bony abnormalities who present with TOS, the further correction of the bony abnormality will depend on whether there are coexisting compressive neurological symptoms which require bony decompression in addition to correction of the arterial problem. The often bilateral nature of TOS and the developmental abnormalities that go with it would require that the contralateral side be examined in patients who present with ATOS so that if necessary pre-emptive treatment can be advised.

16.4 Venous Thoracic Outlet Syndrome [VTOS]

VTOS, also known as Paget–Schroetter syndrome, may produce intermittent symptoms of venous obstruction with activity-related or positional exacerbation, but it more commonly presents acutely with the symptoms of subclavian vein thrombosis which include heaviness, swelling, cyanosis and discomfort. Subclavian vein thrombosis is not as common as major lower limb thrombosis but nonetheless can produce pulmonary embolism and post-thrombotic syndrome complex [14]. The majority of subclavian vein thrombosis is secondary to a recognisable underlying cause. Increasingly these are iatrogenic as increased use of central lines for chemotherapy, haemodialysis, parenteral nutrition, long-term antibiotic and other medications becomes more common. It may also follow radiation treatment and local trauma or malignancy. In patients with no associated recognised precipitating factor in their medical history, the thrombosis is considered a primary event, a proportion of whom will have a thrombophilia, but the majority of whom will be found to have venous compression associated with TOS.

The later consequences of secondary subclavian vein thrombosis are often not severe. In contrast between 30 and 80% of patients having Paget–Schroetter syndrome with thrombosis due to TOS will have significant disabling symptoms in the aftermath of the thrombosis [15]. In part this is due to the nature of the venous obstruction being compressive and in part due to the higher demands put on the limb by the younger, more active patients with VTOS. Persisting symptoms after venous thrombosis may not all be from venous obstruction, but the perivenous inflammation may worsen symptoms of a NTOS [16]. The introduction of catheter-directed venous thrombolysis allowed the opportunity to set back the clock by dissolving the occlusive thrombus. Through this practice we have learned that the thrombosis is not in a normal vein but in a vein which has shown signs of scarring and stenosis from recurrent intermittent compression. Venous thrombolysis has also allowed the opportunity following successful clot lysis to examine the subclavian vein for positional compression, and the identification of a subgroup of patients who do not have TOS and who like those with secondary axillosubclavian thrombosis can be treated with anticoagulation [17]. An additional logistical problem is that not all patients with axillosubclavian thrombosis due to VTOS will present to the vascular service in the acute phase of their illness. It may be that they are treated with initial anticoagulation and only subsequently referred. Trans-catheter thrombolysis is more successful early in the clinical course and is unlikely to be helpful if there has been thrombosis present for several weeks [14]. Those patients presenting acutely or during the first weeks are the best candidates for thrombolysis, though thrombolysis may be worth implementing between 2 and 6 weeks. After 6 weeks the chances of successful lysis diminish [18]. Thrombolysis in the acute or early subacute phase, if successful, offers the opportunity to undertake positional venography which will confirm the compressive component in those with venous TOS and create circumstances in which the patients can undergo decompression of the thoracic outlet. Patients presenting after 6 weeks and those who fail thrombolysis are usually anticoagulated and given consideration to whether they will undergo decompression as there is evidence to suggest that decompression is still beneficial in these individuals and often associated with late recanalisation [19].

The timing of decompression has been the subject of some debate. Machleder [20] initially recommended anticoagulation for 3 months followed by decompression, but the introduction of early decompression showed that good results could be obtained safely without that delay [21].

Surgical decompression can be achieved by three different approaches. The trans-axillary approach provides good access to the first rib but poor access to the medial part of the vein and the scalenus muscles. Supraclavicular and para-clavicular approaches allow good exposure of the proximal vein and access to the scalene muscles for scalenectomy, but the supraclavicular approach offers poor exposure of the medial vein, and the addition of an infra-clavicular incision is a useful addition to provide good medial access to the rib in order to decompress the costa-clavicular space. An alternate infra-clavicular approach allows similar anterior costa-clavicular decompression and resection of the anterior half of the first rib but poorer access for scalenectomy and neurolysis. Almost all surgeons recommend comprehensive venolysis at the time of decompression in order to free the subclavian vein from the surrounding fibrous tissue which has developed as part of the repeated trauma from the compression [22].

There are a number of alternate approaches to managing residual vein abnormality after successful decompression and venolysis. Some favour an intraoperative surgical venoplasty; others, intraoperative venography with immediate balloon venoplasty [21]; and others, post-operative anticoagulation venography at 2 weeks with balloon venoplasty at that time of any residual stenosis [20]. All have produced acceptable results.

Following successful decompression and optimising venous outflow, venous duplex scanning is a reliable way of following the ongoing venous patency, and this combined with the clinical pattern of symptoms should allow identification of individuals who require further venographic assessment. An algorithm for the management of axillosubclavian thrombosis is shown in Fig. 16.3.

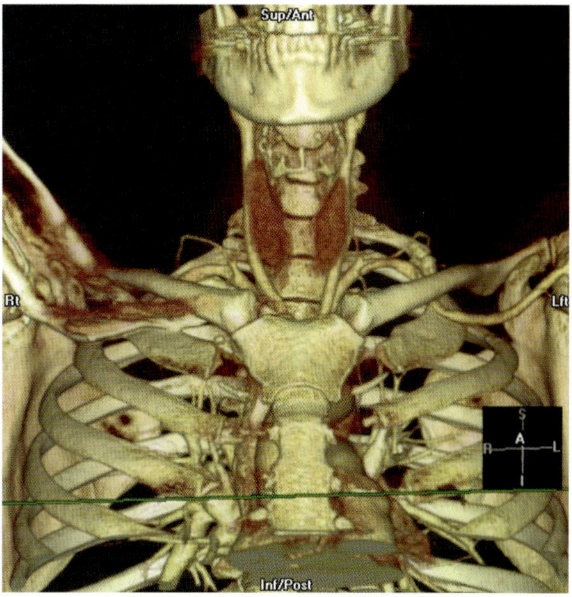

Fig. 16.1 A reconstruction of a CT angiogram showing the subclavian artery arching across the first rib in a patient with a well-formed cervical rib and a pseudarthrosis with the first rib

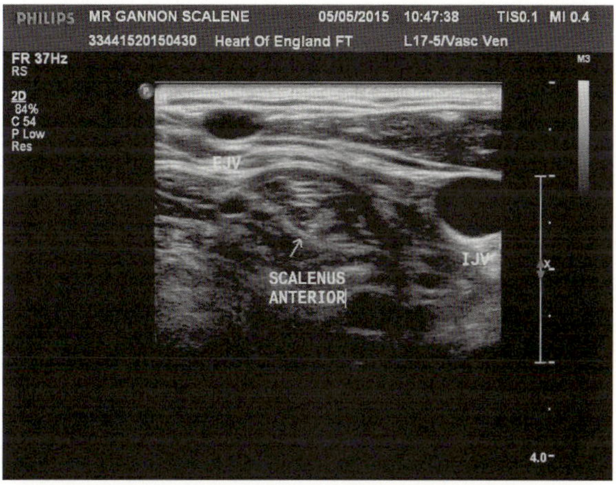

Fig. 16.2 Ultrasound scan of the supraclavicular fossa clearly showing the scalenus anterior muscle between the internal and external jugular veins

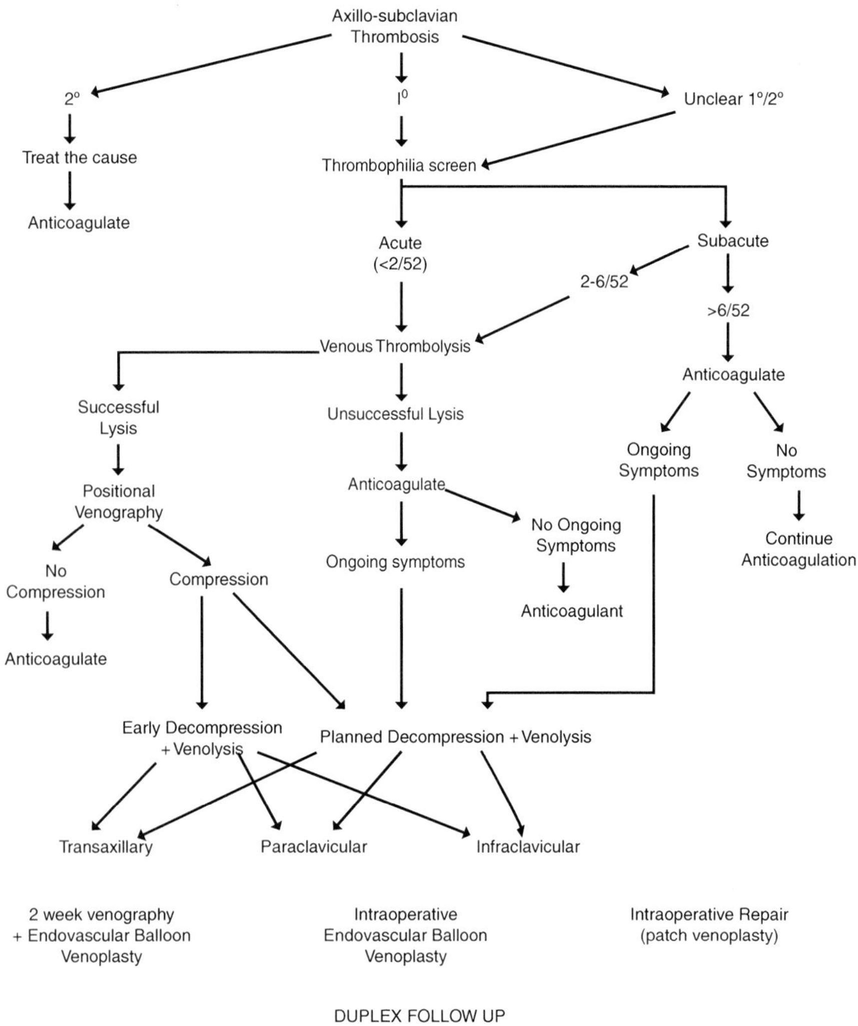

Fig. 16.3 An algorithm for the management of axillosubclavian thrombosis

References

1. Sanders RJ, Hammond SL, Rao NM. Diagnosis of thoracic outlet syndrome. J Vasc Surg. 2007;46:601–4.
2. Sanders RJ. Thoracic outlet syndrome: a common sequelae to neck injuries. Philadelphia: JB Lippincott; 1991.
3. Roos DB, Owens JC. Thoracic outlet syndrome. Arch Surg. 1966;93:71–4.
4. Warrens H, Heaton JM. Thoracic outlet syndrome: the lack of reliability of clinical assessment. Ann R Coll Surg Engl. 1987;69:203–4.
5. Machanic BI, Sanders RJ. Medial antebrachial cutaneous nerve measurements to diagnose neurogenic thoracic outlet syndrome. Ann Vasc Surg. 2008;22:248–54.

6. Gage M. Scalenus anticus syndrome: a diagnostic and confirmatory test. Surgery. 1939;5:599–601.
7. Christo PJ, Christo DK, Carinci AJ, Freischlag JA. Single CT guided chemodenervation of the anterior scalene muscle with botulinum toxin in neurogenic thoracic outlet syndrome. Pain Med. 2010;11:504–11.
8. Torriani M, Gupta R, Donahue DM. Sonographically guided anesthetic injection of anterior scalene muscle for investigation of neurogenic thoracic outlet syndrome. Skelet Radiol. 2009;38:1083287.
9. Axelrod DM, Proctor MC, Geisser ME, Roth RS, Greenfield LJ. Outcomes after surgery for thoracic outlet syndrome. J Vasc Surg. 2001;33:1220–5.
10. Hooper T, Denton J, McGallard K. Thoracic outlet syndrome: a controversial clinical condition. Part 2 non-surgical and surgical management. J Man Manip Ther. 2010;18:132–8.
11. Vanti C, Natalini L, Romeo A, et al. Conservative treatment for thoracic outlet syndrome. Eur Med Phys. 2006;42:1–16.
12. Landy GJ, Moneta GL, Taylor WM, Edwards JM, Porter JM. Long term functional outcome of neurogenic thoracic outlet syndrome in surgically and conservatively treated patients. J Vasc Surg. 2001;33:312–9.
13. Marine L, Valdes F, Mertens R, et al. Arterial thoracic outlet syndrome: the 32 year experience. Ann Vasc Surg. 2013;27:1007–13.
14. Illig K, Doyle A. A comprehensive review of Paget-Schroetter Syndrome. J Vasc Surg. 2010;51:538–47.
15. Donayne CE, White G, Mehringer SM, Wilson SE. Pathogenesis determines late morbidity in axillosubclavian vein thrombosis. Am J Surg. 1986;152:179–84.
16. Thomson RW, Schneider PA, Nelkan NA, Skiolerbrand CG, Stoney RJ. Circumferential venolysis and paraclavicular thoracic outlet decompression for 'effort thrombosis' of the subclavian vein. J Vasc Surg. 1992;16:723–32.
17. Schanzer A, Messina L. Chapter 125: Thoracic outlet syndrome: venous. In: Rutherford's vascular surgery. 7th ed. p. 1910–1.
18. Urschel HC, Razzak MA. Paget-Schroetter syndrome: what is the best management. Ann Thorac Surg. 2000;69:1663–1668; discussion 1668–9.
19. Guzzo JL, Chang K, Demos J, Black J, Freischlag JA. Pre-operative thrombolysis and venoplasty affords no benefit in patients following first rib resection and scalenectomy for subacute and chronic subclavian vein thrombosis. J Vasc Surg. 2010;52:658–63.
20. Machleder HI. Evaluation of a new treatment strategy for Paget-Schroetter syndrome: spontaneous thrombosis of the axillary-subclavian vein. J Vasc Surg. 1993;17:305–17.
21. Schneider DB, Dimuzio PJ, Martin ND, Gordon RL, Wilson MW, Laberge JM. Combination treatment of venous thoracic outlet syndrome: open surgical decompression and intra-operative angioplasty. J Vasc Surg. 2004;40:599–603.
22. Molina JE. Approach to the confluence of the subclavian and internal jugular vein without claviculectomy. Semin Vasc Surg. 2000;13:10–9.

Pectus Excavatum

17

Babu Naidu

Abstract

Pectus excavatum (PE) or funnel chest is a dorsal deviation of the sternum and most commonly the third to seventh rib or costal cartilages, resulting in a concave depression of the anterior chest wall. Depending on the severity of PE, deviation of the thoracic organs and spinal deformities (such as scoliosis in 15–21% of patients) may also be present. PE is the most common congenital chest wall abnormality and has an incidence of 1 in 260 births among white infants, 1 per 1400 births among black infants and 1 in 500 in 'other' infants. Males are more commonly affected, with a male to female ratio of 4 to1. Autopsy records report PE in 1 of 800 cases. Survival analysis indicates that PE patients tended to die earlier. However, PE patients who survived past the age of 56 years tended to live longer than matched controls.

Keywords

Pectus · Ravitch · Nuss

Pectus excavatum (PE) or funnel chest is a dorsal deviation of the sternum and most commonly the third to seventh rib or costal cartilages, resulting in a concave depression of the anterior chest wall. Depending on the severity of PE, deviation of the thoracic organs and spinal deformities (such as scoliosis in 15–21% of patients) may also be present. PE is the most common congenital chest wall abnormality and has an incidence of 1 in 260 births among white infants, 1 per 1400 births among black infants and 1 in 500 in 'other' infants. Males are more commonly affected, with a male to female ratio of 4 to1. Autopsy records report PE in 1 of 800 cases. Survival analysis indicates that PE patients tended to die earlier. However, PE

B. Naidu
Heart of England NHS Foundation Trust and University of Birmingham, Birmingham, UK

D. Parikh, P.B. Rajesh (eds.), *Tips and Tricks in Thoracic Surgery*,
https://doi.org/10.1007/978-1-4471-7355-7_17

patients who survived past the age of 56 years tended to live longer than matched controls.

A positive family history is present in up to 40% cases. Family tree analysis has shown that inheritance can be been autosomal dominant or recessive or X-linked or multifactorial in different families. A third present in infancy but the majority do not notice the depression until the pubertal growth spurt.

Although the exact aetiology of PE is unknown, abnormal mechanical forces during growth are thought to contribute to its development. This is supported by co-presentation with congenital diaphragmatic hernia, following costal cartilage graft harvesting, accompanying upper airway obstruction and in untreated infants with spinal muscular atrophy.

Histologically cartilages removed at surgery appear unremarkable, but mechanical deformation properties of the cartilages, electron microscopic findings and abnormal collagen content have also been reported. Indeed there is an association of PE in patients with a connective tissue disorder, namely, Marfan syndrome (5–8%), Ehlers-Danlos syndrome (3%) and Sprengel's deformity (0.6%).

Surprisingly the earliest reported cases come from a report from Hungary of 2 PE sternums found in a collection of 48 breast bones in graves dated from the tenth to the sixteenth centuries.

Sauerbruch, one of the pioneers of thoracic surgery, reported a case in 1913 of PE treated surgically by excision of a section of the anterior chest wall, including the left fifth to ninth costal cartilages and adjacent sternum. Preoperatively the patient was incapacitated by severe dyspnoea and palpitations, which resolved following surgery. At this time surgical treatment carried significant risk of death. Ravitch's modification more than 20 years later led to wider adoption; the technique included bilateral subperichondrial costal cartilage resection, sternal fracture, complete detachment of the sternum from its attachments below the second or third costal cartilage and placement of a substernal bone graft. Gross noted good correction with only division of the costal cartilages in two places and sternal osteotomy, and Welch reported excellent results without cutting through the intercostal bundles or rectus muscle attachments. Internal support was suggested later and included either homologous rib (Dorner, 1950), curved steel bar through sternum (Wallgren & Sulamaa, 1956) or shorter bar posterior to the sternum (Adkins & Blades, 1961). More recently used support materials include titanium miniplates (our preferred technique), Dacron vascular graft strut, bioabsorbable substernal mesh band. The use of silicone implants for primary correction is not advisable as it does not correct the underlying chest deformity. The sternal turnover technique has not been widely adopted across the world except in Japan because of fear of sternal necrosis and/or infection.

In a small number of reports, following modified Ravitch surgery, concern grew over cases where costal cartilages were replaced with bony, inflexible scar leading to poor results. At around that time, the 10-year experience of a new 'minimally invasive' technique was described (Nuss, 1988) using an internal stainless steel brace and no costal cartilage resection or sternal osteotomy reliant on flexible pliable Pediatric and adolescent skeleton and remodelling of the chest. The technique has since been modified to include the use of video-assisted thoracoscopy, stabilisation of the bar by absorbable suture or bar attachments and special instruments to facilitate dissection. Most recent prospective studies demonstrate that repair by either Nuss or open operation can be achieved with good outcomes and minimal complications.

17.1 Assessment of the Adult and Adolescent Patients with PE

The journey of referral by primary and secondary care physician is usually fraught with difficulty for the patient. Many patients are told that it is a 'cosmetic' operation, that nothing can be done and that surgery involves a high risk of death and routine prolonged admission to intensive care. Barriers to referral are set to increase as the strains on health-care resources aim to push this condition into a group perceived to be of 'low clinical value'. This is far from the truth as many young lives are transformed by this surgery allowing them to live and contribute to society fully. Even consultation with cases of minor severity is important: Reassuring patients that they can carry on with life without concern or worry is worthwhile. The other end of the information spectra is the wide number of pectus forums. Whilst some of them provide valuable support and information for the patient, a number are misinformative.

Tip

One way to deal with this gap in information is to develop your own bespoke patient information. A website which highlights indications for, what to expect and pictures before and after, and videos of patient experience of surgery is a valued resource. With this approach we have found that patients who use our website (www.pectus.co.uk) tend to be more satisfied after the surgery. Also keeping an album of anonymised photos pre- and post-surgery of treated patients not only serves as part of the clinical records but allows patients considering surgery to understand what they can expect from repair of their pectus.

A thorough history and examination is essential as is a frank discussion about expectations for surgery. Success of the surgery relates to how the patient feels about his physical status and the appearance of the repair not the clinicians perception of it. There are times when the cosmetic result of the surgery is not perfect from the surgeon's perspective but the patient is very pleased with the result.

Tip

In our clinical practice, we see patients and their families twice before the decision to undergo major surgery is made. The consultation is summarised in writing to the patient to be clear about the expectation of surgery. 'Improving the look of the chest but never making it perfect.... the more severe usually the more satisfied with surgery.... trading one look for scars' are all useful phrases. The recurrent underestimate in a young person's mind of what suffering they have to undergo with the surgery specifically around pain requires special attention in the consent procedure.

Symptoms broadly speaking are twofold physical or psychosocial, and both need to be explored thoroughly.

Compression of the thoracic organs may result in chest pain, fatigue, dyspnoea on exertion, recurrent respiratory infections, asthma symptoms, palpitations or syncopal episodes. It's important in sedentary individuals to elicit whether behaviour is triggered by limitation in exercise capacity or not. It's not unusual in patients who do not complain of any limitation in physical activity to find after surgery that they are able to do more. This is backed up with evidence; meta-analysis of studies showed that cardiovascular function increased by greater than one half standard deviation following the surgical repair of pectus excavatum despite including studies that measured change in the deconditioned early post-operative period. Direct cardiac compression may result in reduced cardiac output due to a reduction in stroke volume. The degree of severity of PE, however, does not correlate directly with functional impairment perhaps because of the way we define severity. In some PE patients with a deep chest (increased anteroposterior distance), the heart may never be compressed despite severe sternal depression. Improvements in cardiac function especially during exercise (including ejection fraction and right ventricular systolic and diastolic indices) have been reported both in the early post-operative period and long-term following surgical correction. Mitral valve prolapse, as a direct result of cardiac compression, is more prominent than in an age-matched population (17% PE vs. 1% normal population). Dysrhythmias, including first degree heart block, right bundle branch block or Wolff-Parkinson-White syndrome, may be present in up to 15% of patients. Congenital heart disease is present in 2% of patients with PE. Thus a thorough examination of the cardiovascular system is warranted.

The body of evidence showing impairment in spirometry and improvement with surgery has also become clearer in recent years. Both spirometry (measurement of air flow out of the chest on exhalation at rest) and plethysmography (measurement of lung volumes) are usually reduced by approximately 10–20% of the predicted values. For forced vital capacity, forced expiratory volume (FEV) in 1 s and FEV 25–75%, 26%, 32% and 45% of patients, respectively, are in the abnormal category that is below 80% predicted values; with a normal distribution, only 16% should be less than 80% predicted. As these are otherwise healthy patients usually without concurrent pulmonary disease, with pliable chest walls and large physiologic reserve, the abnormal respiratory function may only be unmasked by formal exercise testing. In older patients with symptoms that seem out of proportion with their pectus, other causes should be sought.

Chest wall motion capture technology has enabled a more detailed valuation of the effects of PE on respiratory mechanics. In summary, the bellow action of the ribcage is impaired with PE. Normally, the sternum should move up and down like an old-fashioned water pump, with PE the lower end of the sternum is fixed and the patients compensate by increasing abdominal breathing. This pattern is corrected following repair. This idea is supported by the finding that patients with the more severe depression are more likely to have a restrictive pattern of spirometry.

Technical Tip

One caveat to modest changes in primary PE is the observation of significant restrictive lung function that can occur in recurrent PE with spirometry values about half of predicted values.

17.1.1 Psychosocial

It is important to document the effects of PE in these patients in terms of mental health—anxiety and depression, self-esteem, quality of life and body image. The key is to try and discern how much or many of these symptoms are ascribable to PE. This can at times be difficult to assess for surgeons and if there is any doubt, specialist psychological help is required. Increasingly with financial constraints on the health systems, we must quantify the baseline and any improvement. Using psychometrically validated testing tools is essential in this respect. Studies have shown consistently that there is marked improvement in psychosocial functioning following surgery; interestingly this is independent of the severity of the PE. There can be an apathy of clinicians towards these symptoms which present in a person's life just when they are establishing an independent identity and interacting with others. This deformity reduces capacity to do those things and is very significant within these young people's lives. The Medical community support surgical treatment of syndactyly, revision of burn scars, cleft lip and other conditions where the justification is 'cosmetic'; PE is no different in actual fact and reasons to correct are far more established.

Tip

We prefer to use more than one tool as all aspects may not be covered adequately in just one questionnaire. Our current practice is to institute at the first clinic visit the Patient Health Questionnaire (PHQ-9) screening, diagnosing, monitoring and measuring mental health and the generalised anxiety disorder (GAD-7) in addition to the Nuss questionnaire. In our experience these questionnaires have value in assessing patient's symptoms and bringing out issues that sometimes can be difficult to elicit in consultation. It's also important to discern if there are significant underlying mental health issues that may not improve following surgery. In these cases, there should be a low threshold to seek a formal psychological consultation.

Examination should note the variant concavities of the anterior chest wall listed in frequency order: focal or cup-shaped deformity, broad, shallow, saucer-shaped deformity, long furrow or trench deformity, (which is usually asymmetrical) or mixed pectus carinatum and excavatum. The body habitus of a tall, thin patient with forward-drifting hunched shoulders in an attempt to hide their PE is common. In these patients, it's important to stress the importance of the preoperative programme of physiotherapy of back straightening exercises. This is especially important because if patients maintain a poor posture following surgery, this may contribute to recurrence. Any asymmetry of the PE and associated sternal tilt as well as costal flaring should be documented. This is especially important as sometimes costal flaring may be more troublesome to the patient rather than the dip in the sternum itself.

In women especially note any asymmetry in breast tissue: this can become more marked following correction. Failure of bra's to fit correctly is not an uncommon complaint in female patients.

Tip

Performing a Valsalva manoeuvre, getting the patient to push their chest forward having taken a deep breath in gives an idea of the flexibility of the chest which plays a role in deciding which type of operation would suit the patient.

Note must be taken to the quality of the skin, specifically how well the skin heals from old scars and other coexisting skin conditions such as acne. These can be an indicator of risk for hypertrophic scar formation. Finally features of connective tissue disorders, scoliosis (fixed or reversible), joint laxity and striae may also be present. The presences of scoliosis should also include a test to see if it's fixed or not. Heart murmurs should be excluded, particularly mitral valve prolapse. Nickel allergy occurs in 2% of the population and may be suggested by the absence of wearing a metal backed watch or jewellery. Formal allergy test should be performed if history suggestive and plan for titanium implants rather than stainless steel if the test is positive.

17.2 Investigations

Chest radiograph may demonstrate a concavity in the anterior chest wall. Computed tomography (CT) and magnetic resonance imaging (MRI), however, are better at demonstrating bony and cartilaginous deformities, with the cephalocaudad extent of the depression more easily visualised and cardiac or pulmonary compression and displacement.

Radiological imaging is also important to aid the planning of surgical intervention. In recurrent PE calcification following open repair can be a marker of fixity of the chest.

The Haller radiographic index is defined as the internal lateral transverse thoracic diameter divided by the anteroposterior diameter (shortest distance from the back of the sternum to the front of the vertebral body) (Fig. 17.1). A Haller index

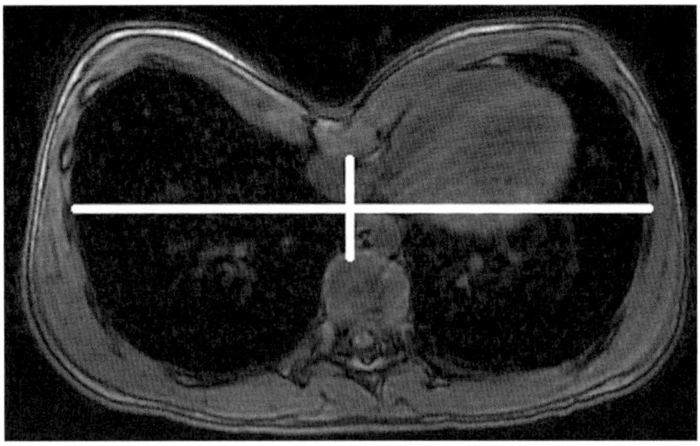

Fig. 17.1 Axial computed tomography image demonstrating the calculation of the Haller index by dividing the internal lateral transverse thoracic diameter by the anteroposterior diameter

above 3.2 represents severe PE, though as mentioned before, the morphology of the chest may not be captured fully by a single measure. The deep depression in a barrel-shaped chest may have little physical compression of the heart. Review of the CT scan with the patient and family before surgery is a useful exercise as it helps to communicate the extent of deformity and its effects as well as potential complications of surgery. MRI may be used instead of CT to reduce radiation exposure, but because more claustrophobic and longer scanning times may not suit all.

If a patient has physical symptoms, then our recommendation is to perform baseline echocardiography and lung spirometry. There is a trend to perform these tests in all patients undergoing surgery though this practice has recently been challenged.

17.3 Criteria for Surgical Repair

Only around half of patients presenting to the surgical team are offered surgery. Minor cases of pectus should be reassured and discouraged from surgery. A programme of physiotherapy can be helpful, and there are reports of some patients who have been successfully treated with vacuum bell devices.

Generally speaking the criteria for offering surgical treatment in patients with severe pectus (Haller index greater than 3.2) should be guided by the presence of psychosocial or physical symptoms. There is a trend for some surgeons to encourage treatment in asymptomatic patients with evidence of cardiac compression on CT or paradoxical motion with deep inspiration, restrictive pulmonary function test, mitral valve prolapse and bundle branch block.

Evidence to recommend major surgical treatment in the asymptomatic patient is sparse though most patients with severe pectus do have symptoms.

No effective validated conservative methods have been described for the treatment of severe PE; surgery remains the only therapeutic option. The most common surgical options include:

(a) Open repair—modified Ravitch procedure (Fig. 17.2)
(b) Minimally invasive repair—Nuss procedure (Fig. 17.3)

The timing of surgical intervention, however, remains controversial. Performing the Nuss or Ravitch procedure before the pubertal growth spurt may necessitate redo surgery as the patient grows the pectus may recur. In the UK, the optimal age for minimally invasive repair is thought to be between 14 and 18.

Choice of operation depends on the flexibility of the chest, patient choice and expertise of the surgeon. Valsalva manoeuvre can assist with this decision. In general Ravitch is offered in patients who are older when the flexibility of the chest reduces and in patients with combined PE and carinatum defects, pouter pigeon deformity with anterior displacement of the manubrium and posterior displacement of the body of the sternum and significant sternal torsion. Prior to surgery, patients are instructed on maintaining good posture and exercises to perform before and

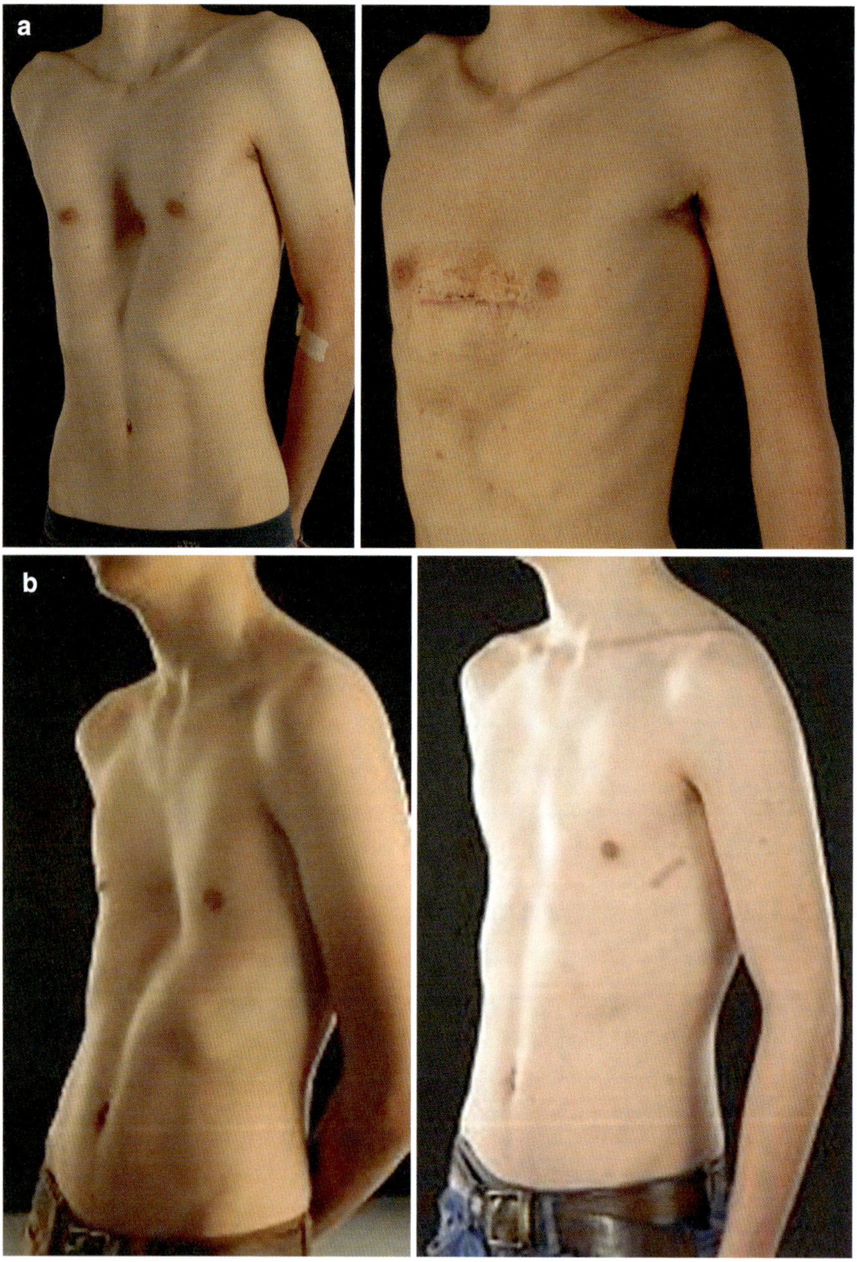

Fig. 17.2 Pectus excavatum, before and after operative repair using (**a**) a modified Ravitch (**b**) Nuss procedure

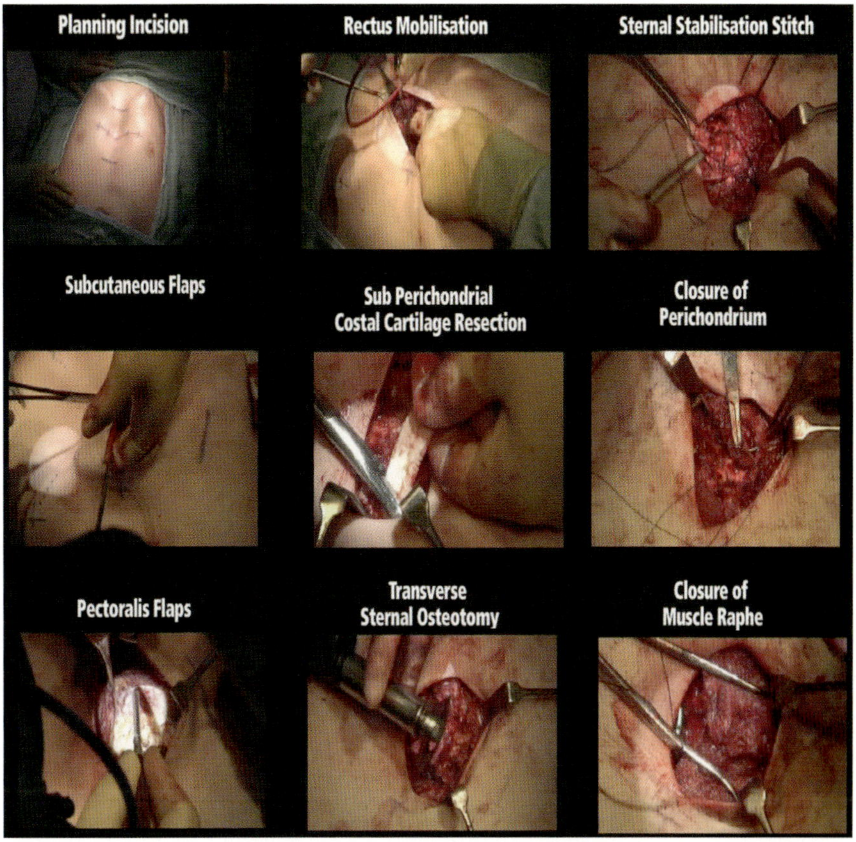

Fig. 17.3 Operative images demonstrating the modified Ravitch procedure

after surgery. They must understand what to expect before and after surgery, and a clear list of dos and don'ts after surgery is valuable in facilitating a complication-free patient journey.

17.4 Modified Ravitch Repair

Careful planning of the incision and extent of resection is required before starting the procedure (Fig. 17.4). The principle of the surgery is to dissect tissues to reach the desired position of the chest wall in a tension-free manner. Placing a transverse incision (our preference) in the midpoint cephalocaudad of the extent of cartilage excision facilitates exposure and limits the size of the incision. This may not always be at the deepest point of the PE.

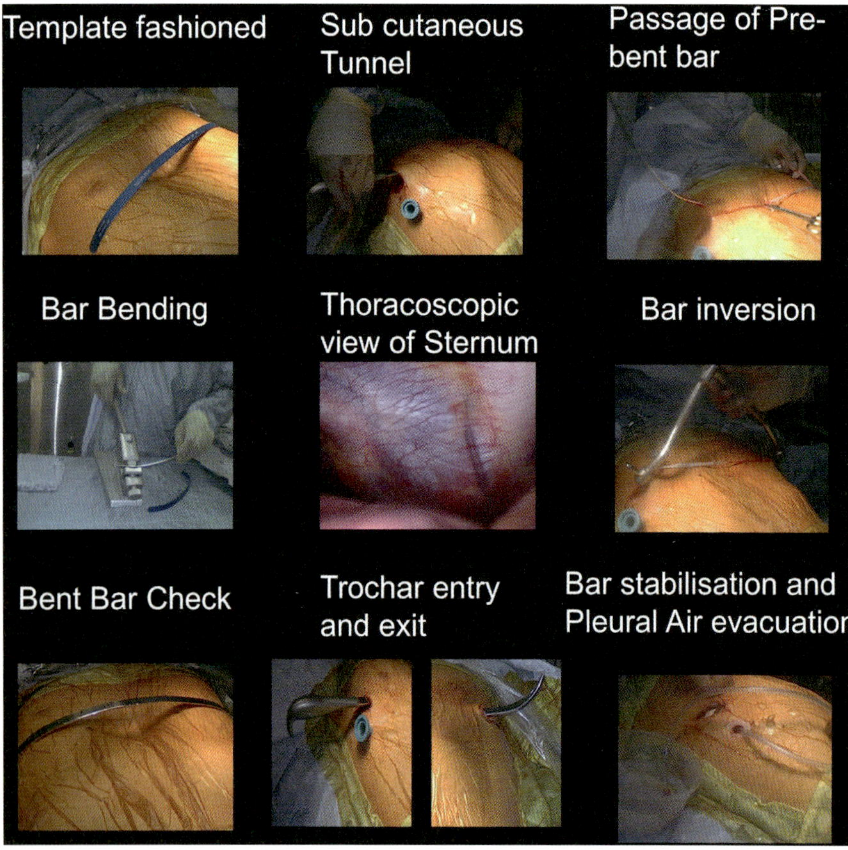

Fig. 17.4 Operative images demonstrating the Nuss procedure

A 6–8 cm transverse skin incision is made, and elevation of subcutaneous and then pectoralis and rectus muscle flaps to the extent of the deformity is performed. It's important when raising these flaps in a thin individual not to button hole the skin nor extend dissection under the nipple which can lead to denervation. The muscle flaps are elevated until they can oppose to the midline without excessive tension. Bilateral subperichondrial resection of deformed cartilages, transverse sternal osteotomy and xiphisternum excision if required are performed as required to allow the sternum to return to a 'neutral' or desired position. Minimal cartilage excision (1–3 cm) adjacent to the sternum followed by multiple chondro-/osteotomies more laterally allow the shape of the chest to be achieved from the outset with good stability rather than excision of larger sections of cartilage which then rely on regrowth of cartilage. This technique can also be used to deal with costal flaring. Anecdotally with this technique, the drainage of serosanguinous fluid is diminished, and it aids faster recovery and discharge from hospital. Scoring the perichondrium at the site of excision in a wide 'H' allows the perichondrium to be pushed off the underlying cartilage. Getting in the right plane results in a relatively bloodless dissection. Going round the back of the cartilage can be precarious as damage to the internal mammary artery or worse the heart may occur if the elevator slips. Thus the technique is always to ensure the direction of pressure, and dissection is away from the deeper structures, i.e. outwards. Once dissection round the back of either the lower or upper edge is done, lifting up with the elevator whilst dissecting the other side with a second elevator facilitates dissection. Once around the cartilage in a subperichondrial plane, this can be extended along its length by using a 'Doyen' costal elevator and applying lateral traction which strips away the perichondrium. It is best to leave all cartilages in situ and complete the dissection as once a cartilage is removed the dissection of the next cartilage is impaired by the lack of resistance provided by the surrounding cartilages. Once all dissected the medial ends are released with either lateral traction with a Doyen costal elevator or dislocated anteriorly at the junction with sternum either with sharp or blunt dissection. At this point the 'fingers of cartilage' overly the sternum. The shortening of these should be done following the osteotomy and repositioning of the sternum.

The osteotomy of the anterior table of the sternum is performed at the point that the sternum starts to dip down and the cartilages below this point are the ones excised. Thus the importance of planning before the skin incision is made where this point is going to be. The idea is to allow the sternum distally to pivot and thus attain the desired position with minimal substernal dissection. Wedge excision osteotomy is used to elevate the distal sternum in cases of excavatum. In cases where there is sternal torsion, more bone is removed from the side which dips more. The sternum is then fixed in the desired 'neutral position'. Our preferred options are to do this with either heavy absorbable sutures in symmetric cases or in more complex or asymmetric cases with a small titanium 'H' sternal plate.

With the first technique, two heavy absorbable sutures (looped '1' polydioxanone (PDS)) are placed across the osteotomy to hold the sternum in place. Slight asymmetric tilt in the sternum can also be corrected by the differential positioning of the two sternal tables at each end of the osteotomy by these two sutures. An additional heavy suture is placed through the distal body of the neutrally placed sternum and later secured to the overlying pectus muscle raphe for additional stability.

Self-tapping screw with the 'H' plate makes insertion easy requiring little additional equipment. The plate can be bent to the desired position to correct for the tilt. Size of screws is determined by a depth gauge. Attachments of the perichondrium and other soft tissue tethering the sternum are divided.

At this point the pre-dissected cartilages are shortened to allow reattachment to the sternum with heavy absorbable sutures. Always removing a little more than you think is required so that the cartilages once re-approximated to the sternum are under slight tension. But prior to this further lateral osteochondrotomies/osteotomies are made to recontour the rib cage. Usually these are made at the angle where the rib suddenly bends. Sometimes multiple osteochondrotomies are required to straighten the rib. The perichondrium is re-approximated where possible. In this 'minimal cartilage' excision technique, the rib cage contour is intact, and minimal regrowth is required to remodel the shape of the chest as compared to a traditional Ravitch operation.

Tip

The pectoralis and rectus muscles are re-apposed in a midline 'Mercedes' sign raphe. Thus the importance of freeing up enough of the muscle in the initial dissection to allow a tension free apposition. At this stage, the body of the sternum is fixed to this raphe using the previously placed suture. Submuscular and subcutaneous drains are placed to allow adequate drainage of blood. The skin may look rather bruised after all the dissection, but this settles down within a few weeks. The midline ridge of the opposed pectus muscles is also noted by patients which again flattens over a few months.

Previously we have used metal bars to support the repair, but fracture and displacement led us away from this technique. Others have used slings of mesh or graft to support the repair.

17.5 Nuss Operation

Our preference is to use a pre-bent bar which is based on the CT scan dimensions. These nowadays do not cost any more than the bars which are bent at the time of surgery, and they require less readjustment once 'inserted'. In patients with nickel allergy, a prebent titanium bar should be used.

There are three commonly used patient positions: supine with either both arms abducted at the shoulders to approximately 70°, taking care to protect the patient from brachial plexus injury; elevating the torso and extending the arms posteriorly, but this can lead to overextension of the chest during the surgery; or finally flexing the left shoulder and elbow anteriorly and holding it above the head, but there are anecdotal reports of brachial plexus injury with this position too. Our preference is for the first position.

Thoracoscopy is used to guide bar placement usually from the right side. In patients with severe PE, it may be necessary to use bilateral thoracoscopy because the heart is displaced to the left, which impedes visibility from the right. Care must be taken during insertion because of the displaced heart. Generally the scope is inserted one space below the incision, and a 30° scope is preferred as it allows for looking 'round the corner'. It can also be inserted through the incision or even superior to the incision site. Following entering the pleural cavity with a blunt small clip to induce a pneumothorax, we direct the trocar insertion in a superior direction to avoid the diaphragm. Carbon dioxide (CO2) insufflation pressure is useful in collapsing the lung and facilitating mediastinal dissection. Pressures are kept low between 5 and 6 mmHg. Leakage increases once the trocar and then bar are inserted thus higher flow rates may be required at this time.

The bar is usually sited at the deepest portion of the pectus unless this is inferior to the body of the sternum. A bar placed at this point will not be seated below the bone (just xiphisternum) and on removal is associated with high recurrence rates. Two small lateral thoracic incisions at the anterior axillary line provide good access to the thoracostomy entry and exit sites. Incisions that run parallel to the ribs require the least amount of subcutaneous dissection and are less likely to cause a keloid reaction. Vertical incisions in the mid or posterior axillary lines can give poor access to the anterior chest wall and tend to cause keloid formation. The exact position usually at the deepest portion of the pectus is guided by placing the pre-bent bar at the site of insertion and centering the incision 1 cm distal to the tip of the bar to compensate for the internal rather than external positioning. Equally if not using a pre-bent, the site of skin incision is marked, and a malleable guide is downsized 2 cm and fashioned to the desired contour of the chest then used as a template to bend the bar using the table top bar bender. It is important to slightly overcorrect the deformity to prevent buckling of the anterior chest wall and to decrease the risk of recurrence. The bar should therefore be semicircular with only a 2- to 4-cm flat section in the middle to support the sternum. If the deepest point of the deformity is inferior to the body of the sternum, two bars may be required: one under the sternum and the other under the deepest point of the depression. When placing two or more bars, making a separate incision for each bar facilitates bar stabilisation and bar removal after 3 years. Two bars may also be used in older patients who have less compliant chests with wide-type defects to achieve a better cosmetic result. In mature female patients, the incisions should be placed in the inframammary crease between the 6- and 9-o'clock positions, and this gives an excellent cosmetic result.

A subcutaneous pocket 360° around the incision is made to make room to seat the stabiliser, and this is followed by a subcutaneous or submuscular tunnel slightly wider than the bar heading to the sternum to the point of entry into the chest and slightly beyond, thereby preventing tethering of the skin once the bar is inserted. It's important to ensure that the dissection does not button hole the skin and use of long thin retractor can be useful. If the correct plane is followed, there should be minimal bleeding. The thoracic entry and exit sites are just medial to the pectoral ridge externally and so is close to the sternum to prevent disruption of the intercostal muscles. Three trocar or introducer sizes are usually available for adults; the medium or larger size is appropriate. The trocar is inserted through the tunnel with the curve pointing downwards, and this is pushed through into the pleural cavity under direct thoracosopic vision. The trocar is flipped so that the tip is now pointing up to the sternum. The trocar tip should always be kept in view during the tunnelling, and in a pawing action is passed from right to left chest cavity hugging the sternum to the point of exit of the bar. The trocar tip is pushed or delivered up through intercostals and then is pushed through the subcutaneous tunnel to appear through the contralateral skin incision. During this whole process, it will be noted how the sternum has been lifted upwards. Thus the trocar is used to dissect the plane between the sternum and pericardium under direct vision and is exteriorised via the left incision. When the trocar is in position across the mediastinum, it is lifted numerous times in an anterior direction gently lifting the patient's torso off the operating table taking care not to hyperextend the neck. Pulling the sternum and anterior chest wall out of their depressed position loosening up the ligaments helps reduces pressure on bar and risk of displacement. A nylon tape is tied to the trocar end and passed to the other side of the chest as the trocar is withdrawn. The tape is used to guide the inverted pre-bent bar (with the convexity facing posteriorly) through the chest. The inverted bar is then turned 180° (with the convexity now facing anteriorly) to push the sternum forward. The bar should sit snugly on chest. If there is a wide gap, the bar will have to be flipped back and the bar ends bent with a hand bar bender until the desired position is achieved. A second bar should be inserted if the repair is suboptimal after insertion of the first bar. In patients with asymmetric deformities, an asymmetrically placed bar may give more lift on the side of the asymmetric deformity. The correction always looks better whilst the patient is lying flat on the operating table than it does when the patient resumes normal posture because the normal thoracic lordosis is eliminated on the operating table. To prevent the bar from rotating, it may be held in place on one or both sides with a stabilising plate, which is fixed to the surrounding soft tissues with sutures. Some surgeons advocate using sutures around the ribs, with either stainless steel wire or heavy nonabsorbable material placed under thoracoscopic guidance. In our practice we have not had any need for this additional step if both ends of the bar are stabilised. Air from the pleural cavity is expelled from the thoracoscopy incision prior to extubation.

Tip

Failed previous repairs may be amenable to successful retreatment; patient expectation of the patients should be managed appropriately as cosmetic result is far less predictable. Rigidity of the chest following Ravitch is a poor prognostic indicator. Generally in patients with previous Ravitch repair with mobile chest, Nuss repair is a good option. Whilst in redo Nuss, one may encounter adhesions that preclude or make surgery dangerous. Patients should be warned of this possibility.

The pain following Nuss surgery is more severe that Ravitch thus patients usually receive an epidural and thus should be warned of the very low risk of paralysis. Though pre-emptive analgesia is desirable, we have not found it practical as patients proceed directly to the operating room from an open admission area on the day of surgery. Following surgery, paracetamol/acetaminophen, non-steroidal anti-inflammatory analgesics with proton pump inhibitor cover, low-dose benzodiazepines for muscle relaxation and anxiolysis are all prescribed prophylactically. On the second post-operative day, long-acting morphine oral agents are commenced and the epidural discontinued on the morning of the third post-operative day. Antibiotics are administered preoperatively at the time of induction of anaesthesia and continued for 5 days post-operatively to reduce the risk of wound and prosthesis-related infection. Following surgery patients are encouraged to mobilise early after surgery and undergo a rigorous physiotherapy regime. Certain activities are restricted, for example, pulling yourself out of the bed using the upper limbs. Patients are restricted from participating in severe physical activities for 6 weeks, at which time they may recommence aerobic activities, and competitive non-contact sports may be resumed at 3 months post repair and contact usually at 6 months.

Early post-operative complications include, pneumothorax requiring chest tube, surgical site infection (SSI), pneumonia, haemothorax, pericarditis, pleural effusion (requiring drainage), temporary paralysis, cardiac perforation in the case of Nuss and of course death.

SSI requires vigorous treatment consisting of wound drainage, cultures and appropriate intravenous antibiotics, followed by long-term oral antibiotics. Usually the bar does not have to be removed until planned with this approach.

Pericarditis with Nuss may be related to undiagnosed nickel allergy and presents with persistent central chest pain, malaise, lethargy, and a pericardial friction rub. The presence of echocardiographically confirmed pericardial fluid may warrant a short course of prednisone. If symptoms recur a longer course of steroids and finally replacement of the bar with a titanium bar may be required after confirmation of aetiology by nickel allergy testing. Nickel allergy may also present late with erythema of the anterior chest wall or inflammation and drainage at the incision sites. Cardiac perforation is a potential risk and can be reduced by the diligent use of thoracoscopy, if necessary bilaterally and preoperative planning by reviewing of position of the heart in relation to sternum especially in patients with severe asymmetry and/or depressions. In these cases placement of bar 1 or 2 intercostal spaces superior to the deepest point and leaving the introducer in place to keep the sternum elevated whilst creating the second tunnel may minimise the risk of injury.

Tip

In severe cases for Nuss, we routinely elevate the sternum. There are several techniques described to do this, and our preference is the Johnson et al. technique that describes the use of a scope in the right hemithorax as a subxiphoid incision is made and a plane between the pericardium and posterior sternum is created using digital dissection under vision of the thoracoscope. Using the finger, a retractor such as a Langenbeck is inserted beneath the sternum, and it is lifted creating a gap between the pericardium and sternum which improves visibility and safety. Other techniques include placement along both subcutaneous tunnels to the hinge point of a Langenbeck retractor which are then lifted; the use of the vacuum bell device, without its hand pump and directly connected to a wall vacuum source; and the crane technique, elevating the depressed sternum, by means of wire sutures threaded through the sternum to a retracting system mounted over the operating table.

Bar displacement if minor less than 20° displaced can be observed. Displacement immediately after surgery, severe or progressing, may require surgical revision. Overcorrection resulting in pectus carinatum is rare but can occur after correction of severe asymmetric defects and in patients with Marfan syndrome and may be treated with earlier bar removal and/or external brace. Persistent pain may be caused by bar displacement, stabiliser dislocation, bar being too tight or too long, sternal or rib erosion, infection or allergy. An anterior and lateral chest radiograph, full blood cell count, ESR, CRP level and nickel allergy testing will identify the cause and allow appropriate treatment.

There is a trend to the use of shorter bars and two stabilisers in a more medial position to reduce the risk of complications. Our experience is limited in this, but we have not found a huge advantage in these modifications.

Systematic review and meta-analysis of 13 comparative studies suggest no difference in total complication rate between Nuss and Ravitch procedures in the Pediatric populations, but in the adult subgroup, the Ravitch group experienced significantly fewer complications, for both overall and early complications, but this subgroup was very small. In the adult subgroups, reoperations were significantly higher in Nuss patients compared to Ravitch patients. However in our own series spanning 20 years, we did not find this perhaps because of shorter follow-up with Nuss technique. We did demonstrate that if a patient developed an immediate post-operative complication, they had a significantly increased chance of late recurrence.

Recommended Reading

1. Brochhausen C, Turial S, Muller FKP, Schmitt VH, Coerdt W, Wihlm J-M, Schier F, Kirkpatrick CJ. Pectus excavatum: history, hypotheses and treatment options. Interact Cardiovasc Thorac Surg. 2012;14:801–6.
2. Jayaramakrishnan K, Wotton R, Bradley A, Naidu B. Does repair of pectus excavatum improve cardiopulmonary function? Interact Cardiovasc Thorac Surg. 2013;16:865–71.
3. Kelly RE. Pectus excavatum: historical background, clinical picture, preoperative evaluation and criteria for operation. Semin Pediatr Surg. 2008;17:181–93.
4. Nuss D, Kelly RE, Croitoru DP, Katz ME. A 10-year review of minimally invasive technique for the correction of pectus excavatum. J Pediatr Surg. 1998;33:545–52.
5. Nuss D, Kelly RE. Indications and technique of Nuss procedure for pectus excavatum. Thorac Surg Clin. 2010;20:583–97.
6. Pilegaard HK, Licht PB. Routine use of minimally invasive surgery for pectus excavatum in adults. Ann Thorac Surg. 2008;86:952–7.
7. Ravitch MM. The operative treatment of pectus excavatum. Ann Surg. 1949;129:429–44.
8. Robicsek F, Watts LT. Pectus carinatum. Thorac Surg Clin. 2010;20:563–74.
9. Kanagaratnam A, Phan S, Tchantchaleishvili V, Phan K. Ravitch versus Nuss procedure for pectus excavatum: systematic review and meta-analysis. Ann Cardiothorac Surg. 2016;5(5):409–21. Review.
10. Tikka T, Kalkat MS, Bishay E, Steyn RS, Rajesh PB, Naidu B. A 20-year review of pectus surgery: an analysis of factors predictive of recurrence and outcomes. Interact Cardiovasc Thorac Surg. 2016;23(6):908–13. Epub 11 Aug 2016.

Sternal Cleft

18

Dakshesh Parikh

Abstract

Sternal cleft is a rare congenital chest wall anomaly as a result of failure of fusion of the sternum in the midline. Types of sternal defects described are complete or partial depending on the degrees of separation. Diagnosis is clinical with an obvious visible anterior chest wall defect sometimes associated with paradoxical respiration. Investigations are essential to rule out associated anomalies. Early neonatal surgery approximating the sternal halves is feasible due to their compliant chest wall and can result in good outcome in some selected cases without causing any cardiovascular and respiratory compromise. Late presentations of this anomaly require careful surgical planning. A number of innovative sternal cleft reconstruction options are available to bridge the defect that may be selected depending on the size/width of defect and without causing cardiorespiratory compromise.

Keywords

Complete sternal cleft · Partial sternal cleft · Pentalogy of Cantrell · Sternal reconstruction · Sliding chondrotomy

18.1 Introduction

Sternal clefts are a rare congenital anomaly where the fusion of the two sternal halves during sixth to tenth week of gestation does not come together leaving either a complete or partial defect [1, 2]. In partial clefts either the upper or lower half of

D. Parikh, MBBS, MS, FRCS (Ped.), MD
Department of Pediatric Surgery, Birmingham Women's and Children's Hospital NHS FT, Birmingham, UK
e-mail: dakshesh.parikh@nhs.net

D. Parikh, P.B. Rajesh (eds.), *Tips and Tricks in Thoracic Surgery*,
https://doi.org/10.1007/978-1-4471-7355-7_18

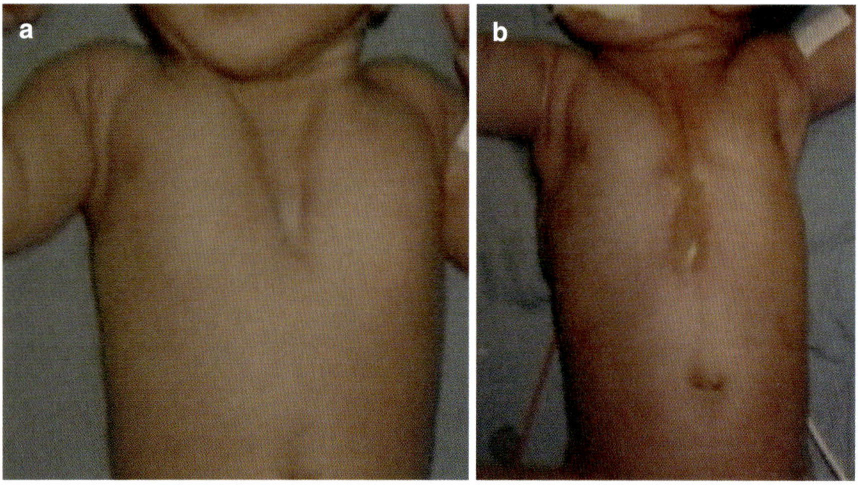

Fig. 18.1 (**a**) Superior sternal cleft in an infant. (**b**) Appearance following primary repair in the same infant

the sternum does not come together in the midline leaving the corresponding portions of the heart and great vessels exposed under the skin [3, 4]. Superior sternal clefts are common affecting the manubrium and upper sternum creating either a broad "U-" or narrow "V-" shaped defect (Fig 18.1a) [5]. Isolated inferior sternal cleft is less common and is generally associated with other developmental abnormalities such as ectopia cordis, combinations of defects that occur in the pentalogy of Cantrell, omphalocele, intracardiac defects and anterior diaphragmatic hernia [5, 6] (Fig. 18.2). In contrast, complete sternal cleft is very rare with parallel sternal bars and diversification of the rectus abdominis muscle [5] (Fig. 18.3). Rarely a small defect with a missing sternebrae is also described. Sternal clefts are also associated with craniofacial haemangiomas.

The reconstructive surgery is carried out in order to protect the mediastinal vital organs from injury and to counteract paradoxical ineffectual respiratory movements that may be responsible for breathlessness on exercise, recurrent chest infections and cyanotic episodes and for cosmetic reasons.

18.2 Technical Tips and Tricks

18.2.1 Preoperative Assessment

- A through clinical examination and appropriate investigations to rule out associated anomalies (up to 72% as per published reports) should be carried out [7]. The specific investigations in order to exclude cardiac anomalies, non-cutaneous visceral haemangiomas, ocular and posterior fossa abnormalities and vascular dysplasias of the vertebrobasilar systems should be performed as some anomalies may require earlier attention than the repair of the sternal cleft [4, 7]. Radiological investigations such as chest CT scan with intravenous contrast and 3D recon-

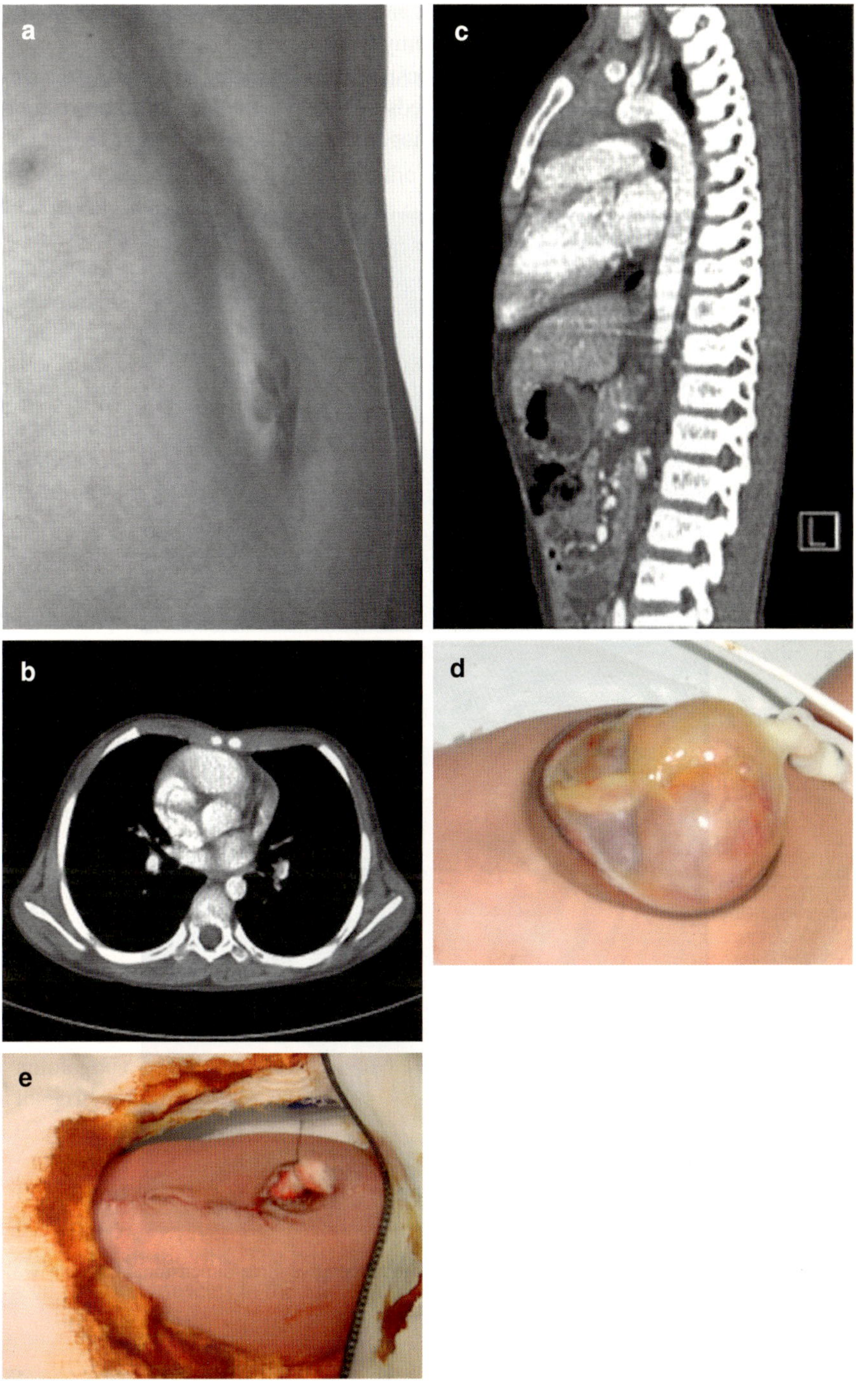

Fig. 18.2 (**a**) Inferior sternal cleft in an older child with a previously repaired exomphalos. (**b**) Axial CT scan in the same child demonstrating separation of the inferior sternal bars. (**c**) Sagittal CT scan in the same child demonstrating the inferior sternal bony defect. (**d**) Inferior sternal cleft associated with exomphalos major in a neonate. (**e**) Appearance following primary repair in the same neonate

Anterior Mediastinal Tumours

19

Mohammed Abdel Aziz and Pala B. Rajesh

Abstract

The mediastinum contains a number of organs and structures of various origins, and thus it can be the host of many pathologies and tumours including benign and malignant. Managing a patient with mediastinal tumour must begin with multidisciplinary approach. Treating mediastinal tumours varies between watchful waiting, surgery, chemotherapy, radiotherapy, hormonal therapy and a combination of all these modalities, and thus accurate diagnosis is crucial in management. Knowledge of correlation between patient demographics and type of tumours, commonest tumours in various compartments of the mediastinum, biochemistry testing in relation to certain tumours and radiological characteristics of the mediastinal tumours can provide focused examination and increase the yield of accurate diagnosis.

In this chapter, we will discuss the various sections and divisions of the mediastinum as well as the most common primary tumours within each division. We will examine the common sites, clinical presentation, radiological feature and management of the common mediastinal tumours. This chapter will provide various tips in diagnosing and tricks in the surgical resection of these tumours.

Keywords

Mediastinum · Tumours · Thymoma · Mediastinal cyst · Pericardial cyst · Germ cell tumour · Teratoma · Seminomatous and nonseminomatous tumours · Lymphoma · Benign hamartomatous malformations · Neurogenic tumours · Surgery · VATS resection

M.A. Aziz, M.B., ChB., F.R.C.S. CTh. • P.B. Rajesh, FRCS Ed (CTh), FRCS Eng, FETCS (✉)
Regional Department of Thoracic Surgery, Birmingham Heartlands Hospital, Birmingham, UK

D. Parikh, P.B. Rajesh (eds.), *Tips and Tricks in Thoracic Surgery*,
https://doi.org/10.1007/978-1-4471-7355-7_19

19.1 Introduction

The mediastinum refers to the space and structures within the thorax bounded by the thoracic inlet superiorly, the diaphragm inferiorly, the sternum anteriorly, the spine posteriorly and the pleural spaces bilaterally. There are my classifications and division systems of the mediastinum, the commonest of which divides the mediastinum to three compartments: the anterior mediastinum governs the space behind the sternum to the anterior pericardium; the middle mediastinum or visceral compartment comprises the space and structures between the anterior surface of the pericardium and posterior aspect of the pericardium, tracheal bifurcation and pulmonary vessels; and the posterior mediastinum refers to the paravertebral sulcus and is the space along the thoracic vertebrae [1].

Knowing the structures in each compartment can increase the diagnostic yield based on the origin of the tumours. The anterior mediastinum contains the thymus, fat and lymph nodes. The middle mediastinum contains the heart, pericardium, ascending aorta, brachiocephalic vessels, main pulmonary vasculature, trachea and main bronchi. The posterior mediastinum contains the oesophagus, descending thoracic aorta, autonomic ganglia and nerves, azygous vein and lymphatic duct [2].

The distribution of tumours within the mediastinum varies amongst different age groups and amongst different compartments of the mediastinum. The location of the tumour within the mediastinum is important when narrowing the diagnosis (Table 19.1).

TIP: Thymic tumours, neurogenic tumours and cystic masses account for 60% of all tumours within the mediastinum, while lymphomas, germ cell tumours and granulomatous disease account for 30% of all tumours [2].

TIP: Based on the distribution of common tumours, the majority of anterior mediastinal tumours will be thymic in origin, middle mediastinum will be cystic in nature and neurogenic in the posterior mediastinum.

Symptoms from mediastinal tumours can be broadly classified into localised or systemic. Local symptoms are those related to mass effect or invasion of the tumour into surrounding structures, and this group includes cough, dyspnoea, diaphragmatic paralysis, Horner's syndrome and dysphagia. Systemic symptoms are related to hormones, cytokines and autoimmune disease associated with the mediastinal

Table 19.1 Differential diagnosis of mediastinal mass according to location [12]

Anterior	Middle	Posterior
Thymoma	Lymphoma	Neurogenic tumour
Teratoma, seminoma	Bronchogenic cyst	Bronchogenic cyst
Lymphoma	Pericardial cyst	Diaphragmatic hernia
Parathyroid adenoma	Metastatic cyst	Meningocele
Goitre	Systemic granuloma	Paravertebral abscess
Lipoma		Enteric cyst
Lymphangioma		
Aortic aneurysm		

tumours such as symptoms of hypercalcaemia, myasthenia gravis and red cell aplasia.

19.2 Anterior Mediastinal Tumours

19.2.1 Thymoma

Thymoma is the most common tumour in the anterior mediastinum affecting men and women equally [3]. The most common age group affected by this tumour is over 40 years old, and two thirds of patients are asymptomatic and diagnosed as incidental findings on radiological investigations. Localised symptoms usually include cough, dyspnoea and chest pain.

Thymoma is associated with various systemic diseases including myasthenia gravis, red cell aplasia, hypogammaglobulinaemia and systemic lupus erythematosis [1]. Myasthenia gravis is the most common systemic disease associated with thymoma. Thirty to 50% of patients with thymoma have myasthenia gravis, and 15% of patients with myasthenia gravis have thymoma. Ten and 1% of patients with thymoma have hypogammaglobulinaemia and pure red blood cell aplasia, respectively.

19.2.2 Diagnosis

Although thymic tumours can exhibit various radiological characteristics including the presence of calcification or necrosis, the thymic tumour commonly appears to be well defined, capsulated and lobulated within the superior aspect of the anterior mediastinum arising from one of the thymic lobes (Fig. 19.1). If associated with

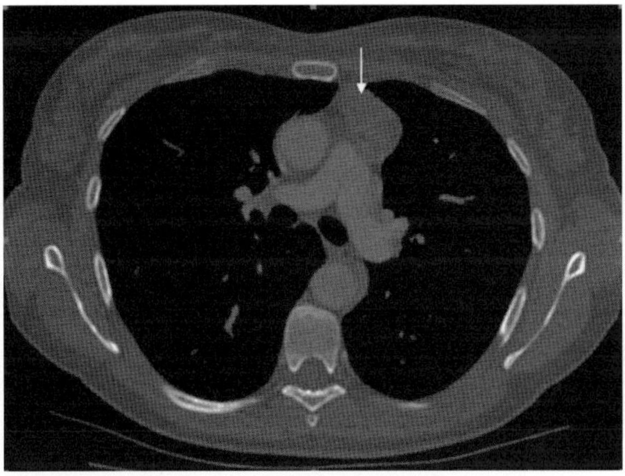

Fig. 19.1 The common appearance of thymic tumour on CT scan (arrow)

myasthenia gravis, biochemical serum testing will reveal high levels of anti-acetylcholine receptor antibody [2].

In the presence of atypical radiological findings especially with features of other anterior mediastinal tumours such as heterogeneity within the tumour or calcification and presence of local lymphadenopathy, surgical or fine needle biopsy is crucial to confirm the diagnosis.

19.2.3 Treatment

Surgery is the mainstay for treating this neoplasm, and several aspects have been identified to influence the prognosis and survival such as completeness of resection and stage of the disease at operation [4]. Neoadjuvant chemotherapy should be considered in patients with advanced thymoma [1, 5].

The association between thymic tumours and myasthenia gravis led to the role of thymectomy in the management of myasthenia gravis.

TIP (the role of thirds): When consenting patients with myasthenia gravis undergoing total thymectomy, one third of patients will be cured, one third will have reduction in their symptoms and one third will not experience any change in their symptoms.

19.2.4 Surgical Technique

Surgical approach to thymectomy can vary based on the size, stage of the tumour and presence of invasion to surrounding organs and structures. Median sternotomy is the most common approach and has the advantage of providing clear surgical view. The thymic tissue, surrounding capsule and any mediastinal fat or structure involved should be removed with an en bloc resection (Fig. 19.2).

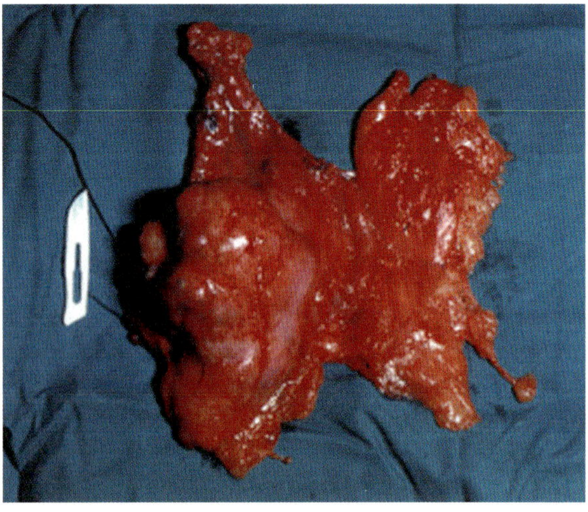

Fig. 19.2 Complete resection of the thymus including the superior and inferior horns. *RSH* right superior horn, *LSH* left superior horn, *RIH* right inferior horn, *LIH* left inferior horn

TRICK: The superior horns can be completely removed at their origin with the aid of traction of the body of the thymus distally towards the feet, and the use of small 'peanut' swab on Roberts forceps and soft tissue attachment of the superior horns can be gently teased away. It is important to securely ligate thymic vein/veins draining into brachiocephalic vein and arterial supply usually from inferior thyroidal or from subclavian artery. Recurrence can be avoided by carefully skeletonising the pericardial fat and making sure the superior horns into the neck is excised.

TRICK: In bulky tumours where visualisation of the phrenic nerve can be challenging, trace it distally near the diaphragm and follow its track upwards towards the tumour.

19.2.5 Germ Cell Tumours (GCTs)

Tumours derived from germ cells that failed to migrate during early embryonic life. GCTs present in early adulthood, and the anterior mediastinum is the most common extragonadal site for these tumours. They represent 10–15% of anterior mediastinal tumours [1–3].

GCTs can be benign or malignant and broadly divided into three subgroups: benign teratoma, seminoma and embryonal tumours (yolk sac carcinoma, choriocarcinoma, teratocarcinoma). Men and women are affected equally; however, over 90% of malignant GCTs affect men than women [6].

19.2.6 Diagnosis

The majority of patients with benign GCTs are asymptomatic, and tumours are found incidentally on radiological testing. Symptoms are common in patients with malignant GCTs and include dyspnoea, bronchial spasm and cough. The most common CT finding is well-circumscribed tumour within the anterior mediastinum in young adult, which is heterogeneous in nature and often contains calcification [1, 6].

TIP: These tumours commonly produce serological markers such as α-Feto proteins (AFP), human chorionic gonadotropin (HCG) and lactate dehydrogenase (LDH) and should be part of preoperative biochemistry investigations in young adults presenting with mediastinal tumour [3].

TIP: Gonadal external examination should be considered in young adults with CT findings of anterior mediastinal tumour suspicious of GCTs.

19.2.7 Mediastinal Teratoma

Teratoma is a benign tumour and is the most common (60–70%) of all mediastinal GCTs. It occurs most frequently in children and young adults and the majority are asymptomatic. Some tumours attempt organ transformation and can contain the teeth, skin, hair, pancreatic tissue, and cartilage/bone (Fig. 19.3). Complete excision

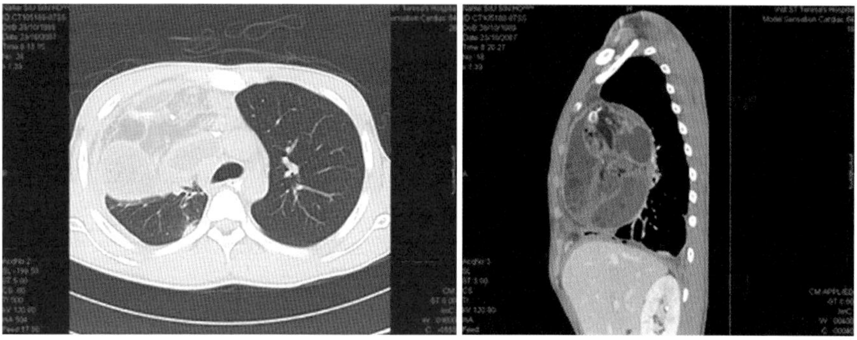

Fig. 19.3 CT scan of mediastinal teratoma; complex heterogeneous tumour with cystic and solid areas

is the treatment of choice for these tumours, but as all GCTs within the mediastinum, they are usually large and adherent to surrounding organs [2, 6].

TIP: Trichoptysis is a pathognomonic sign for teratoma and indicates attempt of organ transformation of the tumour.

19.2.8 Seminomatous and Nonseminomatous Tumours

Malignant germ cell tumours are much more common in males and usually symptomatic. The treatment of seminomatous or nonseminomatous tumour within the anterior mediastinum differs, and hence accurate diagnosis is crucial. As testicular seminomas, mediastinal seminomas are extremely sensitive to radiotherapy and are the mainstay of treating these tumours as compared to chemotherapy with nonseminomatous tumours especially that both of these malignant tumours are usually large and adherent to surrounding vital structures within the mediastinum [1, 2, 6].

TIP: The presence of elevated levels of α-feto proteins excludes the diagnosis of pure seminomas.

19.2.9 Surgical Technique

Surgery is reserved for benign teratoma and residual seminomatous and nonseminomatous tumours post radiotherapy and chemotherapy, respectively. Teratomas are usually quite large and invade the surrounding structures at the time of presentation. Thoracosternotomy and pericardiectomy may be necessary for complete excision of the tumour.

19.2.10 Mediastinal Lymphoma

Lymphomas contribute to 15% of all mediastinal tumours, only 10% of which are primary lymphomas affecting the mediastinum and not part of systemic disease [3, 7].

Nodular sclerosing Hodgkin's lymphoma (HL), primary B-cell lymphoma and lymphoblastic lymphoma are the most common histological types affecting the anterior mediastinum. It usually occurs over the age of 50 years, although HL has a bimodal distribution and also occurs in early adulthood [3].

19.2.11 Diagnosis and Treatment

The majority of patients are symptomatic and exhibit constitutional symptoms (fever, lethargy, night sweats and weight loss) and symptoms of local invasion such as chest pain, cough and dyspnoea.

Radiologically on CT scan, the tumour usually represents soft tissue density or smooth or lobular well-demarcated mass that may have cystic/low-density areas [8].

TIP: The presence of lymphadenopathy and mediastinal mass should prompt the diagnosis of mediastinal lymphoma.

Chemotherapy and radiotherapy are the treatment of choice for mediastinal lymphoma. The use of chemotherapy or radiotherapy depends on the histological subtype and stage of the disease. Early stage (I–II) of HL with bulky tumour is treated with chemotherapy followed by radiotherapy but chemotherapy alone to later stages of HL (stages III–IV).

19.3 Middle Mediastinal Tumours

19.3.1 Mediastinal Cysts

Mediastinal cysts represent 12–18% of all mediastinal masses, and 48% of which are located within the middle mediastinum [9], usually present in the third to fourth decade of life. They are usually congenital in origin and result from abnormal budding or division of the foregut during development. They are referred to based on their origin as bronchogenic cyst, oesophageal cyst and gastroenteric cyst (alimentary) [9, 10].

19.3.2 Diagnosis

Thirty-six to 40% of mediastinal cysts are symptomatic. Symptoms usually have gradual onset and develop with the enlargement of the lesion. Symptoms usually are retrosternal chest pain, shortness of breath, cough and sepsis if the cyst becomes infected [9, 11].

The majority of mediastinal cyst subtypes have the same radiological features being smooth oval in shape containing homogenous fluid attenuation with no evidence of infiltration to adjacent structures.

TIP: Symptoms of gastroenteric cysts may have sudden change in characteristics followed with symptoms of severe inflammatory reaction as they are at higher risk of rupture and haemorrhage when containing functional gastric or pancreatic mucosa.

TIP: Radiological location of the cyst may indicate the aetiology and subtype. Seventy percent of bronchogenic cyst is located usually near the carina and paratracheal region, majority of duplication cyst near the oesophagus, and majority of pericardial cyst located within the cardiophrenic space [11].

19.3.3 Treatment

Surgical approach to mediastinal cysts may vary based on the size and location of the cyst. Surgical approach includes posterior-lateral thoracotomy, axillary thoracotomy or video-assisted thoracoscopic procedure. The aim is to completely excise the cyst however in certain difficult circumstances when the mass is adherent to critical structures within the mediastinum; decision to de-roof the cavity and drain it may be acceptable.

19.3.4 Bronchogenic Cyst

Bronchogenic cyst is the result from abnormal budding of the laryngotracheal tree. It is lined with epithelial cells representing its origin (ciliated columnar epithelium) and contains cartilaginous plates and mucus glands [1, 10, 11]. This subtype represents 60% of all mediastinal cysts and most commonly presents within the middle mediastinum (Fig. 19.4).

TIP: The presence of air is strong indicative of communication between the cyst and tracheobronchial tree. Careful bronchoscopy must be undertaken prior to surgery to assess its proximity to central structure and for surgical planning.

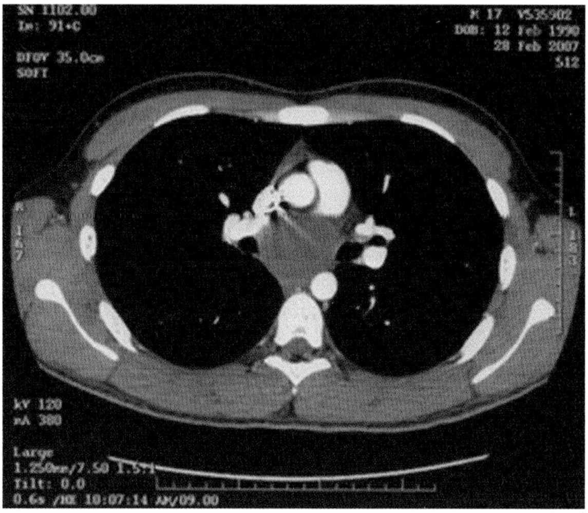

Fig. 19.4 Bronchogenic cyst within the middle mediastinum

19.3.5 Gastroenteric Cyst

Usually lined with epithelium from the alimentary tract (squamous, columnar, gastric or small intestinal epithelium), it accounts for 5–10% of mediastinal cysts. The majority are located centrally and adjacent to the oesophagus (duplication cysts), and with this relation, symptoms of dysphagia may be present with large-sized cysts [10].

19.3.6 Pericardial Cyst

These types of cysts are not related to abnormalities of the foregut. Although the majority of pericardial cysts are considered to be congenital in origin due to abnormal fusion of the pericardial recess during development, they can also be acquired. The majority of pericardial cysts are asymptomatic, and surgical intervention is not indicated unless symptoms develop that may include cardiac compression. They commonly present in the fourth to fifth decade of life [3, 10].

TIP: Central well-demarcated cyst within the right cardiophrenic angle is strongly indicative of pericardial cyst.

References

1. Sellke FW, de Nido PJ, Swanson SJ. Sabiston & Spencer surgery of the chest, vol. I. Amsterdam: Elsevier; 2010.
2. Strollo DC, Rosado de Christenson ML, Jett JR. Primary mediastinal tumors. Part 1: tumors of the anterior mediastinum. Chest. 1997;112(2):511–22.
3. Duwe BV, Sterman DH, Musani AI. Tumors of the mediastinum. Chest. 2005;128(4):2893–909.
4. Wilkins KB, Sheikh E, Green R, Patel M, George S, Takano M, et al. Clinical and pathologic predictors of survival in patients with thymoma. Ann Surg. 1999;230(4):562.
5. Lucchi M, Melfi F, Dini P, Basolo F, Viti A, Givigliano F, et al. Neoadjuvant chemotherapy for stage III and IVA thymomas: a single-institution experience with a long follow-up. J Thorac Oncol. 2006;1(4):308–13.
6. Nichols CR. Mediastinal germ cell tumors. Clinical features and biologic correlates. Chest. 1991;99(2):472–9.
7. TW Shields. General thoracic surgery. Mediastinal germ cell tumors. 2009.
8. Collins J, Stern EJ. Chest radiology, the essentials. Philadelphia: Lippincott Williams & Wilkins; 2007.
9. Takeda S, Miyoshi S, Minami M, Ohta M, Masaoka A, Matsuda H. Clinical spectrum of mediastinal cysts. Chest. 2003;124(1):125–32.
10. Strollo DC, Rosado-de-Christenson ML, Jett JR. Primary mediastinal tumors: part II. Tumors of the middle and posterior mediastinum. Chest. 1997;112(5):1344–57.
11. Juanpere S, Cañete N, Ortuño P, Martínez S, Sanchez G, Bernado L. A diagnostic approach to the mediastinal masses. Insights Imaging. 2013;4(1):29–52.
12. Crapo JD, Glassroth J, Karlinsky J, King TE. Baum's textbook of pulmonary diseases. Philadelphia: Lippincott Williams & Wilkins; 2004.

Thymic Pathology and Myasthenia Gravis

20

Calvin S.H. Ng and Anthony P.C. Yim

Abstract

From a historical perspective, myasthenia gravis (MG) was first described in 1672 by an Oxford clinician, Sir Thomas Willis, who noted a patient with temporary loss of speech [1]. It wasn't until two and a half centuries later in 1911 that the first thymectomy was performed by Ferdinard Sauerbruch in Zurich on a 21-year-old woman with hyperthyroidism and MG. Thymectomy was performed in an attempt to treat her hyperthyroidism, and following surgery both conditions showed improvement temporarily. In 1934, Mary Walker recognized clinical similarities between MG and curaré poisoning and hence introduced the anticholinesterase treatment, physostigmine, producing significant improvement in muscle strength for a MG patient. This was an important discovery implicating the pathogenesis of MG at the neuromuscular junction. Later in 1944, Alfred Blalock at Johns Hopkins reported improvement in MG patients following resection of *normal* thymus and also introduced this as a surgical therapy for this condition. Clinical use of edrophonium was introduced around 1950 and later taken over by the more popular pyridostigmine. John Simpson first proposed in 1960 that MG might be an autoimmune disease, which was later confirmed in 1973 by Patrick and Lindstrom through animal studies by immunizing rabbits with purified acetylcholine receptors. It is now common knowledge that MG is an autoimmune disorder of the postsynaptic nicotinic acetylcholine receptor, characterized by weakness and fatiguability of voluntary muscles. The ocular muscles are frequently involved, rendering ptosis and diplopia the most common modes of presentation. Despite the discovery of the condition centuries ago, considerable controversies still remain over its diagnosis, natural history, and therapy both medical and surgical. Nevertheless, thymectomy is now an established

C.S.H. Ng (✉) • A.P.C. Yim
Division of Cardiothoracic Surgery, Department of Surgery, The Chinese University of Hong Kong, Shatin, NT, Hong Kong
e-mail: calvinng@surgery.cuhk.edu.hk

D. Parikh, P.B. Rajesh (eds.), *Tips and Tricks in Thoracic Surgery*,
https://doi.org/10.1007/978-1-4471-7355-7_20

therapy in the management of generalized MG in conjunction with medical treatment. A meta-analysis of 28 controlled studies has previously shown that MG patients undergoing thymectomy were twice as likely to attain medication-free remission, 1.6 times as likely to become asymptomatic, and 1.7 times as likely to improve. Different demographics and baseline characteristics however existed between groups [2]. A recent randomized prospective trial investigating the role of thymectomy for myasthenia gravis has shown improved clinical outcomes over a 3-year period in patients with nonthymomatous myasthenia gravis [3]. Uncertainties remain over the role of thymectomy for patients with purely ocular symptom and those with late onset of disease.

Keywords
Myasthenia gravis · Single Port · Thymectomy · Thymoma · Uniportal · Video-assisted thoracic Surgery (VATS)

20.1 Introduction

From a historical perspective, myasthenia gravis (MG) was first described in 1672 by an Oxford clinician, Sir Thomas Willis, who noted a patient with temporary loss of speech [1]. It wasn't until two and a half centuries later in 1911 that the first thymectomy was performed by Ferdinard Sauerbruch in Zurich on a 21-year-old woman with hyperthyroidism and MG. Thymectomy was performed in an attempt to treat her hyperthyroidism, and following surgery both conditions showed improvement temporarily. In 1934, Mary Walker recognized clinical similarities between MG and curaré poisoning and hence introduced the anticholinesterase treatment, physostigmine, producing significant improvement in muscle strength for a MG patient. This was an important discovery implicating the pathogenesis of MG at the neuromuscular junction. Later in 1944, Alfred Blalock at Johns Hopkins reported improvement in MG patients following resection of *normal* thymus and also introduced this as a surgical therapy for this condition. Clinical use of edrophonium was introduced around 1950 and later taken over by the more popular pyridostigmine. John Simpson first proposed in 1960 that MG might be an autoimmune disease, which was later confirmed in 1973 by Patrick and Lindstrom through animal studies by immunizing rabbits with purified acetylcholine receptors. It is now common knowledge that MG is an autoimmune disorder of the postsynaptic nicotinic acetylcholine receptor, characterized by weakness and fatiguability of voluntary muscles. The ocular muscles are frequently involved, rendering ptosis and diplopia the most common modes of presentation. Despite the discovery of the condition centuries ago, considerable controversies still remain over its diagnosis, natural history, and therapy both medical and surgical. Nevertheless, thymectomy is now an established therapy in the management of generalized MG in conjunction with medical treatment. A meta-analysis of 28 controlled studies has previously shown that MG patients undergoing thymectomy were twice as likely to attain medication-free remission, 1.6 times as likely to become asymptomatic, and 1.7 times as likely to improve. Different demographics and baseline characteristics however existed between groups [2]. A recent randomized prospective trial investigating the role of thymectomy for myasthenia gravis has shown improved clinical outcomes over a 3-year period in patients with nonthymomatous myasthenia gravis [3]. Uncertainties remain over the role of thymectomy for patients with purely ocular symptom and those with late onset of disease.

Several surgical approaches to thymectomy exist. The most commonly adopted surgical approach to thymectomy is via a median sternotomy. Other open thymectomy techniques include the transcervical incision [4], the combined median sternotomy with transcervical incision (T-incision), and the partial sternotomy (involving either the upper [5] or lower [6] sternum). The thoracoscopic approach to thymectomy was first reported by Sugarbaker from Boston and also the Belgium group in 1993 [7, 8]. Subsequently, several variants have evolved including video-assisted thoracic surgery (unilateral) thymectomy [9, 10] and the bilateral thoracoscopic approach combined with a cervical incision (video-assisted thoracoscopic extended thymectomy, VATET) [11, 12]. More recently, endoscopic robot-assisted thymectomy has also been reported with good immediate and intermediate results; however, long-term data is pending [13]. The trend in single-port (uniportal) VATS surgery has also fueled the development of single-incision VATS thymectomy through the subxiphoid or lateral approach [14, 15].

The low procedural morbidity and mortality, improved cosmesis, and lesser degree of access trauma and postoperative pain associated with minimal invasive techniques have made VATS thymectomy increasingly popular. With increasing long-term data to support equivalent efficacy compared to conventional open techniques, the VATS approach is slowly being accepted as the standard in total thymectomy for non-thymomatous MG. However, in the absence of randomized controlled trials comparing the different surgical approaches to thymectomy in the treatment of MG, there is unlikely to be a universal consensus on the optimum surgical approach. Furthermore, patient heterogeneity, the fluctuating nature of the disease, and different classification systems and practice guidelines can add complexity and difficulty to the interpretation of outcomes following thymectomy.

This chapter reviews our technique on VATS thymectomy from the right-side approach, with additional perspectives on our more novel technique of single-incision VATS thymectomy. We discuss the perioperative management in our institution and criteria for patient selection and reports on our long-term results and those in the literature, as well as provide a glimpse into the future. Tips and tricks in preoperative, intraoperative, and postoperative stages of patient management are shared.

20.2 Tips and Tricks in Preoperative Preparation

1. Patient Selection
   (a) In general, it is well accepted that thymectomy should be offered to young patients with generalized MG. Nevertheless, in patients with purely ocular symptoms of MG, uncertainties remain over the role of thymectomy.

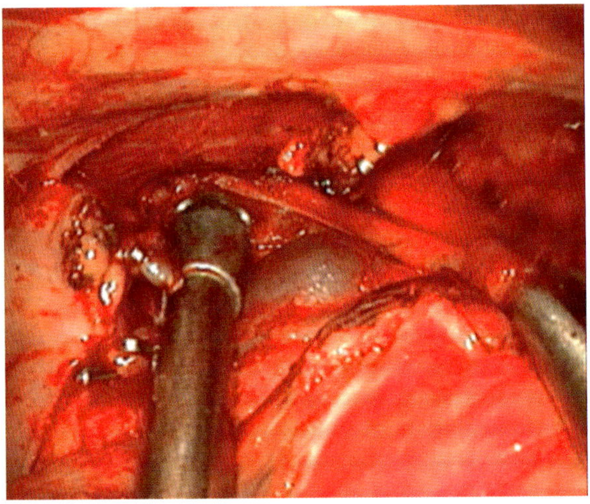

Fig. 20.6 The superior horn can be "taken down" using blunt dissection by sucker and mounted pledget with gentle traction

(e) The right internal mammary vein is found just superior to the brachiocephalic vein-superior vena cava junction. In most cases, it is divided to facilitate exposure of the right superior horn. Due to the relatively large caliber of the internal mammary vein, double clipping with endoclip is recommended for secure hemostasis (Fig. 20.5).

(f) After opening up the fascial attachments with sharp and diathermy dissection, the superior horns can be freed with gentle and deliberate inferior traction on the thymus, mainly using blunt dissection with mounted pledget (Fig. 20.6). The positions of the thoracoscope and inferior instrument port may be exchanged to allow better reach toward the superior parts of the thymus, particularly when conventional instruments are used.

(g) In small children with large hyperplastic thymus and relatively small thoracic cavity, we have found it useful to retract part of the gland out of an anteriorly placed wound, which can create more room for instrumentation and dissection.

(h) It is noteworthy that the left superior horn may very occasionally pass behind, instead of in front, of the brachiocephalic vein. This anatomical variation can be tackled using similar blunt dissection technique as above.

3. Completion of Procedure

(a) The thymus is preferably removed in a protective plastic bag through the most anterior port which has the widest intercostal space and inspected for completeness.

(b) The thymic bed, in particular the area around brachiocephalic veins and superior vena cava junction, should be inspected for hemostasis.

(c) Tube thoracostomy is placed through the anteroinferior port to the thymic bed. The lung is then reinflated under direct vision. Some surgeons do not apply suction to the tube thoracostomy, while others omit drain placement altogether.

(d) In single-port VATS thymectomy, the tube thoracostomy is usually placed at the anterior aspect of the wound. The deep muscle layer needs to be closed with individual stitches either side of the tube thoracostomy prior to routine closure with continuous sutures to reduce risk of wound complications.

20.5 Tips and Tricks: Postoperative Management

1. Early extubation should be encouraged following surgery. The patient can resume full diet when fully awake from the general anesthesia, unless impaired by bulbar weakness from MG.
2. Chest physiotherapy and incentive spirometry are important. Regular checks on oxygen saturation and bedside spirometry should be performed in the early postoperative period to give warning of respiratory muscle weakness.
3. Early resumption of preoperative medications for control of MG is needed, and the neurologists in our institute are consulted to review the patient's MG prior to hospital discharge.

20.6 Results at Our Institution

We have attempted 88 VATS thymectomies using the right-sided approach. Two patients required "conversion" by extending the incision from an anterior port to 4–5 cm for control of bleeding from branch of brachiocephalic vein in our early experience (conversion rate of 2.3%). Four cases were not related to MG, and there were seven thymomas. Therefore, 77 VATS thymectomies were successfully performed for non-thymomatous MG (NTMG). Complete follow-up data was available for 86 patients (2 lost to follow-up).

In the NTMG group, there were 40 females with mean age 33.2 (range 9–75). The mean duration of MG disease till the VATS surgery was 29.1 months (range 2–204 months). Prior to thymectomy, all patients were treated with anticholinesterase, and 61% of cases were also receiving steroid therapy. Preoperatively, 18 patients were in stage I; 24, stage IIA; 7, stage IIB; 11, stage IIIa; 5, stage IIIb; 3, stage IV; and 9, stage V according to the Myasthenia Gravis Foundation of America (MGFA) classification. Mean operative duration was 126 min (range 52–183), and there was no surgical mortality. All patients except eight cases were extubated within 24 h. The risk factors for late extubations were postoperative pneumonia and preoperative mechanical ventilation for MG. Other potential postoperative complications not encountered in our series include wound infection, hypocalcemia, pneumothorax, surgical emphysema, intercostal neuralgia, and phrenic nerve palsy. The median postoperative hospital stay was 3 days. The final pathology results were 47 hyperplastic thymus, 12 atrophic thymus, and 18 normal thymus. After median follow-up of 133 months (range 2–262 months), 64 patients (86%) experienced some improvement. Complete stable remission (CSR) was found in 24.3%, MM2 improvement in 21.6%, and MM3 improvement in 39.1% according to the MGFA postintervention status classification. The status of 12.2% of MG patients remained unchanged, and two died of MG. One of the two deaths occurred in an elderly 73-year-old man who despite successful surgery had gradual progression of his MG and after 8 months died of respiratory failure. This was clearly a case of "thymectomy failure," which was not related to any particular surgical approach but to the unpredictable natural history in patients with "late-onset" MG. The other mortality occurred in a 46-year-old woman who had MM2 improvement following VATS thymectomy but at 22 months postoperatively suffered from pneumonia which she eventually succumbed.

The number of patients experiencing postoperative CSR increased tentatively at 15 months following surgery and then more rapidly increased at around 119 months to 72% at 10 years follow-up. Based on the relatively delayed response, the true benefits of thymectomy for MG require more prolonged surveillance. Using univariate analysis, the only factor associated with statistically significant probability of CSR was disease duration of ≤12 months, hence strengthening the argument for surgery to be performed early following the diagnosis of MG [24].

20.7 Discussion and Published Literature

Currently, there are still uncertainties over the optimal treatment of MG, and furthermore, the best surgical approach to thymectomy for this condition remains controversial. In general, most will agree that an important consideration is achieving completeness of thymectomy for MG. In the 1980s, the Columbia-Presbyterian group advocated "maximal" thymectomy [25] involving a combination of median sternotomy with cervical incision to achieve en bloc thymectomy and anterior mediastinal exenteration, which includes mediastinal pleura from the level of the thoracic inlet to the diaphragm, pericardial fat pad, and all the mediastinal fat as the definitive surgical treatment for MG. However, this very radical surgical approach did not result in significantly different clinical improvements when compared with sternotomy alone [26] or the less invasive transcervial approaches [4, 27, 28]. Another interesting observation from detailed autopsy study identified ectopic thymic tissue in areas (like the retrocarinal fat) which are not accessible via a median sternotomy [29]. The proponents of maximal approaches stress the importance of removing as much mediastinal soft tissue as possible to avoid leaving behind ectopic thymus; however, these remnants have never been conclusively shown to be clinically relevant, and even the most radical surgical approach does not result in a remission rate greater than 40%. Furthermore, a majority of ectopic thymus tissue is actually microscopic, which may even be missed by radical thymectomy [30]. Studies that have compared sternotomy and VATS thymectomy using the bilateral approach for the amount of thymic tissue removed have shown similar results [12].

Broadly speaking, there are basically only two minimally invasive approaches to thymectomy so far—one is the standard VATS approach and its variants including single-port or robotic-assisted; the second is the transcervical approach with or without video assistance. The VATS approach is similar to the transcervical approach in that both are associated with minimal chest wall trauma, low postoperative morbidity, shorter hospital stay, and [31, 32], perhaps more importantly, improved patient acceptance for surgery earlier in the disease compared with the transternal approach [32]. Only rarely is conversion from VATS to sternotomy required, reported to be between 2.6 and 5.5%. We have no conversions to sternotomy because we have been able to tackle intraoperative complications through a mini-thoracotomy by extending one of the anterior ports. The authors have favored the VATS approach over the transcervical for several reasons. Firstly, VATS offers a more panoramic view of the hemithorax, and there is ample room for instrument manipulation and dissection. In comparison, the transcervical approach has only one incision, which may be more prone to crowding and "sword fighting" of instruments. It is noteworthy that during single-port VATS thymectomy, some of the problems associated with instrument crowding can and do occur. However, the correct use of single-port VATS instruments as described above can be crucial in minimizing crowding and fencing. Secondly, if a technical complication like bleeding occurs, it may be easier to control it using the VATS approach than the transcervical approach. Also, the thymus, being largely an anterior mediastinal structure, can be more directly approached through the chest than the neck. However, it should be noted that the transcervical approach can be quicker and obviates the need for double-lumen tube intubation, with certain centers even performing it as an outpatient procedure, with associated cost savings [32]. Video assistance provides a wide, magnified operative field, as well as allows the other team members to learn and appreciate the progress of the VATS procedure. Some transcervical thymectomy surgeons have also used video assistance, mainly for educational purposes, rather than surgical necessity [32]. VATS may also be a helpful approach for completion thymectomy in patients with refractory myasthenia gravis who have already undergone resection by prior transcervical or transternal approach, with the potential advantage of avoiding previously dissected tissue planes and facilitating the search for residual thymic tissue. Interestingly, it has been shown that in patients who did not benefit initially from a transcervical or transternal approach, VATS completion thymectomy can be performed to remove residual thymic tissue resulting in subsequent improvement of symptoms [30, 33]. We believe that we are performing the same operation thoracoscopically compared with the transternal approach by examination of the thymic beds and the resected specimens [19]. The cosmetic appearance of the surgical scars is seldom used to argue for a particular surgical approach. However, thymectomy may be a notable exception considering that the majority of patients are young female and the superior cosmetic appearance of VATS should be considered. In addition, it has been shown that the pulmonary function is significantly better preserved in the immediately postoperative period followed by a faster recovery after VATS compared to the median sternotomy approach to thymectomy for MG in a small randomized prospective study [34]. Such an advantage can contribute toward earlier extubation and potential reduction in the incidence of postoperative pulmonary infections.

However, even among the surgeons performing VATS thymectomy, there is controversy over the exact technique and, in particular, whether the thymus should be approached from the left or right. Mineo et al. [35] from Rome advocated a left-sided approach and the use of pneumomediastinum to facilitate dissection. They believe from the left, the dissection maneuvers are safer because the superior vena cava lies out of the surgical field, thus reducing risk of accidental injury. In addition, the removal of perithymic fatty tissue around the left pericardiophrenic angle and aortopulmonary window can be performed more readily from the left [35]. On the other hand, we advocate the right-sided approach for the following reasons [36]. First, the superior vena cava, easily identified from the right, provides a clear landmark for further dissection of the innominate veins. Second, the confluence of the two innominate veins to form the superior vena cava is an area most difficult to dissect well. This could be more easily accomplished from the right. Third, from the ergonomic standpoint, it is easier for right-handed surgeons performing VATS to start at the inferior poles and work cephalad from the right side. Furthermore, it allows greater maneuverability of instruments in the wider right pleural cavity, particularly in patients with cardiomegaly. The ultimate surgical goal of thymectomy is to completely remove the gland and the anterior mediastinal tissue. The laterality of approach remains largely the surgeon's preference, which is ultimately influenced by his/her experience and training.

In our institution, patients who underwent thoracoscopic thymectomy had significantly less analgesic requirement and shorter hospital stays compared with a historical group who underwent transternal thymectomy [19]. Collective early experience on 33 patients from four centers (Columbia Hospital in Dallas, University of Pittsburgh, Southern Illinois University, and our own) has been previously reported [37]. In this multicenter series, clinical improvement was observed in 88% of patients who underwent thoracoscopic thymectomy after a mean follow-up of 23 months. Subsequently, meta-analysis comparing nine published series performed by other approaches showed no difference in clinical improvement after thymectomy between series [25, 27, 37–40]. More recent studies on minimal invasive thymectomy for MG with more long-term results are presented in Table 20.1. Our CSR rate of 24.3% is comparable to many other studies, particularly with Savcenko et al. [41] who used the same MGFA criteria and similar operative approach as us. Nevertheless, the CSR rate is quite varied between series ranging from 13 to 59%, which can be accountable at least in part by several plausible factors. A review conducted by the American Academy of Neurology reported that the more severe the degree of MG, the larger would be the magnitude of improvement following thymectomy [2]. In our patient cohort, 36.8% of subjects were MGFA stage III–V compared to 55.47% in the series by Mantegazza et al. [42]. Thus, the lower rate of CSR in our series may in part be due to the greater proportion of patients with milder disease (stage I–II). Of note, the percentage of patients on anticholinesterase and immunosuppressive drugs was greater at 100% and 61%, respectively, as opposed to 46.5% and 53.5% in the study by Mantegazza [42]. Interestingly, 100% of patients in Tomulescu's series were receiving steroid therapy preoperatively, with 40% requiring additional treatment with anticholinesterase [43]. This perhaps reflects a different medication prescription practice and management strategy among neurologists, the impact on outcome of which is difficult to qualify. A higher

Table 20.1 Summary from selected publications on various minimal invasive approaches to thymectomy for myasthenia gravis

Author	Publication year	Approach	No. of patients	Mean follow-up (months)	Remission (%)	Improvement (%)
Yu [48]	2012	VATS	67	40	37.5	81.5
Meyer [31]	2009	VATS	48	72	34.9	95.4
Tomulescu [43]	2006	VATS	105	36.4	59.5	97.2
Manlulu and Yim [24]	2005	VATS	36	69	22.2	91.6
Savcenko [41]	2002	VATS	36	53	14	83
Wright [45]	2002	VATS	26	19.5	27	81
Mineo [35]	2000	VATS	31	40	36	96
Zielinski [49]	2004	TC-Sx-VATS	25	24	32	83.3
Hsu [50]	2004	SxVATET	15	18.5	37	NA
Shiono [12]	2009	VATET	30	48	44	NA
Mantegazza [41]	2003	VATET	159	72	33.3	NA
Shrager [32]	2006	TC	151	83	37.1	79.5
de Perrot [44]	2003	TC	120	48	41	NA
Shrager [28]	2002	TC	78	54.6	39.7	NA
Calhoun [4]	1999	TC	100	63.6	35	85
Uchiyama [51]	2001	Infrasternal mediastinoscopy	21	15.5	13.3	86.7

NA not available, *SxVATET* subxiphoid video-assisted thoracoscopic extended thymectomy, *TC* transcervical thymectomy, *TC-Sx-VATS* transcervical subxiphoid videothoracoscopic, *VATET* video-assisted thoracoscopic extended thymectomy, *VATS* video-assisted thoracoscopic surgery percentage of patients on medical therapy also translate into a greater number of patients needed to be weaned off medication before achieving CSR; this clearly has implications on rates of CSR and improvement if an aggressive medication weaning practice was adopted postoperatively. It has been postulated that shorter disease duration results in better outcomes after surgery; therefore, earlier thymectomy could theoretically lead to improved results. In our patient population, the mean preoperative duration of disease was 29.1 months compared with 14.8 months in a series reported by Mineo [35] and 10 months in the study by de Perrot [44]. The timing of surgery in our institution may reflect a delayed surgical referral pattern or prolonged medical treatment, hence, accounting for a lower rate of CSR. Achieving earlier referrals for thymectomy in MG patients have been continuously addressed through better communication with the neurologists, and we have seen MG disease duration till surgery slowly dropping when compared with our previous series. Undoubtedly, differing methods of disease classification and outcome reporting render comparisons between thymectomy studies difficult. To a certain extent, the effect of nonstandardized classification systems becomes readily apparent not only when attempting to establish initial disease severity but moreover when defining a specific outcome such as CSR. For example, duration of CSR according to the MGFA classification is twice as long as the criteria utilized by de Perrot [44] and Shrager [28]. Of note, other authors did not specify the time interval in their definition of remission [35, 45]; this clearly has implications on the overall rate of CSR as there will be more patients achieving remission given a limited duration.

Finally, in the past, great concerns have been raised regarding using the VATS approach for thymoma with or without associated MG. We are careful in restricting this technique to small, completely encapsulated thymoma (Masaoka [46] stage I), although some studies purport acceptable safety and outcomes even for stage II disease [47]. Clinical judgment is of paramount importance in thymic surgery, and any sign of tissue plane invasion should be a strong indicator for conversion to an open dissection [16]. However, it should be noted that there is some evidence to suggest that MG patients with thymoma who undergo VATS thymectomy tend to do less well from their symptoms at least in the early postoperative period [48].

20.8 Conclusion and Future

VATS thymectomy is a safe operation in experienced hands and is a viable alternative technique to open thymectomy for different thymic pathologies. The right-sided approach to the thymus is preferred by us because visualization of the venous anatomy for dissection is essential and clearer from the right; however there is currently no consensus on the ideal laterality for performing VATS thymectomy. Studies so far have shown that VATS approach produces long-term results comparable to other conventional surgical techniques for thymectomy for myasthenia gravis, in terms of complete stable remission from MG and symptomatic improvement. The added advantages of the VATS approach include less postoperative pain, shorter hospital stay, better preserved pulmonary function in the early postoperative period, and superior cosmesis which are important considerations, especially for myasthenia patients many of whom are young females.

The minimal invasive approach would lead to wider acceptance by MG patients and their neurologists, resulting in earlier and more referrals which should further improve clinical outcomes.

The future development of single-port (uniportal) VATS thymectomy, better instrumentation (energy devices and endoinstruments) and camera systems (such as 3-dimensional thoracoscopes), as well as image-guided VATS (iVATS) thymectomy performed in the hybrid operating theatre may further improve outcomes for patients undergoing VATS thymectomy. The role of these advanced techniques and modalities will require further investigation.

References

1. Pascuzzi R. The history of myasthenia gravis. Neurol Clin. 1994;12:231–42.
2. Gronseth GS, Barohn RJ. Practice parameter: thymectomy for autoimmune myasthenia gravis (an evidence-base review). Report of the Quality Standards Subcommittee of the American Academy of Neurology. Neurology. 2000;55:7–15.
3. Wolfe GI, Kaminski HJ, Aban IB, Minisman G, Kuo HC, Marx A, et al. MGTX study group. Randomized trial of thymectomy in myasthenia gravis. N Engl J Med. 2016;375(6):511–22.
4. Calhoun RF, Ritter JH, Guthrie TJ, Pestronk A, Meyers BF, Patterson GA, Pohl MS, Cooper JD. Results of transcervical thymectomy for myasthenia gravis in 100 consecutive patients. Ann Surg. 1999;230:555–9.
5. Milanez de Campos JR, Filomeno LTB, Marchiori PE, Jatene FB. Parital sternotomy approach to the thymus. In: APC Y, Hazelrigg SR, Izzat MB, et al., editors. Minimal access cardiothoracic surgery. Philadelphia: WB Saunders; 2000. p. 205–8.
6. Granone P, Margaritora S, Cesario A, Galetta D. Thymectomy in myasthenia gravis via video assisted infra-mammary cosmetic incision. Eur J Cardiothorac Surg. 1999;15:861–3.
7. Sugarbaker DJ. Thoracoscopy in the management of anterior mediastinal masses. Ann Thorac Surg. 1993;56:653–6.
8. Coosemans W, Lerut TE, Van Raemdonck DE. Thoracoscopic surgery: the Belgian experience. Ann Thorac Surg. 1993;56:721–30.
9. Yim APC. Paradigm shift in surgical approaches to thymectomy. ANZ J Surg. 2002;72:40–5.
10. Yim APC, Low JM, Ng SK, Ho JK, Liu KK. Video-assisted thoracoscopic surgery in the paediatric population. J Paediatr Child Health. 1995;31:192–6.
11. Novellino L, Longoni M, Spinelli L, Andretta M, Cozzi M, Faillace G, Vitellaro M, De Benedetti D, Pezzuoli G. "Extended" thymectomy without sternotomy, performed by cervicotomy and thoracoscopic techniques in the treatment of myasthenia gravis. Int Surg. 1994;79:378–81.
12. Shiono H, Kadota Y, Hayashi A, Okumura M. Comparison of outcomes after extended thymectomy for myasthenia gravis: bilateral thoracoscopic approach versus sternotomy. Surg Laparosc Endosc Percutan Tech. 2009;19:424–7.
13. Bodner J, Wykypiel H, Greiner A, Kirchmayr W, Freund MC, Margreiter R, Schmid T. Early experience with robot-assisted surgery for mediastinal masses. Ann Thorac Surg. 2004;78:259–65.
14. Ng CSH, Lau KKW, Gonzalez-Rivas D, Rocco G. Evolution in surgical approach and techniques for lung cancer. Thorax. 2013;68:681.
15. Suda T, Sugimura H, Tochii D, Kihara M, Hattori Y. Single-port thymectomy through an infrasternal approach. Ann Thorac Surg. 2012;93:334–6.
16. Yim APC, Kay RLC, Izzat MB, Ng SK. Video-assisted thoracoscopic thymectomy for myasthenia gravis. Semin Thorac Cardiovasc Surg. 1999;11:65–73.

17. El-Dawlatly AA, Ashour MH. Anesthesia for thymectomy in myasthenia gravis: a non-muscle-relaxant technique. Anaesth Intensive Care. 1994;22:458–60.
18. Yim AP. Minimizing chest wall trauma in video assisted thoracic surgery. J Thorac Cardiovasc Surg. 1995;109:1255–6.
19. Yim APC, Kay RLC, Ho JKS. Video-assisted thoracoscopic thymectomy for myasthenia gravis. Chest. 1995;108:1440–3.
20. Ng CS, Wong RH, Lau RW, Yim AP. Minimizing chest wall trauma in single-port video-assisted thoracic surgery. J Thorac Cardiovasc Surg. 2014;147:1095–6.
21. Ng CSH, Wong RHL, Lau RWH, Yim APC. Single port video-assisted thoracic surgery: advancing scope technology. Eur J Cardiothorac Surg. 2014. pii: ezu236. [Epub ahead of print]. https://doi.org/10.1093/ejcts/ezu236.
22. Ng CSH, Rocco G, Wong RHL, Lau RWH, Yu SCH, Yim APC. Uniportal and single incision video assisted thoracic surgery- the state of the art. Interact Cardiovasc Thorac Surg. 2014. pii: ivu200. [Epub ahead of print]. https://doi.org/10.1093/icvts/ivu200.
23. Ohta M, Hirabayasi H, Okumura M, Minami M, Matsuda H. Thoracoscopic thymectomy using anterior chest wall lifting method. Ann Thorac Surg. 2003;76:1310–1.
24. Manlulu A, Lee TW, Wan I, Law CY, Chang C, Garzon JC, Yim A. VATS thymectomy for nonthymomatous myasthenia gravis. Chest. 2005;128:3454–60.
25. Jaretzki A III, Penn AS, Younger DS, Wolff M, Olarte MR, Lovelace RE, Rowland LP. "Maximal" thymectomy for myasthenia gravis. Results. J Thorac Cardiovasc Surg. 1988;95:747–57.
26. Olanow CW, Wechsler AS, Sirontkin-Roses M, Stajich J, Roses AD. Thymectomy as primary therapy in myasthenia gravis. Ann N Y Acad Sci. 1987;505:595–606.
27. Cooper JD, Al-Jilaihawa AN, Pearson FG, Humphrey JG, Humphrey HE. An improved technique to facilitate transcervical thymectomy for myasthenia gravis. Ann Thorac Surg. 1988;45:242–7.
28. Shrager JB, Deeb ME, Mick R, Brinster CJ, Childers HE, Marshall MB, Kucharczuk JC, Galetta SL, Bird SJ, Kaiser LR. Transcervical thymectomy for myasthenia gravis achieves results comparable to thymectomy by sternotomy. Ann Thorac Surg. 2002;74:320–6.
29. Fukai I, Funato Y, Mizuno T, Hashimoto T, Masaoka A. Distribution of thymic tissue in the mediastinal adipose tissue. J Thorac Cardiovasc Surg. 1991;101:1099–102.
30. Pompeo E, Nofroni I, Iavicoli N, Mineo TC. Thoracoscopic completion thymectomy in refractory nonthymomatous myasthenia. Ann Thorac Surg. 2000;70:918–23.
31. Meyer DM, Herbert MA, Sobhani NC, et al. Comparative clinical outcomes of thymectomy for myasthenia gravis performed by extended transsternal and minimal invasive approaches. Ann Thorac Surg. 2009;87:385–91.
32. Shrager JB, Nathan D, Brinster CJ, et al. Outcomes after 151 extended transcervical thymectomies for myasthenia gravis. Ann Thorac Surg. 2006;82:1863–9.
33. Ng J, Ng CSH, Underwood MJ, Lau KKW. Does repeat thymectomy improve symptoms in patients with refractory myasthenia gravis? Interact Cardiovasc Thorac Surg. 2014;18:376–80.
34. Rückert JC, Wlater M, Müller JM. Pulmonary function after thoracoscopic thymectomy versus median sternotomy for myasthenia gravis. Ann Thorac Surg. 2000;70:1656–61.
35. Mineo TC, Pompeo E, Lerut TE, Bernardi G, Coosemans W, Nofroni I. Thoracscopic thymectomy in autoimmune myasthenia gravis: results of left sided approach. Ann Thorac Surg. 2000;69:1537–41.
36. Yim APC. Thoracoscopic thymectomy: which side to approach? Ann Thorac Surg. 1997;64:584 [Letter].
37. Mack MJ, Landreneau RJ, Yim AP, Hazelrigg SR, Scruggs GR. Results of video-assisted thymectomy in patients with myasthenia gravis. J Thorac Cardiovasc Surg. 1996;112:1352–60.
38. DeFilippi VJ, Richman DP, Ferguson MK. Transcervical thymectomy for myasthenia gravis. Ann Thorac Surg. 1994;57:194–7.
39. Mulder DG, Graves M, Hermann C. Thymectomy for myasthenia gravis: recent observations and comparisons with past experience. Ann Thorac Surg. 1989;48:551–5.

40. Nussbaum MS, Rosenthal GJ, Samaha FJ, Grinvalsky HT, Quinlan JG, Schmerler M, Fischer JE. Management of myasthenia gravis by extended thymectomy with anterior mediastinal tumor. Surgery. 1992;112:681–8.
41. Savcenko M, Wendt GK, Prince SL, Mack MJ. Video-assisted thymectomy for myasthenia gravis: an update of a single institution experience. Eur J Cardiothorac Surg. 2002;22:978–83.
42. Mantegazza R, Baggi F, Bernasconi P, Antozzi C, Confalonieri P, Novellino L, Spinelli L, Ferro MT, Beghi E, Cornelio F. Video-assisted thoracoscopic extended thymectomy and extended transternal thymectomy (T-3b) in non-thymomatous myasthenia gravis patients: remission after 6 years of follow up. J Neurol Sci. 2003;212:31–6.
43. Tomulescu V, Ion V, Kosa A, Sgarbura O, Popescu I. Thoracoscopic thymectomy mid-term results. Ann Thorac Surg. 2006;82:1003–8.
44. de Perrot M, Bril V, McRae K, Keshavjee S. Impact of minimally invasive trans-cervical thymectomy on outcome in patients with myasthenia gravis. Eur J Cardiothorac Surg. 2003;24:677–83.
45. Wright GM, Barnett S, Clarke CP. Video-assisted thoracoscopic thymectomy for myasthenia gravis. Intern Med J. 2002;32:367–71.
46. Masaoka A, Monden Y, Nakahara K, Tanioka T. Follow up study of thymoma with references to their clinical stages. Cancer. 1981;48:2485–92.
47. Ye B, Tantai JC, Ge XX, Li W, Feng J, Cheng M, Shi JX, Zhao H. Surgical techniques for early-stage thymoma: video-assisted thoracoscopic thymectomy versus transsternal thymectomy. J Thorac Cardiovasc Surg. 2014;147:1599–603.
48. Yu L, Zhang XJ, Ma S, Li F, Zhang YF. Thoracoscopic thymectomy for myasthenia gravis with and without thymoma: a single-center experience. Ann Thorac Surg. 2012;93:240–4.
49. Zielinski M, Kuzdzal J, Szlubowski A, Soja J. Transcervial-subxiphoid-videothoracoscopic 'maximal' thymectomy-operative technique and early results. Ann Thorac Surg. 2004;78:404–10.
50. Hsu CP, Chuang CY, Hsu NY, Chen CY. Comparison between the right side and subxiphoid bilateral approaches in performing video-assisted thoracoscopic extended thymectomy for myasthenia gravis. Surg Endosc. 2004;18:821–4.
51. Uchiyama A, Shimizu S, Murai H, Kuroki S, Okido M, Tanaka M. Infrasternal mediastinoscopic thymectomy in myasthenia gravis: surgical results in 23 patients. Ann Thorac Surg. 2001;72:1902–5.

Posterior Mediastinal Tumors

21

Keith S. Naunheim and Melanie A. Edwards

Abstract

The posterior mediastinum begins at the posterior pericardium and ends at the anterior longitudinal ligament. The thoracic inlet and diaphragm, respectively, form the superior and inferior extent, and the pleural reflections comprise the lateral margins. Within this space lies the oesophagus, descending thoracic aorta, thoracic duct, azygos and hemiazygos veins, nerve roots, sympathetic nerves, and proximal intercostal nerves and vessels [1]. The pathologic processes found in the posterior mediastinum vary according to age; 50–75% of posterior mediastinal tumors are of neurogenic origin in infants and adults (up to 95%), while lymphoma is more common in adolescents. Most tumors found in adults originate from the peripheral nerve sheath and are benign [2]. In the pediatric population, posterior neurogenic tumors comprise a greater proportion of all thoracic tumors, and up to 60% are malignant [1, 3].

Keywords

Mediastinal neoplasm · Mediastinal cyst · Neurilemmoma · Ganglioneuroma Neuroblastoma · Thoracoscopy · Thoracic surgery · Video assisted

K.S. Naunheim, M.D. (✉)
St Louis University School of Medicine, St. Louis, MO, USA
e-mail: naunheim@slu.edu

M.A. Edwards, M.D.
Division of Cardiothoracic Surgery, St Louis University School of Medicine, St. Louis, MO, USA
e-mail: medwar13@slu.edu

D. Parikh, P.B. Rajesh (eds.), *Tips and Tricks in Thoracic Surgery*,
https://doi.org/10.1007/978-1-4471-7355-7_21

21.1 Introduction

The posterior mediastinum begins at the posterior pericardium and ends at the anterior longitudinal ligament. The thoracic inlet and diaphragm, respectively, form the superior and inferior extent, and the pleural reflections comprise the lateral margins. Within this space lies the oesophagus, descending thoracic aorta, thoracic duct, azygos and hemiazygos veins, nerve roots, sympathetic nerves, and proximal intercostal nerves and vessels [1]. The pathologic processes found in the posterior mediastinum vary according to age; 50–75% of posterior mediastinal tumors are of neurogenic origin in infants and adults (up to 95%), while lymphoma is more common in adolescents. Most tumors found in adults originate from the peripheral nerve sheath and are benign [2]. In the pediatric population, posterior neurogenic tumors comprise a greater proportion of all thoracic tumors, and up to 60% are malignant [1, 3].

21.2 Technical Tips and Tricks of Posterior Mediastinal Tumor Resection

21.2.1 Preoperative Evaluation

Many of the lesions found in the posterior mediastinum are discovered incidentally on cross-sectional imaging performed for other indications. Patients can also present with pain, neurologic symptoms, dyspnea, or cough [4]. A computed tomography (CT) scan of the chest with and without intravenous contrast should be obtained to evaluate the proximate relationships, the presence of mediastinal adenopathy, and the vascular enhancement of the mass (Fig. 21.1). Magnetic resonance imaging (MRI) is an important adjunct that is more sensitive than CT for delineating intraspinal extension and should be obtained for all tumors along the paravertebral sulcus (Fig. 21.2). Additionally, MRI characteristics correlate well with pathologic findings and can demonstrate the relationship to surrounding tissues in more detail [5, 6]. Preoperative visualization of the origins and course of the spinal blood supply with either direct or MR angiography has been recommended by some authors for tumors located between T5 and T12 to decrease the risk of spinal cord ischemia [7–12]. 18-Fluorodeoxyglucose

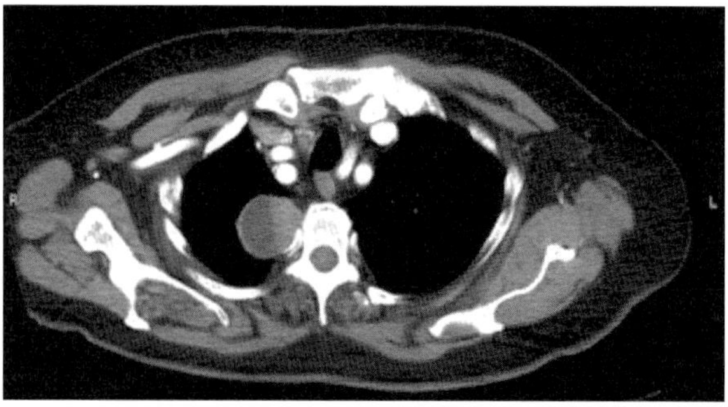

Fig. 21.1 CT scan of a right posterior mediastinal schwannoma

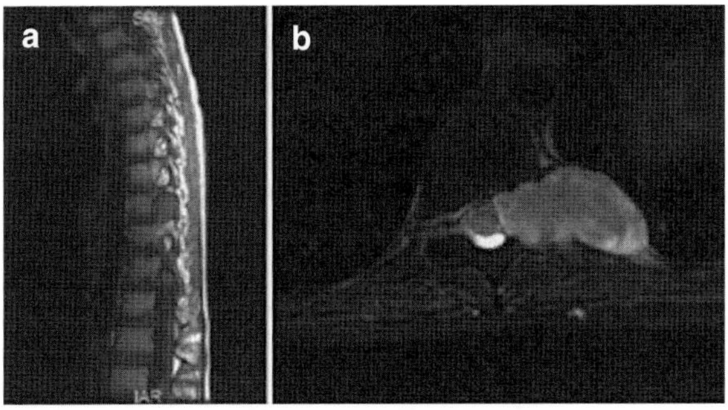

Fig. 21.2 Classic thoracic dumbbell nerve sheath tumor. Note the markedly enlarged neural foramen on the paramedian sagittal image (**a**) and the intra- and extraspinal components on the axial image (**b**) (*From* Binning M, Klimo Jr P, Gluf W, Goumnerova L. Spinal Tumors in Children. Neurosurgery Clinics of North America. 2007;18(4):631–58; with permission)

positron emission tomography (18-FDG PET) scan can also be performed if there is uncertainty about a benign diagnosis. Most posterior mediastinal masses are easily accessed by percutaneous needle biopsy either with ultrasound or CT guidance. Endoscopic transoesophageal ultrasound fine needle aspiration is another diagnostic modality that can be used if malignancy is suspected.

21.2.2 General Considerations

Surgical resection is indicated for most cystic and solid posterior mediastinal lesions. In 1992, Landreneau performed the first video-assisted thoracoscopic surgery (VATS) to remove a posterior mediastinal tumor, and subsequently, VATS has become the preferred approach in adults since the great majority of these lesions are benign [7, 13–20]. Not all tumors are amenable to removal with VATS, however, including larger tumors (>6 cm), locations at the extremes of the hemithorax, tumors in proximity to vital structures, and those with the presence or likelihood of malignancy [14, 20–22].

21.3 Video-Assisted Thoracoscopic Surgery

1. Single-lung ventilation through a double-lumen endotracheal tube assists in creating an unimpeded working space.
2. The patient is positioned in the lateral decubitus position with the table flexed to open up the intercostal spaces and rotated anteriorly to shift the lung away from the operative field.
3. The camera port is positioned in the midaxillary line in the sixth, seventh, or eighth intercostal space depending on the cranio-caudal position of the tumor within the hemithorax, and a 5 mm 30-degree camera is used for visualization. The working ports are positioned so as to create triangular convergence on the

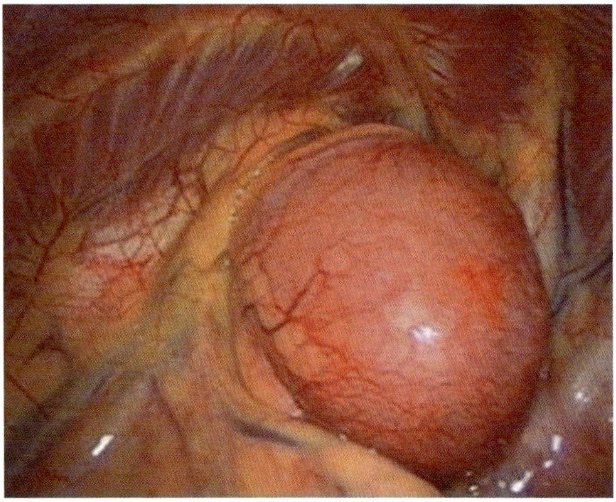

Fig. 21.3 Intraoperative view of a left posterior mediastinal paraganglioma (*From* Ng CS, Yim AP. Technical advances in mediastinal surgery: videothoracoscopic approach to posterior mediastinal tumors. Thoracic surgery clinics. 2010;20(2):297-309; with permission)

area of interest using lower anterior placement to look down up at higher tumors in the hemithorax and a higher placement to look down at lower tumors. The camera position can be moved as needed to provide the necessary views [23].

4. The entire hemithorax is examined, and the tumor is assessed to determine the feasibility of a thoracoscopic resection (Fig. 21.3). Access to the lower hemithorax and costophrenic sulcus can be difficult, especially in larger patients with an elevated hemidiaphragm. A suture for retraction placed in the fibrous portion of the diaphragm can improve visualization in this area, and the use of a laparoscopic triangular or fan retractor supported by the Martin arm retractor system (KLS-Martin, Tuttlingen, Germany) may be necessary. The reverse Trendelenburg position can also be helpful in this regard.
5. Standard thoracic instruments supplemented with laparoscopic graspers are sufficient for these cases. The hook cautery is used to score the pleura around the periphery of the tumor, and a combination of careful sharp and blunt dissection is used to separate the tumor from the adjacent structures. The harmonic scalpel (Ethicon Endosurgery, Cincinnati, OH, USA) is particularly useful, especially for more vascular lesions [7], and the endoscopic bipolar shears (LigaSure, Covidien, Mansfield, MA, USA, or Enseal Ethicon Endosurgery, Cincinnati, OH, USA) provide an alternative energy source. Intercostal vessels and nerves are ligated with an endoscopic clip applicator.
6. A stitch using heavy suture placed into the body of the tumor will help retract larger solid benign lesions that can be difficult to grasp.
7. In the case of a cystic mass, needle aspiration decompresses the cyst in a controlled manner and improves visualization and mobility. If a benign cyst is attached to a vital structure where a complete resection would be potentially dangerous, partial resection followed by fulguration of the remaining cyst wall with either cautery or the argon plasma coagulator is a safe and appropriate alternative [24]. Nonetheless, a complete resection should be attempted if possible, as cyst recurrences have been noted in some series [15].

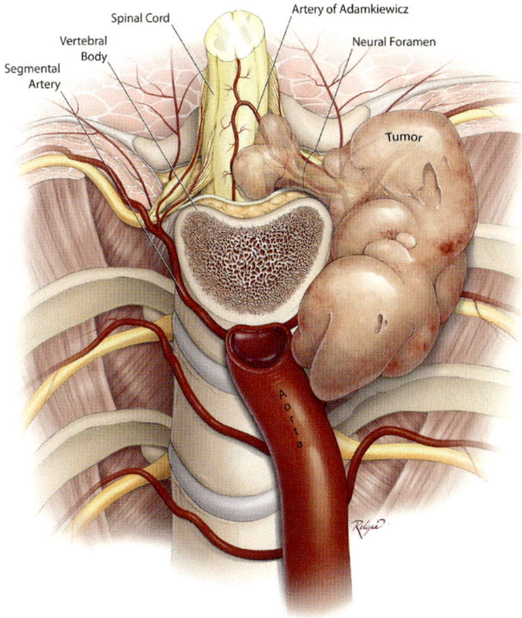

Fig. 21.4 Illustration demonstrating the relationship of a posterior mediastinal tumor to the AKA and the artery's course relative to the anterior spinal artery (*From* Nordin AB, Fallon SC, Jea A, Kim ES. The use of spinal angiography in the management of posterior mediastinal tumors: case series and review of the literature. Journal of pediatric surgery. 2013;48(9):1871-7. Illustration by Katherine Relyea, printed with permission from Baylor College of Medicine)

8. When approaching neurogenic tumors in the lower paravertebral sulcus, special consideration must be given to the location and supply of the artery of Adamkiewicz to avoid a potentially devastating neurologic injury (Fig. 21.4).
9. Once the tumor has been completely freed, it is placed into an endoscopic specimen retrieval bag and removed from the chest through the most anterior port. This incision may need to be enlarged slightly to accommodate a larger specimen. Meticulous hemostasis is obtained with electrocautery, a single chest tube is placed, and the incisions are closed.

21.4 Video-Assisted Thoracoscopic Surgery in Children

Posterior mediastinal tumors in the pediatric population have traditionally been removed through a thoracotomy. The smaller-sized airways and thoracic cavities pose several technical challenges; however, adaptations of the approach have allowed successful resections to be performed even in infants [25–30].

1. Single-lung ventilation can be accomplished with a double-lumen endotracheal tube in older, larger adolescents. For most young children, a single-lumen endotracheal tube is advanced into the contralateral main stem bronchus, or if possible, a bronchial blocker is placed in the operative side. Smaller children and infants are managed without lung isolation, and carbon dioxide is insufflated at low pressures of 3–5 mmHg to collapse the lung.

2. Patients are positioned either prone or lateral with a significant anterior tilt, and the resection is carried out in much the same fashion as in adults [26–28, 30].

21.5 Tips and Tricks That Will Avoid and Deal with Intraoperative Anticipated and Unanticipated Complications

1. Bleeding: If the preoperative imaging suggests a hypervascular or malignant tumor, consideration should be given to an initial thoracotomy approach for better control. Temporary packing with thrombin-soaked gel foam or methylcellulose during VATS dissection can be useful for generalized oozing, but one must avoid leaving these substances in place especially in or near the intervertebral foramen for fear they can swell and exert pressure on the spinal cord. For more robust hemorrhage, an initial attempt to control bleeding thoracoscopically is appropriate, but one should not hesitate to perform a thoracotomy if initial attempts are unsuccessful or if the view is not adequate.
2. Difficult mobilization: Larger tumors can pose a significant challenge, especially when located at the apex. Well-encapsulated benign tumors can be enucleated with an intracapsular dissection to minimize the risk to adjacent arteries and nerves. Once the tumor mass has been removed, the decompressed pseudocapsule can then be safely removed [22, 31]. It should be noted that several series have documented increased conversions and complication rates with larger tumors, so consideration should be given to an initial open approach or converting to a thoracotomy early if difficulty is encountered [14, 22].

21.6 Alternate Methods to Resect Posterior Mediastinal Tumors

1. Thoracotomy: A standard posterolateral thoracotomy is a reasonable and safe approach to posterior mediastinal tumors. Tumors especially suited to this approach include larger masses and dumbbell tumors [4, 9]. Strong consideration must be given to removing malignant tumors through a thoracotomy, as they tend to be more vascular and invasive and may require removal of adjacent structures for a complete resection. As with the VATS approach, the patient is intubated with a double-lumen endotracheal tube and placed in the lateral decubitus position. A posterolateral skin incision is made, dividing the latissimus dorsi and sparing the serratus anterior muscle to enter the chest in the fourth or fifth interspace. Resecting the fourth rib will improve the exposure to apex of the chest, especially when dealing with a large tumor. Both sharp and blunt dissections are again used to mobilize the tumor, while the attached intercostal arteries and nerves are clipped or suture ligated, being mindful of the spinal blood supply as discussed above. Considering the more invasive tendencies of malignant tumors, concomitant chest wall resection may be required with reconstruction of defects that extend below the fourth rib. Either polypropylene or polytetrafluoroethylene (PTFE) mesh is suitable for this application.

2. Robotic resection: While the benefits of using a robotic-assisted thoracoscopic approach to the anterior mediastinum have been described [32, 33], the experience in the posterior mediastinum, especially for lower tumors, is still in evolution [34]. Further study will need to be performed in order to define the role of this technology in the routine management of posterior mediastinal tumors.

21.7 Uncommon Pathology

- Dumbbell Neurogenic Tumor
- The so-called dumbbell neurogenic tumor extending into the intervertebral foramen represents 10% of mediastinal neurogenic tumors, and up to 40% of these patients will be asymptomatic. Akwari found that over 60% arise from the peripheral nerve and 90% are benign [4]. It had been considered a contraindication to the VATS approach due to the risk of catastrophic intraspinal hemorrhage and neurologic complications; however, in recent years, several series have demonstrated the feasibility of thoracoscopy in this setting when combined with neurosurgical support [20, 35–39].
- Collaboration with neurosurgeons is essential to ensuring optimal outcomes with these uncommon tumors. The approach, single- or two-staged, and sequence of laminectomy and thoracotomy or thoracoscopy continue to be the subject of controversy. A two-stage approach can usually be avoided, unless an extensive laminectomy with prolonged operating time and significant blood loss are encountered that would make the addition of a thoracotomy or thoracoscopy unwise in the same setting [40]. Those who advocate performing the thoracic portion first cite the advantages of improved vascular control through ligation of the feeding intercostal vessels and the potential to avoid a laminectomy in some cases of limited extradural intraspinal extension through an enlarged neural foramen [9, 41, 42]. However, traction on the proximal nerve root can lead to avulsion, intraspinal hemorrhage, and cerebrospinal fluid (CSF) leak [43]. Thus, the authors recommend a single-stage combined posterior and anterior approach where the intraspinal component is resected first. Typically, patients are placed in the prone position, and the laminectomy is performed first and then repositioned lateral for the thoracic mobilization [18, 38, 39]. The need to reposition can be avoided by using the lateral position for both portions of the case. The operating table is rotated anteriorly 45° for the laminectomy with the operating microscope allowing simultaneous access to both operative fields if needed [31, 42].
- The patient is secured to a fluoroscopy-compatible table with rolls for support instead of a beanbag that can obscure the fluoroscopic views. The appropriate level is identified with fluoroscopy, and a vertical incision is made centered over that area. A unilateral laminectomy is performed and extended laterally into the involved foramen. If the tumor is intradural, the dura is opened, that portion of the tumor is removed, and the proximal nerve root is ligated. The dura is then closed, the incision is closed over a suction drain, and the thoracic portion of the operation is commenced. Stabilization is usually not required for laminectomy performed at 1–2 levels. The thoracic dissection is then performed as described above. Once the tumor is removed, a Valsalva maneuver is performed to check

for a CSF leak following which, pericardial fat and fibrin sealant can be used to buttress the dural closure [19, 31]. Methylcellulose or gel foam packing should not be left in the foraminal space as these substances can swell, migrate, and lead to delayed neurologic injury [44, 45].

- Malignant peripheral nerve sheath tumor
  Fewer than 5% of the peripheral nerve sheath tumors are malignant [2]. Malignant schwannoma (or neurofibrosarcoma) is more often seen in patients with neurofibromatosis-1 or a history of radiation exposure (Fig. 21.5). These tumors can be large and present with distant metastasis. Complete surgical resection offers the best long-term prognosis but may not be feasible due to local invasion [1, 2, 46].
- Paraganglioma
  Patients with a posterior mediastinal tumor who present with sustained or paroxysmal hypertension, headaches, palpitations, or other metabolic derangements should be evaluated for a paraganglionic tumor with urine or serum catecholamines and metaiodobenzylguanidine (MIBG) scintigraphy [47]. Although a rare tumor, this diagnosis is best made preoperatively as significant intraoperative cardiovascular instability can result from manipulation of the tumor. The presence of a hypervascular, metabolically active lesion should also raise suspicion for a paraganglioma, as asymptomatic patients with functioning tumors have been described [48–50]. If a paraganglioma is diagnosed, patients are treated with preoperative alpha blockade with additional beta blockade added as needed. These tumors have a higher malignant potential and tend to be quite vascular making them more suited for resection through an open approach [51, 52]. Ensure appropriate access for volume infusion and the availability of appropriate alpha agonists and antagonists to treat fluctuations in hemodynamic parameters. The risk of recurrence is higher than in patients with adrenal pheochromocytoma, making long-term follow-up mandatory [53].
- Autonomic ganglion tumors
  These tumors originate from the sympathetic ganglia along the paravertebral sulcus and include ganglioneuroma, ganglioneuroblastoma, and neuroblastoma. The

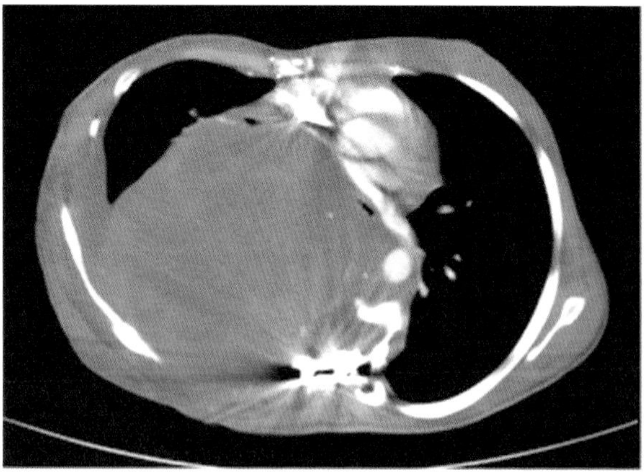

Fig. 21.5 CT scan of a recurrent malignant peripheral nerve sheath tumor, presenting with paralysis

behavior and malignant potential range from the benign ganglioneuroma through the intermediate ganglioneuroblastoma to the highly malignant neuroblastoma. Ganglioneuromas and ganglioneuroblastomas are treated with complete surgical resection. A thoracotomy approach is typically recommended given the higher incidence of malignancy of these tumors, and intraoperative frozen section should be obtained in all cases where a diagnosis of malignancy has not been confirmed. Neuroblastomas are more commonly found in young children and comprise 50% of pediatric mediastinal tumors [1]. Localized tumors are treated with surgical resection, and more advanced disease requires multimodality therapy [1, 2, 46].

21.8 Postoperative Complications and Follow-up

Serious complications after resection of posterior mediastinal tumors are infrequent, and mortality is rare. Kumar performed a review of 231 thoracoscopic posterior mediastinal resections performed in the literature and found a 12% complication rate and no mortalities. Horner's syndrome, paresthesias, neuralgia, hoarseness, CSF leak, pleural effusion, chylothorax, and delayed hemorrhage have been reported in both open and thoracoscopic series [14, 20, 42, 43].

Chylothorax: Persistent or increasing chest tube output should raise suspicion for the development of a chylous fistula, especially after the resection of larger or malignant tumors. Pleural fluid should be sent for triglyceride analysis, and pretreatment with a high fat-containing meal can increase the diagnostic yield. Conservative management with a medium-chain fatty acid diet or total parental nutrition should be instituted once the diagnosis is made. In high-output (>10 cc/kg) chylothoraces, early reoperation and thoracic duct ligation are recommended to decrease the potential nutritional and immunologic morbidity of a prolonged chylous fistula.

CSF leak: Patients with a dural fistula often present with headaches, nausea and vomiting, increased chest tube output, or a pleural effusion. Imaging with MRI or CT myelogram is typically diagnostic. The negative pressure within the pleural space can exacerbate the leak leading to failure of conservative management. Reoperation and buttressed repair of the dura are often required and can be done through a minimally invasive approach in selected cases [44, 54].

Neurologic deficits: Transient paresthesias and Horner's syndrome are often reported in most series and were either present preoperatively or resolved during the follow-up period. Yang and colleagues noted a higher incidence of brachial plexus injuries after VATS resection of tumors located at the apex of the chest when compared to thoracotomy patients [22]. Severe neurologic deficits and paraplegia are rare but have been reported, possibly caused by damage to the anterior spinal artery [8, 10]. As a preventative measure, preoperative angiography has been proposed to visualize the origin of the artery of Adamkiewicz for tumors located between T5 and T12 [7, 9, 10]. Angiography, however, carries some risk, and magnetic resonance angiography (MRA) can correctly identify the course of the artery in 94–100% of cases in a noninvasive manner [55–57]. The use of methylcellulose packing in this region has been associated with neurologic injuries and is not recommended [45].

Follow-up: In several thoracoscopic series, recurrence rates after the resection of benign neurogenic tumors have been low with no recurrences observed by several groups after follow-up ranging from 2 to 35 months [20, 42, 43]. Shadmehr and colleagues surveyed 16 patients after open resection of a dumbbell tumor and found no recurrences at an average 7.5-year follow-up [12].

21.9 Summary

Posterior mediastinal tumors in adults are well suited to the thoracoscopic approach since most of these tumors are benign. Open surgery has been recommended when a patient presents with a large tumor, proven or suspected malignancy, and intraspinal extension (dumbbell tumors). Similarly, in the pediatric population, the thoracotomy approach has been standard; however, recent advances have increased the age range to which thoracoscopic techniques can be applied. Combined posterior and anterior approaches have facilitated the successful minimally invasive resection of selected dumbbell tumors. Malignant and large tumors, however, are still best resected through a thoracotomy.

References

1. Pearson FG, Patterson GA. Pearson's thoracic & esophageal surgery. 3rd ed. Philadelphia: Churchill Livingstone/Elsevier; 2008.
2. Reeder LB. Neurogenic tumors of the mediastinum. Semin Thorac Cardiovasc Surg. 2000;12(4):261–7. https://doi.org/10.1053/stcs.2000.16738.
3. Kelemen JJ, Naunheim KS. Minimally invasive approaches to mediastinal neoplasms. Semin Thorac Cardiovasc Surg. 2000;12(4):301–6. https://doi.org/10.1053/stcs.2000.17919.
4. Akwari OE, Payne WS, Onofrio BM, Dines DE, Muhm JR. Dumbbell neurogenic tumors of the mediastinum. Diagnosis and management. Mayo Clin Proc. 1978;53(6):353–8.
5. Nakazono T, White CS, Yamasaki F, Yamaguchi K, Egashira R, Irie H, et al. MRI findings of mediastinal neurogenic tumors. Am J Roentgenol. 2011;197(4):W643–W52. https://doi.org/10.2214/AJR.10.6119.
6. Sakai F, Sone S, Kiyono K, Maruyama A, Ueda H, Aoki J, et al. Intrathoracic neurogenic tumors: MR-pathologic correlation. AJR Am J Roentgenol. 1992;159(2):279–83. https://doi.org/10.2214/ajr.159.2.1632340.
7. Pons F, Lang-Lazdunski L, Bonnet PM, Meyrat L, Jancovici R. Videothoracoscopic resection of neurogenic tumors of the superior sulcus using the harmonic scalpel. Ann Thorac Surg. 2003;75(2):602–4.
8. Furak J, Geczi T, Tiszlavicz L, Lazar G. Postoperative paraplegia after resection of a giant posterior mediastinal tumour. Importance of the blood supply in the upper spinal cord. Interact Cardiovasc Thorac Surg. 2011;12(5):855–6. https://doi.org/10.1510/icvts.2010.257105.
9. Grillo HC, Ojemann RG, Scannell JG, Zervas NT. Combined approach to "dumbbell" intrathoracic and intraspinal neurogenic tumors. Ann Thorac Surg. 1983;36(4):402–7.
10. Nordin AB, Fallon SC, Jea A, Kim ES. The use of spinal angiography in the management of posterior mediastinal tumors: case series and review of the literature. J Pediatr Surg. 2013;48(9):1871–7. https://doi.org/10.1016/j.jpedsurg.2013.04.029.
11. Shamji MF, Maziak DE, Shamji FM, Ginsberg RJ, Pon R. Circulation of the spinal cord: an important consideration for thoracic surgeons. Ann Thorac Surg. 2003;76(1):315–21. https://doi.org/10.1016/s0003-4975(03)00139-5.

12. Shadmehr MB, Gaissert HA, Wain JC, Moncure AC, Grillo HC, Borges LF, et al. The surgical approach to "dumbbell tumors" of the mediastinum. Ann Thorac Surg. 2003;76(5):1650–4. https://doi.org/10.1016/s0003-4975(03)00882-8.
13. Landreneau RJ, Dowling RD, Ferson PF. THoracoscopic resection of a posterior mediastinal neurogenic tumor. Chest. 1992;102(4):1288–90. https://doi.org/10.1378/chest.102.4.1288.
14. Bousamra IIM, Haasler GB, Patterson GA, Roper CL. A comparative study of thoracoscopic vs open removal of benign neurogenic mediastinal tumors. Chest. 1996;109(6):1461–5. https://doi.org/10.1378/chest.109.6.1461.
15. Demmy TL, Krasna MJ, Detterbeck FC, Kline GG, Kohman LJ, DeCamp MM Jr, et al. Multicenter VATS experience with mediastinal tumors. Ann Thoracic Surg. 1998;66(1):187–92. https://doi.org/10.1016/S0003-4975(98)00378-6.
16. Roviaro G, Varoli F, Nucca O, Vergani C, Maciocco M. Videothoracoscopic approach to primary mediastinal pathology. Chest. 2000;117(4):1179–83. https://doi.org/10.1378/chest.117.4.1179.
17. Zierold D, Halow KD. Thoracoscopic resection as the preferred approach to posterior mediastinal neurogenic tumors. Surg Laparosc Endosc Percutan Tech. 2000;10(4):222–5.
18. Arapis C, Gossot D, Debrosse D, Arper L, Mazel C, Grunenwald D. Thoracoscopic removal of neurogenic mediastinal tumors: technical aspects. Surg Endosc. 2004;18(9):1380–3. https://doi.org/10.1007/s00464-003-9329-9.
19. Kan P, Schmidt MH. Minimally invasive thoracoscopic resection of paraspinal neurogenic tumors. Neurosurgery. 2008;63:ONSE54. https://doi.org/10.1227/01.neu.0000313118.73941.d7.
20. Li Y, Wang J. Experience of video-assisted thoracoscopic resection for posterior mediastinal neurogenic tumours: a retrospective analysis of 58 patients. ANZ J Surg. 2013;83(9):664–8. https://doi.org/10.1111/j.1445-2197.2012.06174.x.
21. Ricci C, Rendina EA, Venuta F, Pescarmona EO, Gagliardi F. Diagnostic imaging and surgical treatment of dumbbell tumors of the mediastinum. Ann Thorac Surg. 1990;50(4):586–9. https://doi.org/10.1016/0003-4975(90)90194-B.
22. Yang C, Zhao D, Zhou X, Ding J, Jiang G. A comparative study of video-assisted thoracoscopic resection versus thoracotomy for neurogenic tumours arising at the thoracic apex. Interact Cardiovasc Thorac Surg. 2015;20(1):35–9. https://doi.org/10.1093/icvts/ivu328.
23. Naunheim KS. Video thoracoscopy for masses of the posterior mediastinum. Ann Thorac Surg. 1993;56(3):657–8.
24. Hazelrigg SR, Landreneau RJ, Mack MJ, Acuff TE. Thoracoscopic resection of mediastinal cysts. Ann Thorac Surg. 1993;56(3):659–60.
25. Fraga JC, Aydogdu B, Aufieri R, Silva GV, Schopf L, Takamatu E, et al. Surgical treatment for pediatric mediastinal neurogenic tumors. Ann Thorac Surg. 2010;90(2):413–8. https://doi.org/10.1016/j.athoracsur.2010.04.086.
26. Fraga JC, Rothenberg S, Kiely E, Pierro A. Video-assisted thoracic surgery resection for pediatric mediastinal neurogenic tumors. J Pediatr Surg. 2012;47(7):1349–53. https://doi.org/10.1016/j.jpedsurg.2012.01.067.
27. Guye E, Lardy H, Piolat C, Bawab F, Becmeur F, Dyon JF, et al. Thoracoscopy and solid tumors in children: a multicenter study. J Laparoendosc Adv Surg Tech A. 2007;17(6):825–9. https://doi.org/10.1089/lap.2007.0043.
28. Lacreuse I, Valla JS, de Lagausie P, Varlet F, Héloury Y, Temporal G, et al. Thoracoscopic resection of neurogenic tumors in children. J Pediatr Surg. 2007;42(10):1725–8. https://doi.org/10.1016/j.jpedsurg.2007.05.030.
29. Partrick DA, Rothenberg SS. Thoracoscopic resection of mediastinal masses in infants and children: an evaluation of technique and results. J Pediatr Surg. 2001;36(8):1165–7. https://doi.org/10.1053/jpsu.2001.25740.
30. Petty JK, Bensard DD, Partrick DA, Hendrickson RJ, Albano EA, Karrer FM. Resection of neurogenic tumors in children: is thoracoscopy superior to thoracotomy? J Am Coll Surg. 2006;203(5):699–703. https://doi.org/10.1016/j.jamcollsurg.2006.07.022.
31. Barrenechea IJ, Fukumoto R, Lesser JB, Ewing DR, Connery CP, Perin NI. Endoscopic resection of thoracic paravertebral and dumbbell tumors. Neurosurgery. 2006;59(6):1195–201; discussion 1201–2. https://doi.org/10.1227/01.NEU.0000245617.39850.C9.

32. Savitt MA, Gao G, Furnary AP, Swanson J, Gately HL, Handy JR. Application of robotic-assisted techniques to the surgical evaluation and treatment of the anterior mediastinum. Ann Thorac Surg. 2005;79(2):450–5; discussion 455. https://doi.org/10.1016/j.athoracsur.2004.07.022.
33. Seong YW, Kang CH, Choi JW, Kim HS, Jeon JH, Park IK et al. Early clinical outcomes of robot-assisted surgery for anterior mediastinal mass: its superiority over a conventional sternotomy approach evaluated by propensity score matching. Eur J Cardiothorac Surg. 2014;45(3):e68–73; discussion e73. https://doi.org/10.1093/ejcts/ezt557.
34. Cerfolio RJ, Bryant AS, Minnich DJ. Operative techniques in robotic thoracic surgery for inferior or posterior mediastinal pathology. J Thorac Cardiovasc Surg. 2012;143(5):1138–43. https://doi.org/10.1016/j.jtcvs.2011.12.021.
35. Negri G, Puglisi A, Gerevini S, Voci C, Zannini P. Thoracoscopic techniques in the management of benign mediastinal dumbbell tumors. Surg Endosc. 2001;15(8):897. https://doi.org/10.1007/s004640042001.
36. Venissac N, Leo F, Hofman P, Paquis P, Mouroux J. Mediastinal neurogenic tumors and video-assisted thoracoscopy: always the right choice? Surg Laparosc Endosc Percutan Tech. 2004;14(1):20–2.
37. Konno S, Yabuki S, Kinoshita T, Kikuchi S. Combined laminectomy and thoracoscopic resection of dumbbell-type thoracic cord tumor. Spine. 2001;26(6):E130–4.
38. McKenna RJ Jr, Maline D, Pratt G. VATS resection of a mediastinal neurogenic dumbbell tumor. Surg Laparosc Endosc. 1995;5(6):480–2.
39. Vallieres E, Findlay JM, Fraser RE. Combined microneurosurgical and thoracoscopic removal of neurogenic dumbbell tumors. Ann Thorac Surg. 1995;59(2):469–72.
40. Heltzer JM, Krasna MJ, Aldrich F, McLaughlin JS. Thoracoscopic excision of a posterior mediastinal "dumbbell" tumor using a combined approach. Ann Thorac Surg. 1995;60(2):431–3.
41. Maeda S, Takahashi S, Koike K, Sato M. Preferred surgical approach for dumbbell-shaped tumors in the posterior mediastinum. Ann Thora Cardiovasc Surg. 2011;17(4):394–6.
42. Ng CS, Wong RH, Hsin MK, Yeung EC, Wan S, Wan IY, et al. Recent advances in video-assisted thoracoscopic approach to posterior mediastinal tumours. Surgeon. 2010;8(5):280–6. https://doi.org/10.1016/j.surge.2010.06.001.
43. Kumar A, Kumar S, Aggarwal S, Khilnani GC. Thoracoscopy: the preferred approach for the resection of selected posterior mediastinal tumors. J Laparoendosc Adv Surg Tech A. 2002;12(5):345–53. https://doi.org/10.1089/109264202320884090.
44. Epstein NE. A review article on the diagnosis and treatment of cerebrospinal fluid fistulas and dural tears occurring during spinal surgery. Surg Neurol Int. 2013;4(Suppl 5):S301–17. https://doi.org/10.4103/2152-7806.111427.
45. Attar S, Hankins JR, Turney SZ, Krasna MJ, McLaughlin JS. Paraplegia after thoracotomy: report of five cases and review of the literature. Ann Thorac Surg. 1995;59(6):1410–5; discussion 1415–6.
46. Saenz NC. Posterior mediastinal neurogenic tumors in infants and children. Semin Pediatr Surg. 1999;8(2):78–84.
47. Wiseman GA, Pacak K, O'Dorisio MS, Neumann DR, Waxman AD, Mankoff DA, et al. Usefulness of 123I-MIBG scintigraphy in the evaluation of patients with known or suspected primary or metastatic pheochromocytoma or paraganglioma: results from a prospective multicenter trial. J Nucl Med. 2009;50(9):1448–54. https://doi.org/10.2967/jnumed.108.058701.
48. Liu L, Mei J, Che G. Asymptomatic paraganglioma of the posterior mediastinum misdiagnosed until operation. Thorac Cardiovasc Surg. 2010;58(5):302–4. https://doi.org/10.1055/s-0029-1185874.
49. Suzawa K, Yamamoto H, Ichimura K, Toyooka S, Miyoshi S. Asymptomatic but functional paraganglioma of the posterior mediastinum. Ann Thorac Surg. 2014;97(3):1077–80. https://doi.org/10.1016/j.athoracsur.2013.06.100.
50. Bouhouch A, Hendriks JM, Lauwers PR, De Raeve HR, Van Schil PE. Asymptomatic pheochromocytoma in the posterior mediastinum. Acta Chir Belg. 2007;107(4):465–7.
51. Ayala-Ramirez M, Feng L, Johnson MM, Ejaz S, Habra MA, Rich T, et al. Clinical risk factors for malignancy and overall survival in patients with pheochromocytomas and sympathetic

paragangliomas: primary tumor size and primary tumor location as prognostic indicators. J Clin Endocrinol Metab. 2011;96(3):717–25. https://doi.org/10.1210/jc.2010-1946.
52. Brown ML, Zayas GE, Abel MD, Young WF Jr, Schaff HV. Mediastinal paragangliomas: the Mayo Clinic experience. Ann Thorac Surg. 2008;86(3):946–51. https://doi.org/10.1016/j.athoracsur.2008.04.105.
53. Spector JA, Willis DN, Ginsburg HB. Paraganglioma (pheochromocytoma) of the posterior mediastinum: a case report and review of the literature. J Pediatr Surg. 2003;38(7):1114–6. https://doi.org/10.1016/S0022-3468(03)00208-2.
54. Kitagawa RS, Satyan KB, Relyea K, Dauser RC, Nuchtern JG, Minifee PK, et al. Video-assisted thorascopic repair of a subarachnoid-pleural fistula in a child after thoracic tumor resection: technical note. Spine. 2010;35(9):E347–50. https://doi.org/10.1097/BRS.0b013e3181d83538.
55. Muraki S, Tanaka A, Miyajima M, Harada R, Watanabe N, Hyodoh H. Adamkiewicz artery demonstrated by MRA for operated posterior mediastinal tumors. Ann Thorac Cardiovasc Surg. 2006;12(4):270–2.
56. Nijenhuis RJ, Jacobs MJ, Jaspers K, Reijnders M, van Engelshoven JMA, Leiner T, et al. Comparison of magnetic resonance with computed tomography angiography for preoperative localization of the Adamkiewicz artery in thoracoabdominal aortic aneurysm patients. J Vasc Surg. 2007;45(4):677–85. https://doi.org/10.1016/j.jvs.2006.11.046.
57. Yoshioka K, Niinuma H, Ehara S, Nakajima T, Nakamura M, Kawazoe K. MR angiography and CT angiography of the artery of Adamkiewicz: state of the art. Radiographics. 2006;26(Suppl 1):S63–73. https://doi.org/10.1148/rg.26si065506.

Part VI

Tracheo-Broncheal Tree

the 1970s revolutionised bronchoscopic examination of the airway [2]. The bronchoscope is an important tool in the armamentarium of a thoracic surgeon; hence a thoracic surgeon must have a clear understanding of both flexible and rigid bronchoscopy, including indications, anaesthetic techniques, instrument options and the management of complications [3]. The bronchoscope has a role in diagnosis and staging and therapeutic and palliative role in the management of patients in a thoracic surgical practice.

22.2 Rigid Bronchoscopy

Rigid bronchoscopes are metallic tubes with a light source, which allow visualisation as well as act as a conduit for ventilation [1, 4]. The scopes are almost always introduced under general anaesthesia. It allows ventilation with jet ventilation based on the Venturi effect. The calibre of the scopes allows instrumentation to perform biopsies and debulking as well as interventions like laser ablation and stenting through the scopes. There are various types of bronchoscopes ranging from simple Negus scopes to the Jackson or Storz ventilating bronchoscopes, which provide separate channels for ventilation and intervention. A range of rigid telescopes is used for inspection of airways viewing with 0-, 30- or 90-degree viewing angle. The 0-degree angle allows wide visualisation of the distal end of the scope, and 90-degree viewing angle is usually used to visualise the upper lobe on the right or the apical segmental orifices of the lower lobe. A fibre-optic bronchoscope may be used in conjunction with rigid bronchoscope.

22.3 Fibre-Optic Bronchoscopy

Flexible bronchoscopy using fibre optics has significantly changed the practice of bronchoscopy [1, 5]. This can be performed either under general anaesthesia or sedation in a spontaneously breathing patient. The scope calibre varies depending on role of bronchoscope from diagnostic to intervention; the balance is in maintaining a smaller size to allow ventilation along the scope at the same time offering adequate channels for biopsy, toileting or interventions like laser. This is particularly important when used through an endotracheal tube. The standard-size scopes are usually 3.5 mm, with a 1.2-mm suction/biopsy port.

22.4 Indications

Indication for bronchoscopy is varied from being a diagnostic tool to an instrument acting as conduit for interventions [1]. The choice of the technique varies according to local practice and expertise; however their utility can be broadly classified as listed in Table 22.1.

Table 22.1 Indications for bronchoscopy

Diagnostic	Staging	Therapeutic	Palliation
Assessment of airway	Fixity and splaying of the carina	Establishing airway	Stenting airways for extrinsic compressions
Assessment of haemoptysis	Assessing tumour extent	Establishing lung isolation in massive haemoptysis	Photodynamic therapy
Biopsy of endoluminal lesions	EBUS of mediastinal nodes in lung cancer	Photodynamic therapy	Laser/cryoablations
Washing and brushing from mucosal lesions		Tracheal dilatation	Palliation of endoluminal malignancy with endoluminal interventions
Transbronchial aspiration and biopsy		Endoscopic resection of endoluminal lesions	
A conduit for endobronchial ultrasound and biopsy (EBUS)		Laser/cryoablations	
Chartis assessment for collateral ventilation in endoscopic volume reduction		Stenting for benign conditions	
		Tracheobronchial toileting	
		Guiding percutaneous tracheostomy	
		Deploying endobronchial valves	
		Deploying endobronchial coils	
		Removal of foreign bodies	

22.5 Instruments

22.5.1 Rigid Bronchoscope

The scope needs a light source, which offers light to the bronchoscope; it requires an adapter to connect to the Sanders jet insufflator which is used to inject oxygen. The scope has fenestrations on the side of the scope to draw air along with the insufflated oxygen using the Venturi principle. The department should have the selection of telescopes to inspect the airway (Fig. 22.1).

22.5.1.1 Adjuncts

A wide-bore rigid suction tube is a usual accompaniment to the bronchoscope to clear secretions. A selection of straight and angled biopsy forceps is available to biopsy the lesions. Some forceps are enabled to incorporate a straight telescope to biopsy with clearer magnified vision. A fibre-optic scope may be used with a rigid scope to perform various interventions.

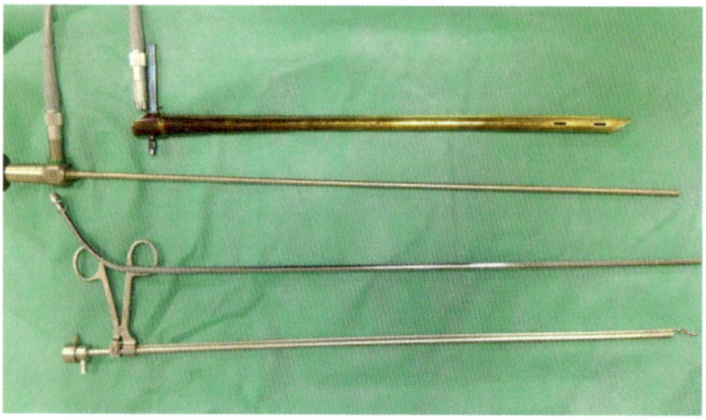

Fig. 22.1 Rigid bronchoscopy kit which includes a rigid bronchoscope, telescope with light cables, suction and biopsy forceps

22.5.2 Fibre-Optic Bronchoscope

Fibre-optic bronchoscopes come with a light source in varying sizes and a suction and biopsy channel. The flexible scope can be used by viewing directly through the eyepiece or by connecting it to a camera and viewing it on a magnified screen. The images and videos can be captured for the record. The interventional bronchoscopes come with a wider interventional channel to allow the deploying device. Most manufacturers make endoscopes in smaller version that has a standard-size suction/biopsy channel. This allows the procedure to be performed through endotracheal tubes.

22.5.2.1 Adjuncts

A port adapter for the endotracheal tube is required when performing a flexible bronchoscopy through an endotracheal tube. Additional adjuncts include biopsy forceps, disposable brushes, basket forceps for foreign body extraction, sputum traps, irrigation catheters and biopsy/injection needles. Endobronchial ultrasonogram (EBUS) uses special scopes, which have an ultrasonic probe. Interventions like laser, cryotherapy, endobronchial valves and coil deployments require specific equipment.

22.6 Anaesthetic Considerations

Flexible endoscopy is mostly performed by the physicians with the aid of a topical anaesthetic and intravenous sedation with established guidelines [5]. The procedure is performed in a dedicated bronchoscopy unit with an endoscopy nurse. Most thoracic surgeons perform the flexible bronchoscopy under general anaesthesia through an endotracheal tube or rigid bronchoscope.

The patients should be monitored with an electrocardiogram, non-invasive blood pressure monitor and pulse oximeter. The patient should be given supplemental oxygen before, during and after the procedure. The choice of the sedative and local anaesthetic agents varies between units with midazolam being the most preferred agent drug because of its sedative and amnesiac effects.

A choice of methods is available for administration of local anaesthesia for bronchoscopy. The procedure is commenced with lidocaine spray of the oropharynx with supplemental lidocaine delivered locally through the bronchoscope on to the vocal cords and trachea. Some surgeons prefer percutaneous supplementation via the cricothyroid membrane or inhaled nebulized lidocaine.

Post procedure patient should be monitored at least for two hours.

Rigid bronchoscopy is performed under general anaesthesia with short-acting agents like propofol. As the procedure is both highly stimulating and painful to the patient, it requires a deep plane of anaesthesia for short periods of time. This also requires total muscular relaxation with bolus doses of relaxants to give 45–60 s of complete relaxation. For bronchoscopy, the surgeon must be ready to intubate the trachea as soon as deep anaesthesia has been reached [3].

22.6.1 Performing the Procedure

22.6.1.1 Flexible Bronchoscopy

Flexible bronchoscopy is usually performed from the right side of the patient with the operator facing the head of the bed in the endoscopy unit; the surgeon stands at the head end when using in conjunction with a rigid scope in theatre. The orientation hence needs to be absolutely correct. The bronchoscope is held in the non-dominant hand (usually left hand), leaving the other hand free to manipulate the scope and perform the instrumentation down the biopsy/suction channel. The choice of transnasal or oral approach depends on the preference of the operator. The advantage of transnasal approach is it offers a stable platform and a more direct approach to the larynx because of the fixation through the nares as opposed to the oral route, which requires flexion of the scope around the tongue and the epiglottis within a short distance. Either way, there is complete visualisation of the airway from the vocal cords down. It must be appreciated that bronchoscopy through an endotracheal tube does not allow visualisation of the larynx or the upper trachea. The inspection of the airway is best performed on the way in to avoid any impact on the airway due to potential scope trauma.

22.6.1.2 Rigid Bronchoscopy

Rigid bronchoscopy is performed from the head of the bed. The patient's head is placed with the neck extended and chin flexed or in an exaggerated sniffing position. This allows access through the oropharynx into the trachea. The frontal teeth are protected with a swab or mouth guard. The rigid scope is passed with the right hand; the thumb and forefinger of the left hand are used as a fulcrum to stabilise the scope and to protect the lips and teeth. In patients with prominent or wobbly tooth, the scope can be passed from the angle of the mouth; however it is important to aim the scope towards midline. The scope is passed beyond the tongue till the epiglottis is visualised. The tip of the bronchoscope is used to hook and elevate the epiglottis, which reveals the vocal cords. Hyperextension of the neck or advancing the scope too far will result in the scope entering the oesophagus. Once the vocal cords are visualised, the scope is rotated 90 degrees to allow the bevelled tip to negotiate the cords with least trauma. The tracheobronchial tree is inspected to the carina by advancing the scope slowly using the thumb and forefinger as a fulcrum. Rotating the patient's head in the opposite direction to straighten the alignment of the bronchus allows the main stem bronchial inspection. The head is turned to the left for right bronchial intubation and vice versa [3, 4].

22.7 Diagnostic Bronchoscopy

Diagnostic bronchoscopy is performed mostly with the flexible bronchoscope by the physicians; however if the patient cannot tolerate sedation or deoxygenates, it is done under a general anaesthesia with or without a rigid bronchoscope.

Once the basics are checked, bronchoscope is introduced observing the cords, trachea for any tracheomalacia and carina for the sharpness.

22.7.1 Flexible Bronchoscopy

- Always ensure the kit is working ensuring that light source, optic connections to the video screen and suction are all working.
- Depending on the procedure, ensure the channels are adequate for biopsy, suction or deploying catheters.
- Ensure the biopsy forceps are working.
- Adequate sedation, local anaesthetic and oxygen are available to last the procedure.
- Sputum traps to collect secretions for microbiology and washing cytology.
- Availability of adequate lubricants.
- An assistant to help and monitor the patient.
- Always check consent and brief the team of procedure.
- Ensure cold saline wash is available if needed.
- Enter the normal side first and then the side with the problem to avoid spilling infection or tumour dissemination.

22.7.2 Rigid Bronchoscopy

- Same as above.
- Ensure the light channels are not blocked.
- Ensure a good fit on the Sanders jet ventilation port and advice anaesthetist to hold to avoid inadvertent injury to the surgeon if the connector comes off whilst jetting.
- Appreciate the difference between endotracheal intubation and bronchoscopy and ensure positioning appropriately.
- Ensure lubrication is on the tip and not all along the scope obliterating the ventilating side holes as this reduces the ventilatory impact and may jet the lubricants into distal airways.

- Have a clear plan regarding the sequence of events both for diagnostics as well as intervention.
- If there was a need for radiological screening, ensure radiographer and radiologist are present and all staff are protected with lead aprons.
- If there was a need for laser, ensure all eyes are protected with laser goggles including patient and the doors are locked and marked 'laser in progress'.

22.7.2.1 Preoperative Bronchoscopy

It is a good practice for the surgeon to perform by the operating surgeons in all patients prior to cancer resection within 6 weeks.

The advantages of performing a preoperative bronchoscopy are as follows:

- To confirm the anatomy particularly the distance of the right upper lobe take off from the carina to enable anaesthetist in planning the correct double-lumen tube placement. A high take off of the upper lobe may require a left-sided tube or a bronchial blocker option.
- To check for any mucosal skip lesions and assess the resection limits in endobronchial tumours, i.e. lobectomy versus sleeve resection.
- Finally to clear the secretions preoperatively.

The surgeon also can assist the anaesthetist with isolation of the lungs by placing an intubation bougie, which can be used to rail road the double-lumen tube.

If the anaesthetist is struggling to get a double-lumen tube, the surgeon can place the DLET on the zero degree telescopes and place it under direct vision using a laryngoscope instead of rigid scope (Fig. 22.2).

22.7.2.2 Biopsy

The biopsies can be done with standard biopsy forceps or a biopsy forceps with a telescope as in a Storz scope. It is essential to ensure the lesion is sampled from the centre after clearing the covering debris. Bleeding can be controlled with pressure with a pledget with or without adrenaline or cold saline lavage. It is important to ensure the pledget is radiopaque and a long string is sutured to the pledget to enable retrieval if it slips. If bleeding is significant, that can be controlled by various adjuncts like cautery, laser or argon beam.

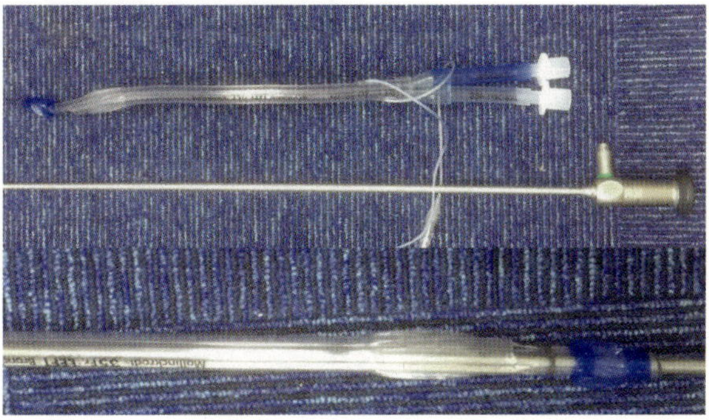

Fig. 22.2 Bronchoscope aiding placement of double lumen tube: The Endotracheal tube is straightened, the zero degree telescope is advanced into the bronchial lumen to the tip. The DLET is placed with the bronchoscope in-situ with a laryngoscope to aid intubation under vision. The bronchoscope guides the placement of the tube into selective bronchus

If a definite lesion is not visualised, it is important to take brush biopsies and washing from various suspicious areas and label them correctly.

22.7.2.3 Assessment of Tracheal Stenosis

Tracheal stenosis either due to benign or malignant causes should be assessed with a bronchoscopy to plan remedial intervention in the same sitting or in a planned setting further. In most causes the bronchoscopy in itself alleviates the narrowing to a certain extent with the bronchoscope acting as a dilator as well.

- Assessment of a tracheal narrowing is best performed under general anaesthesia as mostly the patients have respiratory compromise due to the narrowing.
- The pre-procedural briefing both to the theatre team and anaesthetist is of paramount importance in this setting.
- Plans should be in place to establish an airway including a surgical airway in a patient with critical airway stenosis.
- The muscle relaxant is given only once the surgeon is in a position with all his equipment checked and is ready to place the scope as soon as the patient is paralysed.
- It is useful to start with an adolescent scope to negotiate the narrowing.

The surgeon introduces the scope carefully and inspects the airway if the narrowing will allow the passage of the scope. The scope is advanced beyond the narrowing to the level of the carina. At this point the assistant ties a suture on the bronchoscope at the level of the incisor. The scope is gently pulled back to the distal extent of the narrowing, and the second suture is placed on the scope at the level of incisors. It is important to mark this at the level of the mucosal abnormality than the physical narrowing. The scope is pulled back to the proximal narrowing and to the cords with two further sutures marking the levels. The scope now offers an inverse image of the trachea with the extent of narrowing as well the distance from the cords and trachea which allows planning of further interventions [4] (Fig. 22.3).

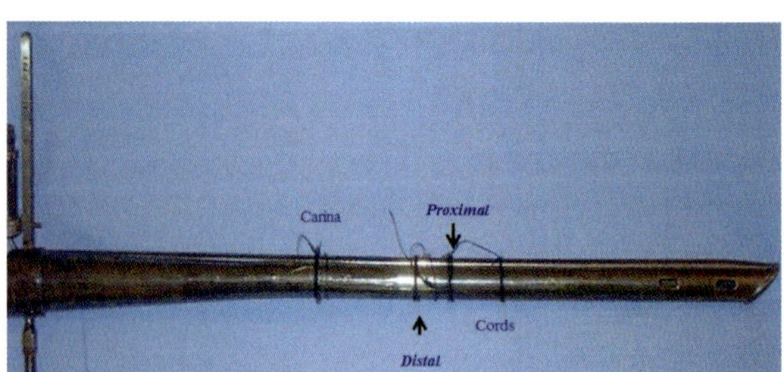

Fig. 22.3 Assessment of tracheal stenosis. The suture closes to the tip marks the cords, followed by proximal stenosis then distal stenosis and finally the carina. The bronchoscope offers an inverse image of the trachea

22.8 Staging with Bronchoscopy

22.8.1 Assessment with Rigid Bronchoscope

A rigid scope assesses the extent of direct invasion based on the site of the tumour; it assesses the presence of sub-carinal nodal extent as evidenced by a splayed carina. The presence of tumour and extrinsic compression can be judged by the lateral bowing of the trachea from midline in mediastinal masses and malignancies.

Moving the scope laterally can assess the fixity of the carina as the fixed carina will offer resistance.

22.8.2 Transbronchial Needle Aspiration and Endobronchial Ultrasound

The fibre-optic bronchoscopes are used for EBUS, and this allows sampling of the various nodal stations. Transbronchial needle aspiration allows sampling of nodes by needle aspiration [6]. The advent of EBUS has added a safety aspect to this with the operator visualising the nodes in real time, whilst biopsy is performed. EBUS is a safe and effective technique for the assessment of hilar and mediastinal lymph nodes in lung cancer [7]. Endobronchial ultrasound has greatly reduced the number of cervical mediastinoscopies due the yield of diagnosis. The technique and tools are beyond the scope of this chapter.

22.9 Therapeutic Bronchoscopy

22.9.1 Tracheobronchial Toilet

Ensure all the necessary kits are available. A rigid bronchoscope and rigid sucker offer the ability to ventilate and clear suction rapidly. The flexible bronchoscope may then be introduced. Once the scope is in, it is important to clear the trachea of any secretions which is collected in the trap. As always the normal side is cleared first with the bronchoscope clearing all lobar orifices. It may be useful to use a flexible bronchoscope to clear sub-lobar bronchial orifices.

22.9.2 Dilation of Tracheal Stenosis

Dilatation of the trachea is one of the most important therapeutic interventions with a rigid bronchoscope. A variety of dilators are available to dilate the trachea.

The Porjees dilator is a silastic dilator, whilst the Chevalier Jackson is a wooden-tipped dilator mounted on a long metallic stem (Fig. 22.4).

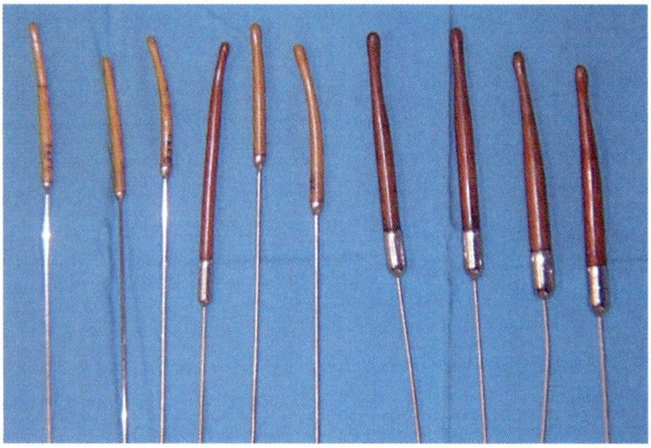

Fig. 22.4 Chevalier Jackson tracheal dilators

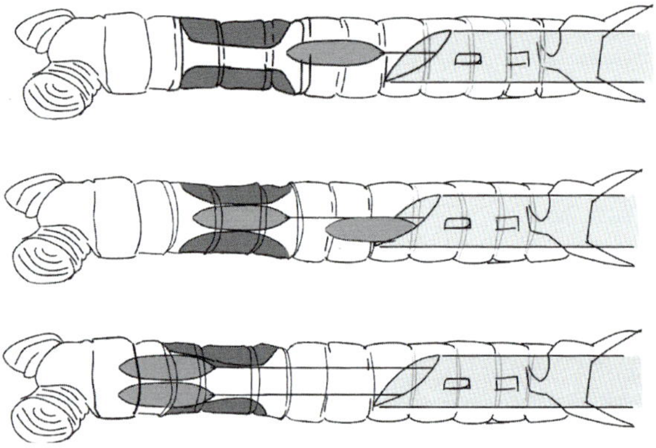

Fig. 22.5 Tracheal dilatation using two dilator to incrementally dilate the stenosis without being limited by the diameter of the bronchoscope

The rigid bronchoscope is placed to secure the airway. The scope is placed proximal to the stenosis. The dilators are introduced in gradually increments with lubrication to gently dilate the trachea. The sizes of the dilators are limited by the size of the scope as the larger the dilator, it obstructs the lumen and affects the jet ventilation.

A useful technique is to introduce the Chevalier Jackson dilator beyond the tip of the scope and past the stenosis. A second dilator is passed similarly beyond the stenosis. The two dilators are gently pulled back together that way it offers a wider dilating diameter and preserves a ventilatory lumen (Fig. 22.5). Once the dilator has dilated the lumen to allow the tip of the bronchoscope, the tip is advanced using the body of the scope as a dilator. Maximum dilatation can be achieved by turning the head to the left and advancing the scope into the right main bronchus.

The scope is left in position for a few minutes to disrupt the fibrotic strands of the stricture with sustained pressure.

Dilatation can be repeated at periodic intervals, and surgery can be reserved to patients with failed serial dilatation.

There are balloon inflatable dilators which can be used in gradual increments to dilate strictures. The balloon dilators can also be used with a flexible bronchoscope.

22.9.3 Ablation of Endobronchial Tumours

Bronchoscopy is an essential technique in obliteration of the endobronchial tumours both for therapeutic and palliative purposes [8]. It is imperative to have preoperative images and an MDT discussion to enable a firm preoperative plan. Depending on the local practice of the unit, there are various options available for the surgeon to deal with endobronchial lesions each with varying mode of action depending on local practice [3, 9] (Fig. 22.6).

Electrocautery uses high-frequency electric current to cause heating which leads to coagulation at lower temperatures or tissue vaporisation at higher temperatures which is used to ablate endoluminal tumours [10]. Electrocautery attached to insulated long forceps can be used to fulgurate and excise tissue as well as control bleeding whilst debulking or resecting tumour. It is important to check the forceps are insulated and only the tip can discharge the current. Argon plasma coagulator is a non-contact mode of electrocautery that causes desiccation and coagulation of exophytic endobronchial tumours and provides rapid haemostasis in haemoptysis arising from visible endobronchial lesions [11]. Laser therapy uses the heat energy from laser light to coagulate and vaporise endobronchial tissue [12]. Most current work is performed using Nd:YAG laser. Laser ablation requires the standard laser precautions including eye protection laser safety training and correct equipment.

Photodynamic therapy (PDT) uses laser light (usually 630 Nm at the red end of the spectrum) which in the presence of sensitiser and oxygen causes tumour cell death by a complex pathway triggered by the release of singlet oxygen [13]. A systemic photosensitiser like haematoporphyrin derivative, which is selectively retained and concentrated in tumour tissue, is used to render the tumour sensitive to light of a given wavelength.

Cryotherapy is a technique used to deep freeze the lesions, arrest bleeding or ablate tumours.

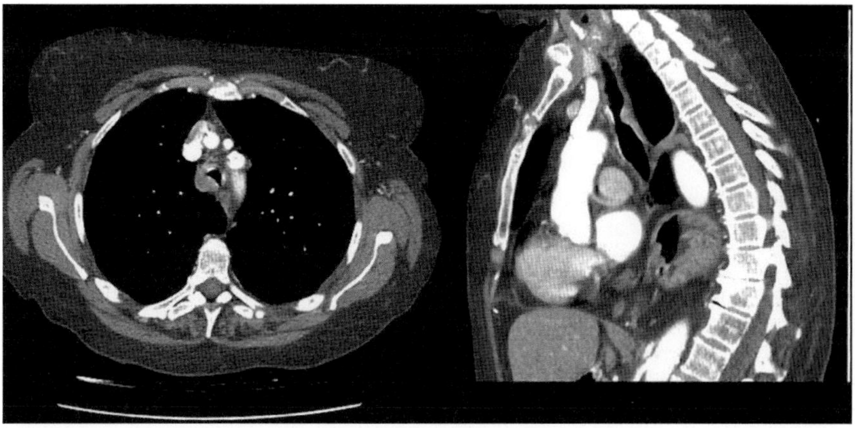

Fig. 22.6 CT demonstrating endotracheal tumour. The cross section and reconstructed image demonstrating the endoluminal component of the tracheal tumour which was laser ablated

Cryotherapy uses extreme cold to cause delayed local destruction of tissue [14]. Standard cryotherapy is performed when the cryoprobe is inserted through the instrument channel of a bronchoscope and applied directly to the target tissue. Freezing and thawing in repeated cycles leading to tissue necrosis ablate the target tissue. A further bronchoscopy is performed to extract and to remove necrotic material. Cryoextraction is performed with probes, which allow removal of the extracted debris of tumour in the same sitting.

Brachytherapy offers localised radiation through bronchoscopy both for curative and palliative malignant conditions [15].

- Electrocautery and laser have to be used cautiously with suspension of jet ventilation when deploying for the risk of the fire hazard.
- The laser fibre is passed through the biopsy channel of the flexible bronchoscope.
- The laser is directed on to the tumour ensuring it is parallel to the bronchial tree to avoid perforation of the bronchial wall.
- It is important to extract the smoke as it impairs vision; sometimes it may be necessary to have an additional suction catheter next to the flexible scope as the flexible scope extraction will be restricted by the laser fibre in the channel. Depending on the size of the endobronchial lesion, sometimes it may be useful to core or debulk the volume and laser the base.
- It is important to document the duration of laser ablation and the energy used in joules in the medical documentation.
- Patients undergoing endobronchial ablation may go into respiratory failure following the procedure due to CO2 retention, smoke injury as well as reperfusion to the lobe which may cause an obstructive hypoxic vasoconstriction. So it is important to offer them immediate post-operative ventilatory support in the immediate post-operative period even if it is palliative laser ablation.

22.9.4 Stenting of the Airway

Tracheobronchial stenting as explained earlier could be done under general anaesthesia or local anaesthesia using either fibre-optic or rigid bronchoscope. It is important to measure the length of the stenosis with the preoperative CT scan and bronchoscopy. Whilst using a rigid bronchoscope, ventilation is continued, and the stent loading devices are introduced into the bronchoscope and placed at the optimum position. They can be repositioned using the biopsy forceps; however metallic uncovered stents will prove to be a challenge especially if there is the tumour bulk. Stents using fibre-optic scope are passed through the biopsy channel. It is advantageous to use fluoroscopic guidance with a C Arm.

The bronchoscope is advanced to the level of the stenosis with the tip of the bronchoscope positioned at the proximal extent of the stenosis. A long metallic sucker is placed on the patient's chest and is advanced to correlate with the bronchoscope tip under fluoroscopic guidance. Once both are in concordance a needle

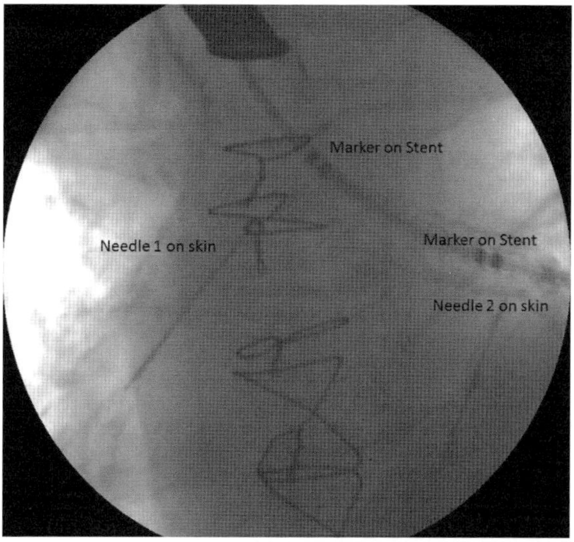

Fig. 22.7 Tracheal stent. Tracheobronchial stenting of the right main bronchus under fluoroscopic guidance. The skin needles mark the proximal and distal extent of the narrowing. The stent markers are aligned to the marker and deployed

is placed on the chest to mark the site. The site is then marked with a needle on the skin. The scope is then passed beyond the stenosis to the distal extent of the stenosis. The procedure is repeated with a second needle placed marking the distal extent of the narrowing. The stent guide wire is passed through the fibre-optic scope and negotiated beyond the stenosis. The stent is loaded onto the guide wire and placed in the optimum position. The radiological markers are aligned to the two needles which are on the skin surface to ensure it is positioned in a satisfactory position (Fig. 22.7). The stent is deployed whilst screening continuously ensuring that the position is accurate.

As the stent is in a satisfactory position, a fibre-optic scope is passed beyond the stent to clear all the secretions. Always ensure that once the stent is in position, save screenshots of placement and immediate post-operative chest radiograph as a benchmark of the position of the stent.

22.9.5 Removal of Foreign Bodies

Foreign body aspiration presents usually with the classical triad of paroxysmal coughing, wheezing and diminished breath sounds on the affected side particularly in children. Acute presentations of foreign bodies may facilitate removal; however chronic presentations usually present with the effects of the obstruction making bronchoscopic removal challenging.

Most foreign bodies are removed with rigid bronchoscopy offering control of the airway enabling ventilation of the patient, whilst the foreign body is removed. Various options are available to the surgeon including sophisticated optical grasping forceps, snares, Dormia stone basket or Fogarty balloon [4]. One scenario where removal is challenging is peanuts as the arachis oil induces a local chemical inflammation making the removal difficult.

22.9.6 Guide to Tracheostomy

Tracheostomy tubes are often placed in the intensive care unit by the Seldinger technique. Bronchoscopy acts as a guide to placing the tracheostomy safely. It has reduced the subglottic placement at the advent of introduction of percutaneous tracheostomy whilst resulted in a complex problem of subglottis stenosis if the patient developed a stenosis.

Points to consider:

- Rigid bronchoscope offers the option of ventilating, whilst the percutaneous tracheostomy is performed. It also offers a rigid support which is useful whilst dilating the trachea.
- A flexible bronchoscope can be introduced through an endotracheal tube.
- The operator has to be careful when introducing the needles to avoid damage to the flexible scope.

22.10 Endobronchial Volume Reduction

Bronchoscopic techniques are constantly evolving to offer a better quality of life for patients with advanced emphysema [16]. Endobronchial valves are deployed bronchoscopically in the treatment of patients with emphysema with severe hyperinflation. The valves are inserted into the target area of the lungs via flexible bronchoscopy under conscious sedation or general anaesthesia. The valves prevent air entering the target lobe whilst allowing air and secretions to exit. The technique includes assessment for collateral ventilation using a special catheter called the Chartis catheter. The valves are preloaded into the deploying device which is passed through the biopsy channel and deployed at the orifice of the target bronchus.

Endobronchial coils use nitinol coils which are believed to improve symptoms by improving elasticity of the lungs [17]. The coils are placed through the bronchoscope. First a guide wire is advanced into segmental bronchus, and the coils are then straightened in the applicator. The coils are then deployed into the bronchus, and once the deployer is removed, the coils assume their curved shape due to the shape memory.

22.11 Rare Utility of Bronchoscopy

A rigid bronchoscope can be used as a tool to establish an airway in the acute setting in the intensive care unit with slipped tracheostomy tubes. The scope allows visualisation of the airway perorally to guide in replacing the tracheostomy tube under vision.

In dire emergency in a patient with a tracheostomy tract, the fibre-optic bronchoscope can be used to visualise the tract to reposition the tracheostomy tube. Alternatively if the rigid scope was available that can be used to enter the trachea through the tracheostomy tract, this establishes an airway to ventilate and buy time for a definitive airway by way of an endotracheal tube or tracheostomy tube.

However the rigid scope into tracheostomy has to be used as with extreme caution in experienced hands only when there is a definitive tract.

22.12 Bronchoscopy Training

Bronchoscopy is an essential skill, which general thoracic surgical trainees need to attain competency. Both rigid and flexible bronchoscopy should be part of training curriculum for thoracic trainees with rigid bronchoscopy as a lifesaving skill in an emergency [3]. Teaching this skill has been a challenging prospect in the part due to the nature of the procedure.

- The trainee needs to understand the anatomy and technical principles with the ability to perform the procedure before the patient desaturates due to hypoxia.
- It is useful to train in non-emergent elective preoperative patients initially to master the technique before performing interventional procedure.
- The recent advent of simulation mannequins enables the surgeon to teach the trainees without patient care getting compromised.
- The surgeon then has to break the procedure into parts and allow the trainee to perform them. The most difficult aspect is getting into the trachea by hooking the epiglottis and negotiating the cords.
- The surgeon should observe the trainee with a teaching scope or the video screen with the new bronchoscopy system.
- The surgeon can assess and feedback to the trainee with a structured procedure-based assessment tool (PBA).

Conclusion

Bronchoscopy is an essential tool in the surgeon's armamentarium. Thoracic surgeons must become expert endoscopists, and it is the ability to perform rigid endoscopy that distinguishes them from their medical counterparts and gives a distinct advantage when performing therapeutic procedures [3]. It is imperative to train thoracic surgical trainees in the art of rigid endoscopy as this is a lifesaving skill, which will be an invaluable skill in their career.

Acknowledgements Late Mr FJ Collins for imparting the wisdom of bronchoscopic techniques to many consultants in the United Kingdom.

Akhash V Rathinam for illustrations.

References

1. Warren W, Faber P. Bronchoscopic evaluation of the lungs and tracheobronchial tree. In: Shields T, LoCicero J, Reed C, Fiens R, editors. General thoracic surgery. Philadelphia: Lippincott Williams & Wilkins; 2009. p. 286–7.
2. Ikeda S, Yanai N, Ishikawa S. Flexible bronchofiberscope. Keio J Med. 1968;**17**:1–16.

combination of well-planned anesthetic airway management, meticulous operative technique, and careful postoperative care.

It is imperative when working on the airway to focus on patient's symptoms as many of the treatment methodologies focus on symptom relief, rather than improvement in any one quantitative endpoint. In addition, a full understanding of the patient's primary underlying disease is needed to coordinate timing of an intervention and to optimize a successful outcome.

Post-intubation tracheal stenosis is now uncommon with the advent of high-volume low-pressure cuff tubes and careful management of the ventilated ICU patient. However, this is still the most common etiology for which tracheal resection and reconstruction are considered. Cuff injuries occur because of prolonged pressure with resultant full-thickness necrosis of the tracheal cartilage. This produces circumferential scar contracture with symptoms typically developing 3–6 weeks after extubation (Fig. 23.1a). Stomal stenosis after tracheostomy occurs when there is a large anterior tracheal defect from the tracheostomy stoma with subsequent anterior scar contracture when the patient is decanulated. This etiology of tracheal stenosis typically results in an "A-frame" appearance, with anterior narrowing and relatively normal posterior membranous wall (Fig. 23.1b).

Tip: While the circumferential scar formation of a cuff-induced tracheal stenosis is readily amenable to tracheal dilatation, a stomal stenosis usually has no benefit from tracheal dilatation. The normal posterior membranous wall is compliant and gives away to the dilating force but then rebounds to its normal position when the dilatation is complete. This prevents any meaningful impact on the area of anterior scar.

Other etiologies of benign tracheal stenosis are trauma, inflammatory, or idiopathic. Patients with a neck or chest injury or operative trauma to the airway may sometimes be undetected at the time of injury but present later because of secondary tracheal narrowing. Severe tracheal infections and a number of collagen vascular diseases may result in acute and chronic inflammation with secondary tracheal stenosis. Idiopathic tracheal stenosis occurs most commonly in women from the third to sixth decade of life, most commonly focused at the level of the cricoid cartilage with varying degrees of subglottic involvement.

Tumors of the trachea are extremely uncommon and present only 0.2% of all malignancies of the respiratory tract. Squamous cell carcinoma and adenoid cystic carcinoma are the two most common tracheal tumors and account for more than two-thirds of all primary tumors of the upper airway. Squamous cell carcinoma is primarily a disease of smokers, and the peak incidence is in the sixth and seventh decades with a male predominance. Patients with adenoid cystic carcinoma have a fairly even age distribution from the third to the seventh decade and are evenly distributed between the sexes. After squamous cell carcinoma and adenoid cystic carcinoma, the most common tracheal tumors are carcinoid and mucoepidermoid tumors. However there is a wide variety of rare tumors with varying degrees of malignancy from both epithelial and mesenchymal origins.

Tip: It is important to understand that virtually all tracheal tumors involve the full thickness of the trachea and may extend into the paratracheal tissue and thus are

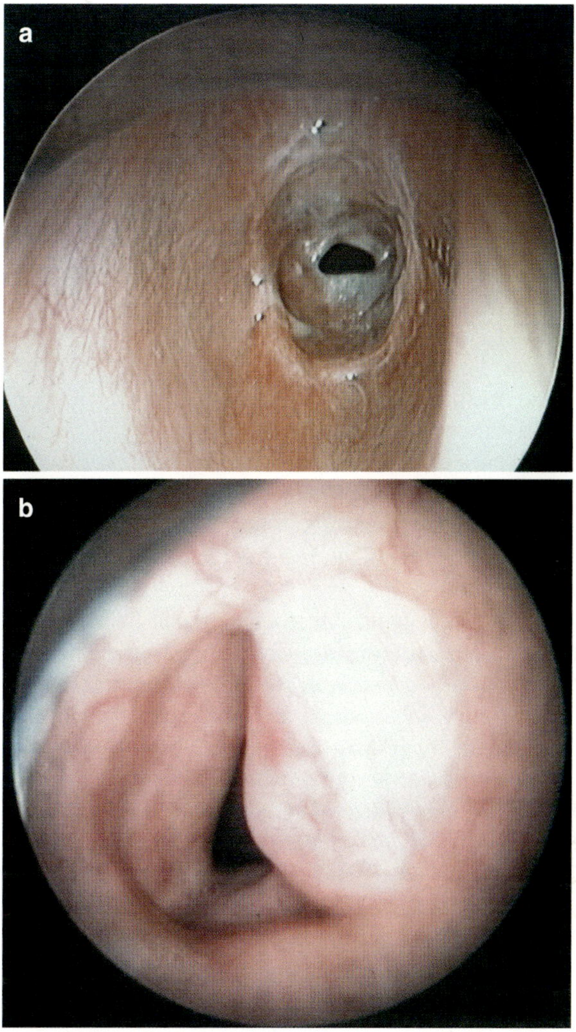

Fig. 23.1 (**a**) Typical circumferential scar formation of a post-intubation tracheal stenosis of cuff etiology. (**b**) Anterior "A-frame" appearance of a post-tracheostomy stomal stenosis with anterior narrowing and a normal posterior membranous wall

extremely unlikely to be cured with endoscopic management. Initial endoscopic management may appear in encouraging because of the long natural history of these tumors, particularly adenoid cystic carcinoma and mucoepidermoid tumors. However, resection with primary reconstruction is the treatment of choice for nearly all tracheal tumors.

The prognosis for untreated tracheal tumors is poor even with benign tumors, due to the risk of airway obstruction. Tumors of the trachea should be considered for resection if they can be removed with less than half of the longitudinal length of the trachea and do not have unresectable local extension into surrounding structures. Radiation plays an important role as an adjunct to surgery, since at best there are narrow surgical margins after tracheal resection and reconstruction for primary tumors. Centers with large experience in these tumors routinely recommend postoperative radiation for both squamous cell and adenoid cystic carcinoma, even in the absence of nodal metastases or positive margins. Fast neutron radiation has had favorable results with minor salivary gland tumors of the head and neck and so is often considered as an alternative treatment for unresectable adenoid cystic carcinoma of the trachea.

23.2 Patient Assessment

23.2.1 Symptoms and Signs

The diagnosis of airway disease can be delayed secondary to the gradual onset of disease process and compensatory mechanisms of the patient. Often symptoms such as dyspnea on exertion can be missed as the patients have either underlying cardiac or pulmonary disorders or slowly accommodate to their gradual worsening of symptoms. Asking patients about concomitant symptoms such as wheezing, problems with clearing secretions, recurrent infections, and stridor can help isolate the airway in a diagnosis.

Tip: Patients with symptomatic tracheal stenosis often have a prolonged history of adult-onset asthma that is refractory to standard therapies. The unusual symptom of stridor associated with an undiagnosed tracheal stenosis is often mistaken for "wheezing" since asthma and associated bronchospasm are far more commonly encountered by primary care physicians.

Symptoms of central airway obstruction can be surprisingly insidious and may often go undiagnosed for a long period of time. Dyspnea on exertion is the primary symptom in patients with a significant tracheal stenosis, but these patients may also present with wheezing, stridor, cough, difficulty clearing secretions, recurrent respiratory infections, or hoarseness. Patients with tracheal or bronchial tumors may also present with any of the previous symptoms but in addition may have hemoptysis. A careful history should elicit evidence of previous neck or chest trauma, prolonged intubation or tracheostomy, or symptoms of primary malignancy or mediastinal malignancy invading other nearby structures. An assessment of the severity of symptoms and their time course is useful for an establishing the etiology and the acuity of the airway pathology. A 50% reduction in the cross-sectional area of the trachea usually results in dyspnea only with significant exertion, while narrowing of the lumen to less than 25% of the cross-sectional area usually produces dyspnea and stridor at rest. Patients may be reasonably compensated in spite of significant stenosis but can have acute life-threatening deterioration with a minor amount of airway edema or secretions. A high index of suspicion in the presence of these symptoms is critical to the diagnosis of central airway pathology.

In some of these patients, the physical exam can be normal or near normal. Usually however, a patient will have a protracted phase of respiration, wheezing, stridor, or weak or hoarse voice from diminished airflow across the vocal cords.

Signs of airflow obstruction may include increased bronchial breath sounds, inspiratory and expiratory vibration over the sternum, the use of accessory muscles of respiration, or signs of retained secretions or obstructive pneumonia. Neck or chest scars may suggest previous trauma or surgical interventions that may be the etiology of current airway pathology.

23.2.2 Preoperative Workup

Quantitative evaluation of the patient should be centered on radiologic and bronchoscopic means. A plain posterior-anterior and lateral chest X-ray often will provide evidence of proximal airway narrowing, while distal lesions are often diagnosed with findings of airway obstruction such as atelectasis and air bronchograms. An overpenetrated view of the trachea with anteroposterior, lateral, and oblique views can further define the presence of a tracheal tumor or stricture. Computed tomography (CT) is very important in the evaluation of airway malignancy, providing the best definition of the size and local extent of the lesion as well as possible involvement in the surrounding structures. Fine-cut helical CT with sagittal and coronal reconstruction also provides a very good definition of tracheobronchial anatomy for benign lesions. Dynamic CT or magnetic resonance imaging (MRI) may provide radiologic documentation of tracheobronchial malacia with evidence of central airway collapse or distal air trapping.

Tip: Spirometry and flow-volume loops are neither sensitive nor specific when diagnosing central airway pathology. They lead little in the decision-making management of these patients and should neither sway a practitioner to delay or proceed with treatment.

Bronchoscopy is critically important for the diagnosis and initial evaluation of tracheobronchial pathology. Bronchoscopy provides the most accurate evaluation of the nature and extent of airway pathology. It allows identification of the anatomic location and diameter of the lesion and its relation to important landmarks such as the cricoid cartilage and carina. It also allows identification of inflammation and erythema as well as evidence of submucosal extension of tumor.

Flexible bronchoscopy is most often performed as an initial method as it is well tolerated under minimal anesthesia and allows for dynamic evaluation of the airway in an awake patient. Due to the fact that flexible bronchoscopy can precipitate airway obstruction in some patients, a practitioner should have an understanding and access to rigid bronchoscopy as well. Rigid bronchoscopy provides the best means for airway control and emergency airway palliation and should be available as a routine management option for physicians evaluating airway obstruction. In cases of critical tracheal obstruction or bronchial obstruction, rigid bronchoscopy with dilatation, core-out of tumor, laser, or stenting provides effective temporary palliation, allowing completion of the medical workup and elective timing of surgical intervention. Rigid bronchoscopy also allows for more flexibility in treatment such as balloon dilation, laser treatment, and debulking of lesions. Rigid bronchoscopy in particular allows for the user to more accurately map out the severity and longitudinal extent of airway lesions as well as their relation to structures such as the carina and vocal cords. Biopsies of lesions can and should be taken, and an evaluation of tissue proximal and distal to the lesion should be assessed when planning a resection.

Tip: Patients with symptomatic central airway obstruction should have their initial bronchoscopy procedure performed in an operating suite with access to rigid bronchoscopy, including anesthesiologists and nurses experienced with interventional bronchoscopy procedures.

Tip: Rigid bronchoscopy allows simultaneously ventilation through the bronchoscope while visualizing the anatomy and initiating therapeutic interventions. This is the safest and most reliable way to assure a safe airway during initial endoscopic assessments.

Trick: Many bronchoscopists prefer intermittent ventilation or high-frequency jet ventilation during rigid bronchoscopy. However, standard ventilation through a side port of the bronchoscope allows ongoing ventilatory support during visualization and therapeutic interventions. This also avoids the noise and aerosolization of blood and secretions that accompany jet ventilation.

Tip: Close coordination with the anesthesiologist allows efficient initiation and pauses in ventilation when the circuit is temporarily open for biopsy, suctioning, or other interventions.

23.2.3 Initial Management

Most patients will present electively or semi-electively with progressive symptoms that lead to the diagnosis of airway pathology. However some patients may present with acute respiratory distress due to acute progression of their stenosis or due to an exacerbating illness such as an upper respiratory tract infection. In these patients, prompt intervention can be lifesaving, and immediate efforts should be made to stabilize the airway.

Tip: Endotracheal intubation may be impossible and even dangerous, precipitating complete airway obstruction. For most patients it is unlikely that emergency tracheostomy or cricothyroidotomy will be effective since the insertion point will be above the critical stenosis. Fiber-optic endoscopy should also be avoided since it can precipitate cough, bleeding, or further mucosal edema leading to complete airway obstruction.

Patients presenting with critical airway stenosis should be placed in a quiet room and given very mild sedation and cool humidified oxygen. Nebulized racemic epinephrine and intravenous steroids help by reducing inflammatory or edematous components of the obstruction. These measures will usually provide a temporary improvement in symptoms, allowing preparation for urgent rigid bronchoscopy for completion of airway evaluation and temporary palliation.

As noted earlier, the ventilating rigid bronchoscope provides the safest and most effective means of airway control and initial stabilization in both benign and malignant tracheobronchial pathologies. Although rigid bronchoscopy has the disadvantage of requiring a general anesthetic, it has the significant advantage of providing ventilation concurrent with airway assessment and allowing the endoscopist to directly secure airway control distal to a critical stenosis. Rigid bronchoscopy also has the advantage of larger instrumentation to facilitate mechanical debridement of endoluminal tissue and aspiration of secretions and blood.

Tip: Rigid bronchoscopy under general anesthesia also assures a more complete team of anesthesiologists and nurses to help manage complications that may arise in the initial management of a critical stenosis.

In patients with benign stenosis, the stenotic area will usually require dilatation before the distal airways can be assessed and a satisfactory stable airway established. Carrot-tipped Pilling oesophageal bougies can be introduced through the rigid bronchoscope to initiate serial dilatation of a very tight stenosis. Less critical stenoses can be progressively dilated with pediatric rigid bronchoscopes. Hydrostatic balloon dilatation is also highly effective. Dilatation allows the bronchoscope to pass into the distal airway to allow distal assessment of disease as well as provide temporary stabilization of the airway so that definitive surgical correction can occur in a semi-elective manner.

Malignant lesions are best managed by initially negotiating the rigid bronchoscope beyond the tumor to achieve adequate distal ventilation and allow assessment of the distal airways. The very nature of manipulating the bronchoscope past the tumor will result in dilatation of the airway, which will provide some immediate short-term palliation. In the vast majority of cases, these maneuvers will provide temporary airway stability to allow completion of the assessment of the patient and decisions regarding optimal management and, if surgery is appropriate, allow this to be performed in a semi-elective fashion.

Trick: If there is an endoluminal component of the tumor, this can be cored out using the tip of the rigid bronchoscope with or without biopsy forceps. This also provides diagnostic tissue for pathologic examination (Fig. 23.2a, b).

23.3 Patient Preparation

Patients virtually never require emergency tracheal resection if one follows the initial management strategies described above. Although patients may present with severe and urgent symptoms, endoscopic palliation is virtually always successful, at least temporarily, allowing for elective or semi-elective planning of tracheal resection and reconstruction.

Tip: Severe central airway obstruction should be dilated or opened with a core-out of tumor to allow clearing of distal secretions and resolution of any pneumonitis before consideration of surgery.

Tip: Mucosal inflammation should be corrected with antibiotics and/or steroids before embarking on tracheal reconstructive surgery.

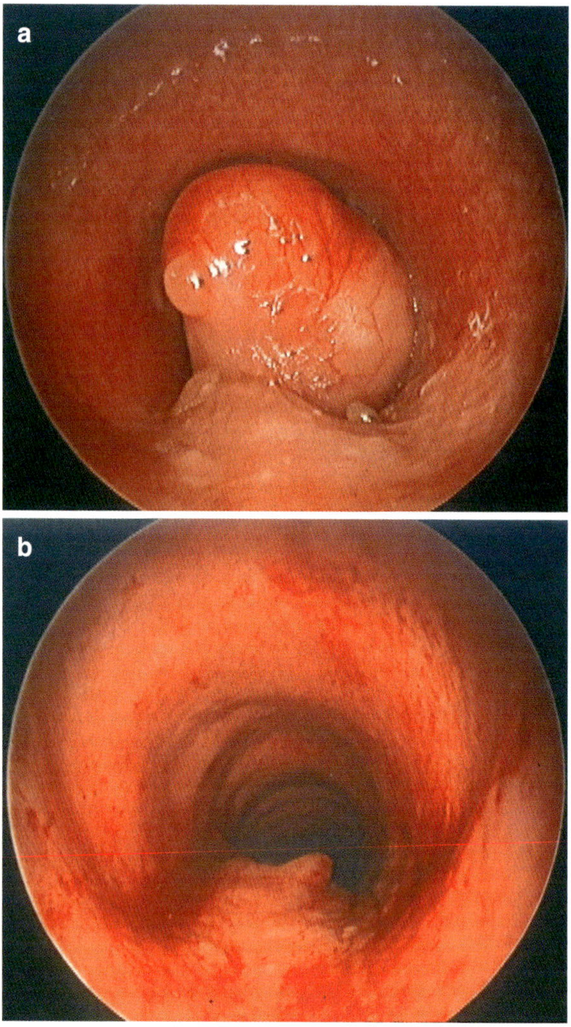

Fig. 23.2 (**a**) Proximal near obstructing tracheal adenoid cystic carcinoma as seen on initial bronchoscopy. (**b**) Tracheal lumen after core-out of endoluminal tumor using the tip of the rigid bronchoscope. This provides immediate stabilization of the airway and a large tissue sample for histologic diagnosis

23.4 Anesthetic Management

Close cooperation between the anesthesiologist and surgeon is critical to the successful management of a tracheal or carinal lesion. The surgeon should be present at the induction of anesthesia with the immediate availability of rigid bronchoscopes for securing the airway if necessary. A mixed inhalation and intravenous anesthetic, maintaining spontaneous ventilation, provides the safest and most controlled induction until a satisfactory airway is established. Cardiopulmonary bypass is virtually never necessary for intraoperative management of central airway resection. Jet ventilation is potentially dangerous if performed through a stenotic lesion. Intraoperatively, it is usually easiest to perform standard ventilation through a sterile endotracheal tube into the distal end of the transected airway (Fig. 23.3a). This does

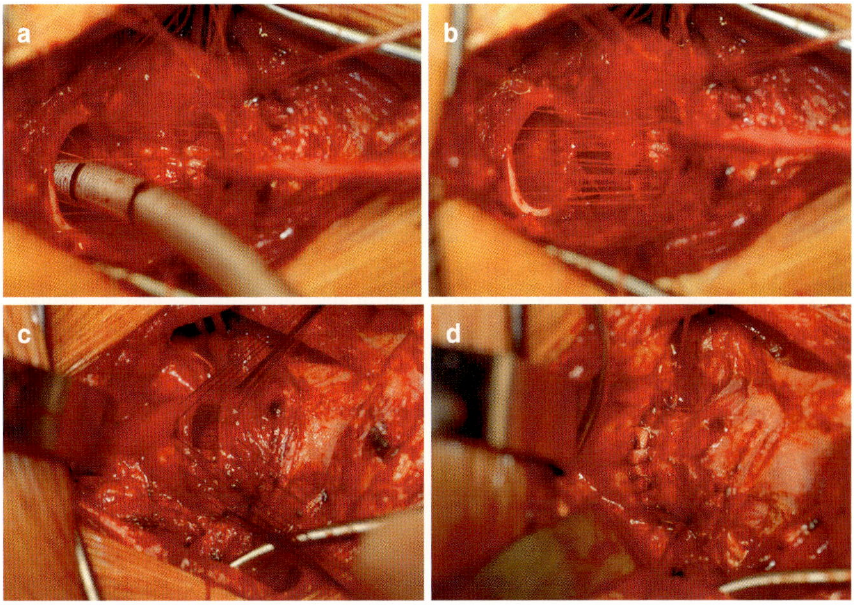

Fig. 23.3 (**a**) Cervical tracheal resection with sterile tracheal tube place in the distal airway for standard ventilation. (**b**) Cervical tracheal resection with all anastomotic sutures placed, before oral endotracheal tube is passed through the open anastomosis into the distal airway. (**c**) Cervical tracheal resection with lateral traction sutures tied, providing approximation of proximal and distal airway for completion of anastomosis. (**d**) Completion of cervical anastomosis

not require additional equipment or experience and has the added advantage of a cuffed tube preventing aspiration of blood into the distal airway.

Trick: Jet ventilation during the airway reconstruction is sometimes useful since it can be delivered through a small catheter with less bulk and rigidity.

Tip: Jet ventilation has the significant disadvantages of allowing aspiration of blood into the distal airways, producing aerosolization of blood around the operative team, and has a higher risk of barotrauma if the catheter becomes lodged in the distal airway.

23.5 Operative Technique

Tracheal resection techniques evolved over the past four decades. Initially, safe length of tracheal resection was limited to 2 cm. Pioneered by Grillo and others [1, 2], tracheal resection and reconstruction were shown to be safe and efficacious up to lengths of 5–6 cm. This is partly due to experience with tracheal stenosis and development of proximal and distal tracheal mobilization allowing for tension-free reconstruction. Furthermore, subglottic [3] and carinal [4] resection techniques were developed for more proximal and distal tumors, respectively.

The process of endoscopic evaluation and stabilization allows for the elective consideration of definitive management with tracheobronchial resection and reconstruction. For benign tracheal lesions, the majority can be resected and primarily reconstructed if they involve less than half of the tracheal length. The primary contraindications for tracheal reconstruction include the need for continued mechanical ventilation, a lesion that cannot be completely excised and primarily reconstructed (approximately half of the trachea), an active infection or inflammatory lesion, or stenosis from an uncontrolled systemic disorder such as Wegener's granulomatosis or sarcoidosis.

In spite of being a major operation, tracheal resection and reconstruction are usually physiologically trivial, with minimal pain, minor fluid shifts, little blood loss, and stable hemodynamics, so that even significant comorbidities are not usually contraindications for surgery. Tracheal resection and reconstruction are a major undertaking however, requiring experience with complex perioperative airway management, judgment regarding the extent of resection, and meticulous attention to the technical details of airway reconstruction. It is obvious that technical or judgment failures are potentially life-threatening. Success with the primary attempt at reconstruction is critical since there are no prosthetic substitutes for the trachea and limitations in the extent of airway resection.

Most benign stenoses are approached through a neck incision and rarely require thoracotomy. Principles of reconstruction include resection to normal airway, minimal dissection beyond the segment to be resected to avoid devascularization, and primary reconstruction without anastomotic tension, utilizing a variety of standard and extended mobilization techniques. In some cases, proximal tracheal stenosis may extend into the subglottic larynx requiring resection of the anterior cricoid cartilage and laryngotracheal reconstruction. Management of tracheal stenosis by tracheal resection and reconstruction produces reliable and durable results with low morbidity and mortality. Successful results are obtained in 94% of patients undergoing tracheal resection for benign stenosis, with a failure rate of 4% and a mortality rate of 2% [1].

Most patients with benign tracheal stenosis can be resected through a low cervical collar incision and do not require a sternotomy or thoracotomy. Distal tracheal or carinal tumors are best approached through a right thoracotomy. A median sternotomy is rarely utilized for airway resection and reconstruction although a manubriotomy is sometimes combined with the neck incision to provide better access for patients requiring more extensive tracheal resection and reconstruction.

Trick: Older patients who may have cervical kyphosis may provide substantial challenges to access to the intrathoracic trachea through a neck incision. These patients are those in whom manubriotomy may provide important added exposure for safe tracheal resection.

Tip: Older or kyphotic patients may also have less degree of tracheal mobility, limiting extent of tracheal resection to 25–30% of length rather than the potential 50% of length usually deemed feasible.

The principles of airway resection and reconstruction are similar for tracheal, carinal, or bronchial pathology. Dissection of the airway is limited to the region to be resected to preserve tracheobronchial blood supply, the pathology must be completely resected to normal airway, and a variety of release maneuvers are utilized to allow a tension-free anastomosis. In most tracheal resections, adequate airway mobilization can be achieved by thorough development of the avascular pre-tracheal plane along with neck flexion, which is maintained through the early postoperative period. Precise placement of interrupted absorbable suture allows an airtight anastomosis, correction of size discrepancy between the distal and proximal airway, and minimal anastomotic granulations if the anastomosis is brought together without tension (Fig. 23.3b–d).

Advances in tracheal reconstructive surgery required a clear understanding of tracheal blood supply. Salassa and colleagues performed a comprehensive and definitive study of tracheal blood supply published in 1977 [5]. These authors described the diverse origin of tracheal blood supply as well as five routes of collateral arterial blood supply. Blood supply originates from the inferior thyroid, subclavian, supreme intercostal, internal mammary, innominate, and superior and middle bronchial arteries. The predominant impacts of these findings are that the tracheal blood supply is segmental and that lateral tracheal blood supply must be preserved in order to maintain airway viability. Interruption of this lateral blood supply and skeletonization of the airway to improve mobility will result in a high incidence of anastomotic complications and the potential for devastating long segment ischemic necrosis of the residual trachea. This knowledge and experience have produced one of the dominant principles in tracheal surgery, i.e., that skeletonization of the proximal and distal tracheal margins should only be performed to the extent needed to complete the anastomosis, usually 5–7 mm.

For benign disease a cervical collar incision is appropriate for all but the most distal lesions. The trachea is encircled while maintaining dissection close to the tracheal wall.

Trick: In most cases it is not necessary, and perhaps more dangerous, to look for the recurrent laryngeal nerves. Instead, dissection tightly against the tracheal wall with care to develop the correct paratracheal plane posteriorly will help avoid recurrent laryngeal nerve injury.

Tip: It is important to prevent aggressive instrument retraction, heavy use of cautery, or indiscriminate grasping with forceps in the tracheoesophageal groove in order to avoid inadvertent recurrent laryngeal nerve injury.

The extent of trachea to be excised is exposed, and the pre-tracheal plane is developed from the cricoid cartilage to the carina and over each anterior mainstem bronchus.

Trick: Development of the pre-tracheal plane is similar to the dissection performed during the initial stages of a mediastinoscopy and can be assisted with the use of the mediastinoscope if desired.

Tip: If a patient has had a previous mediastinoscopy, the paratracheal scarring may make it much more difficult to develop the normal pre-tracheal planes and may limit mobilization of the trachea for a tension-free anastomosis.

Assessment for resection of tracheal tumors requires careful evaluation of the longitudinal and radial extent of tumor, as well as the absence of metastatic disease. As with other solid tumors, surgical treatment requires complete resection, and resection should not be offered to patients with an extent of tumor that cannot be encompassed by tracheal resection and primary reconstruction.

neck flexion up to 35° adds approximately 2.5 cm of resectable trachea beyond the known 2 cm that could be resected prior to the development of airway release maneuvers. This degree of neck flexion is usually comfortable for the patient. If needed, further neck flexion beyond 35° may permit resection of an additional 1–1.5 cm of trachea, but this may be more uncomfortable to maintain for the patient in the postoperative period.

During the exposure and resection of a tracheal lesion via a cervical approach, the neck is maximally extended by the use of a roll underneath the shoulders. When the anastomotic sutures have been placed, but prior to being tied, the shoulder roll can be removed and the neck flexed forward by the anesthesiologist, approximating the proximal and distal tracheal ends for a tension-free anastomosis. The head flexion is not simply an elevation of the head, as for intubation, but is an actual rotation of the head forward, bringing the chin down toward the manubrium.

There are several ways to maintain this position in the postoperative period. Some have developed elaborate neck braces to prevent postoperative neck extension.

Trick: The simplest, least expensive, and probably most effective technique to maintain postoperative neck flexion is to place a guardian suture from the chin to the upper anterior chest. At the completion of the procedure with the neck in the desired position, a heavy suture is placed just posterior to the tip of the chin and deep within the presternal soft tissue at the level at the sternal manubrial junction (Fig. 23.4).

Tip: It is important to not be overzealous in tightness of the suture, positioning the patient in a more flexed position than is necessary, which may be uncomfortable in the postoperative period.

In cases of minimal tracheal length being excised, it may be adequate to allow the head to be in a neutral position, using the guardian suture to prevent postoperative neck extension by the patient. These sutures are effective reminders for the patient during sleep or other unconscious movement, to prevent neck extension beyond the degree determined at time of surgery. There is no scientifically

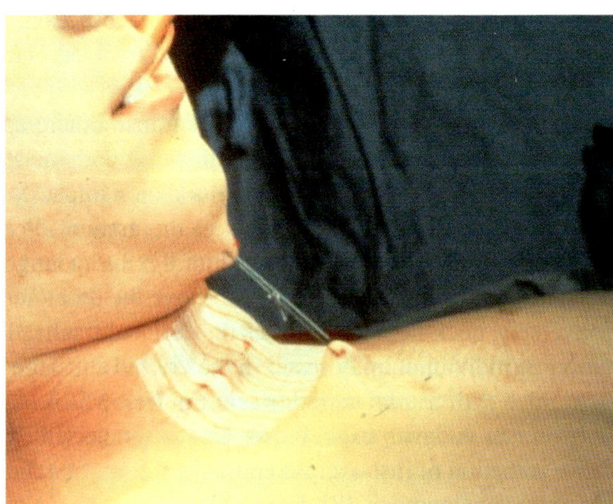

Fig. 23.4 Neck flexion with placement of a chin to chest guardian suture to prevent early postoperative neck extension

established period of time that these guardian sutures stay in place, but the most common practice in major centers is to keep these in place for 7 days postoperatively at which time the suture is removed. At that time the patient is instructed to consciously avoid neck extension—a restriction that they gradually forget simultaneous with a progressive healing that no longer requires movement restriction.

There is a large degree of variability in the range of neck flexion and overall less cervical mobility with advancing age. Previous cervical spine pathology, kyphosis, and advancing age may all diminish the potential benefit desired from neck flexion alone. However, neck flexion combined with pre-tracheal dissection is all that is required to reduce anastomotic tension in the vast majority of airway resective procedures.

When there is still excessive anastomotic tension in spite of the maneuvers of pre-tracheal dissection and neck flexion, two additional selective maneuvers may be employed—laryngeal release and/or hilar release. A laryngeal release maneuver is necessary in approximately 8% of patients undergoing tracheal resection for post-intubation injuries and approximately 15% of patients undergoing resection for tracheal tumors. A laryngeal release may provide 2–3 cm of additional tracheal mobility [9].

Tip: The added mobility of a laryngeal release transmits only to the proximal trachea and does not have much utility in improving mobility for resections in the distal trachea and carina.

Two types of laryngeal release maneuvers have been described, infrahyoid laryngeal release described by Dedo and Fishman and the suprahyoid laryngeal release reported by Montgomery. The infrahyoid laryngeal release involves division of the thyrohyoid muscle along the superior border of the larynx and bilateral division of the superior cornu of the larynx. Sternohyoid and omohyoid muscles are preserved, and the thyrohyoid membrane is divided to allow the larynx to drop away from the hyoid cartilage providing a total caudal laryngeal mobilization of approximately 2–3 cm. Some authors have added division of the inferior constrictor muscles that are attached to the posterior border of the thyroid cartilage to maximize its caudal mobilization. The major complication of this technique is a common occurrence of postoperative odynophagia and aspiration. In the original report of Dedo and Fishman, the return of swallowing function took 3–14 days, but other authors have reported a significant incidence of long-term swallowing difficulties after the infrahyoid laryngeal release.

Montgomery developed the suprahyoid release in which the larynx, cricoid, and proximal trachea are released by dividing the suprahyoid laryngeal suspensory attachments [9]. This technique involves division of the stylohyoid, mylohyoid, geniohyoid, and genioglossus muscles along with bilateral division of the hyoid bone anterior to the digastric muscle attachments. This allows the hyoid and laryngeal apparatus to descend 2–3 cm caudally for similar mobilization as that achieved by an infrahyoid laryngeal release. The supraglottic approach is generally preferred due to fewer problems with postoperative swallowing dysfunction compared to the infrahyoid approach, while yielding similar degrees of proximal tracheal mobilization. However, even patients having the suprahyoid release have a greater problem with postoperative aspiration and swallowing difficulties than those without a laryngeal release, and so this maneuver should only be performed when routine mobilization techniques are inadequate to provide a low tension anastomosis.

Hilar release maneuvers provide significant mobilization of the mainstem bronchi, allowing the carina and distal trachea to be mobilized more cephalad and release anastomotic tension in the lower trachea.

Tip: A hilar release provides little mobility to the upper cervical trachea and so is not often utilized for proximal tracheal resections.

For most distal tracheal or carinal resections, a right hilar release is performed during a right thoracotomy approach, which is the primary approach for most distal airway procedures. However, a right-sided release can also be accomplished through a median sternotomy and with a thoracoscopy if necessary. A left-sided hilar release can also be performed for additional mobility but is less gratifying than a right-sided hilar release since the left mainstem bronchus and hilum are still restricted by the aortic arch.

A hilar release has progressive components depending on the degree of mobilization required. Division of the pulmonary ligament during a right thoracotomy for airway resection should be a routine part of the procedure allowing the hilum to raise in a more cephalad direction. When additional mobilization is required, this can be accomplished by a pericardial release. The primary component of this is a U-shaped incision in the pericardium around the anterior, caudal, and posterior aspect of the inferior pulmonary vein. Division of the pericardial reflection attached to the atrium and vena cava completes this maneuver which allows 2–3 cm of cephalad mobilization of the right hilum and right mainstem bronchus.

When all of the anastomotic sutures are placed and the desired release maneuvers accomplished, the lateral traction sutures are used to pull the proximal and distal ends of the trachea together.

Tip: This step of using the traction sutures to pull the tracheal ends to each other can also be used during the dissection to assess the safe extent of longitudinal resection and the ability to achieve a tension-free anastomosis.

The lateral traction sutures are then tied to accomplish partial airway approximation and allow easier tying of the anastomotic sutures. Anastomotic sutures are then tied in the reverse order that they were placed, finishing with ties behind the trachea that are not possible to visualize and instead are tied by feel.

Tip: We prefer braided absorbable suture for the tactile feedback of knot tightness and to minimize stiff "knot balls" of monofilament.

Trick: If there is some tension anteriorly, an assistant can hold and cross adjacent sutures to take tension off for more meticulous knot approximation.

We place a drain on bulb suction and routinely extubate the patient in the operating room immediately post-op. Early extubation in the operating room allows for ease of re-intubation in a more controlled environment if needed. Removal of the cuffed tube also decreases the chance that the submucosal plexus of feeding arteries will be damaged. A guardian stitch is placed keeping the patient's neck in flexion prior to waking the patient. In cases of inability to resect the entire area or in cases of anastomotic failure after resection, placement of a temporary or permanent "T" tube is the safest method of maintaining a patient's airway.

Trick: In higher-risk anastomoses, such as a laryngotracheal anastomosis or one under some tension, one may anticipate needing to place a postoperative tracheostomy if there are airway complications. If this is anticipated, it is helpful to mark an ideal site on the anterior tracheal wall with a permanent suture in order to minimize the amount of dissection required and to increase the accuracy of stomal placement away from the anastomosis.

23.6 Postoperative Management

Patients are extubated in the operating room, even after complex reconstruction. Most of the postoperative management is similar to routine care after other neck operations or thoracotomy for pulmonary resection, with the unique aspects limited to airway management and the vigilance for the potential complications of airway reconstruction. Careful airway observation is maintained in the early postoperative period, and aggressive pulmonary toilet, including liberal use of bedside bronchoscopy, is important since these patients occasionally have clearing secretions above their anastomosis. Some patients with tracheal resection have problems with postoperative aspiration due to difficulty in elevating the larynx during deglutition. This is usually a self-limited problem but can be more severe in patients who have undergone a laryngeal release.

23.7 Outcomes

Tracheal or bronchial resection remains a neglected choice in the management of airway disease. As complications are feared and the patients often have underlying diseases, many patients, even those with benign processes, are not given the option of resection. However, excellent success is possible with tracheal resection and is an indication for resection as primary management for the majority of patients with anatomically resectable lesions. In the series published by Grillo et al. of 503 patients undergoing tracheal resection for stenosis after tracheostomy, 94% of patients had a good result as graded by the patient [1]. Complications such as wound infection, glottis dysfunction, and innominate hemorrhage were all less than 5%.

Perioperative mortality in tracheal resection series for tracheal tumors is 5% [2, 10]. Tracheoinnominate artery fistula, anastomotic dehiscence, and pneumonia are causes of initial mortality. Oncologic results in patients with resected tumors in the trachea vary depending on tumor type. Five-year survival rates in patients with adenoid cystic carcinoma range from 66% (22) to 75% following resection [2]. In a more recent update of the MGH experience, 5- and 10-year survival in resected adenoid cystic carcinoma patients was 52% and 29% as compared to unresected tumors with 33% and 10% survival, respectively [6]. Patients with tracheal squamous cell carcinoma have less favorable outcomes. Grillo and Mathisen reported a 35% survival rate in 41 patients resected with tracheal squamous cell carcinoma [2]. Ten-year survival falls to 18%; however, only 4.9% of unresected patients are alive at 10 years [6].

23.8 Alternative Interventions for Central Airway Pathology

The choice of endoscopic airway management or surgical resection is made by considering the patient's underlying disease, anatomical considerations, and likely future progress of the disease. Assortments of endoscopic techniques have been developed for the palliation of airway obstruction including dilatation, core-out, debridement, laser, cautery, cryoablation, brachytherapy, photodynamic therapy, and stenting [11]. Although all have reported success, it is best to tailor each application or combination of therapies to the patient as needed for a successful outcome. Dilatation and laser resections are advocated as palliation for benign tracheal bronchial stenosis. In both benign and malignant disease, tracheobronchial stents have been used to palliate the effects of large airway obstruction caused by extrinsic compression, intraluminal disease, or loss of cartilaginous support. Flexible and creative application of each of these techniques, even combined within individual patients, provides the best chance for successful airway palliation.

Patients with unresectable benign stenoses are usually initially managed with dilatation. It is likely that the dilated stenosis will contract again resulting in recurrent symptoms. If the interval between dilatations is sufficiently long, it may be best to perform periodic dilatations as symptoms prescribe. When there is rapid recurrence of stenosis and symptoms in a recalcitrant stricture, airway stenting can provide a longer period of palliation [12]. Expandable metal stents are avoided in patients with benign disease since these stents are usually difficult to remove, may result in inflammatory overgrowth of tissue, and ultimately produce a more complex airway problem in patients with a prolonged natural history. For this reason, solid silicone rubber stents or fully covered expandable stents are preferred since they have minimal tissue reactivity and can be adjusted or removed at any time. The major problems with placement of any stent are the interruption of normal mucociliary clearance and potential clogging or dislodgment of the stent requiring a stent revision.

Unresectable malignant airway stenosis can produce obstruction with both endoluminal tumor and extrinsic compression of the airway. The simplest management of significant endoluminal tumor is a simple mechanical debridement or core-out of the tumor. This can be achieved with the tip of a rigid bronchoscope and/or with biopsy forceps. In slow-growing tumors, this may provide a prolonged period of airway palliation. In cases where endoluminal recurrence occurs rapidly or there is significant extrinsic compression of the airway by tumor, airway stenting provides an important adjunct to the endoluminal core-out procedure [12]. Silicone rubber stents still have an advantage of ease of revision or removal, and, because they are solid, there are no difficulties with tumor ingrowth.

Tip: Expandable stents should be coated rather than a bare metal stent in order to prevent ingrowth of tumor or granulations through the interstices of the stent and subsequent stent obstruction.

There are several other procedures that may help palliate malignant airway obstruction. Systemic chemotherapy or external beam radiation are possibilities if indicated by the tumor histology and the patient's functional status. External beam radiation can be supplemented by endoluminal brachytherapy to achieve higher doses of radiation to the tumor. Cryotherapy and photodynamic therapy are additional management strategies that are popular in some institutions but in most cases add little to the palliation achieved by the techniques described above.

Conclusion

Disorders involving the airway are rare. Except for a handful of thoracic surgeons and pulmonologists with specific interests in the airway, most individuals will see only an occasional patient with tracheal pathology. Because of this, tracheobronchial reconstructive procedures have been frequently regarded as complex operations with high morbidity and mortality. Since the indications are relatively uncommon, airway surgery has been primarily applied in tertiary or quaternary thoracic surgical units. Outside of these centers, there is a widespread lack of familiarity with the indications for, and the results from, airway resection and reconstruction. This may prevent airway resection from being considered as a viable treatment option for many patients. However, tracheal reconstruction may preclude the need for a life-long tracheostomy and allow preservation of laryngeal function in benign strictures while providing treatment with curative intent for primary airway tumors.

The treatment of airway pathology requires a flexible and multimodality approach. When done for palliation or cure, effective management of airway pathology has a great impact on patient's quality and longevity of life. It is important for the practitioner to have a long-term plan for the patient when they begin interventions. Resection and reconstruction either in benign or malignant disease remain the gold standard for treatment.

References

1. Grillo HC, Donahue DM, Mathisen DJ, Wain JC, Wright CD. Post intubation tracheal stenosis: treatment and results. J Thorac Cardiovasc Surg. 1995;109:46–93.
2. Grillo HC, Mathisen DJ. Primary tracheal tumors: treatment and results. Ann Thorac Surg. 1990;49:69–77.
3. Pearson FG, Cooper JD, Nelems JM, et al. Primary tracheal anastomosis after resection of the cricoid cartilage with preservation of recurrent laryngeal nerves. J Thorac Cardiovasc Surg. 1975;70:806–16.
4. Grillo HC. Carinal reconstruction. Ann Thorac Surg. 1982;34:356–73.
5. Salassa JR, Pearson BW, Payne WS. Gross and microscopical blood supply of the trachea. Ann Thorac Surg. 1977;24:100–7.
6. Gaissert HA, Grillo HC, Shadmehr MB, Wright CD, Gokhale M, Wain JC, Mathisen DJ. Long-term survival after resection of primary adenoid cystic and squamous cell carcinoma of the trachea and carina. Ann Thorac Surg. 2004;78(6):1889–97.
7. Heitmiller RF. Tracheal release maneuvers. Chest Surg Clin North Am. 1996;6:675–82.
8. Mulliken JB, Grillo HC. The limits of tracheal resection with primary anastomosis. J Thorac Cardiovasc Surg. 1968;55:418–21.
9. Montgomery WW. Suprahyoid release for tracheal anastomosis. Arch Otolaryngol. 1974;99:255–60.

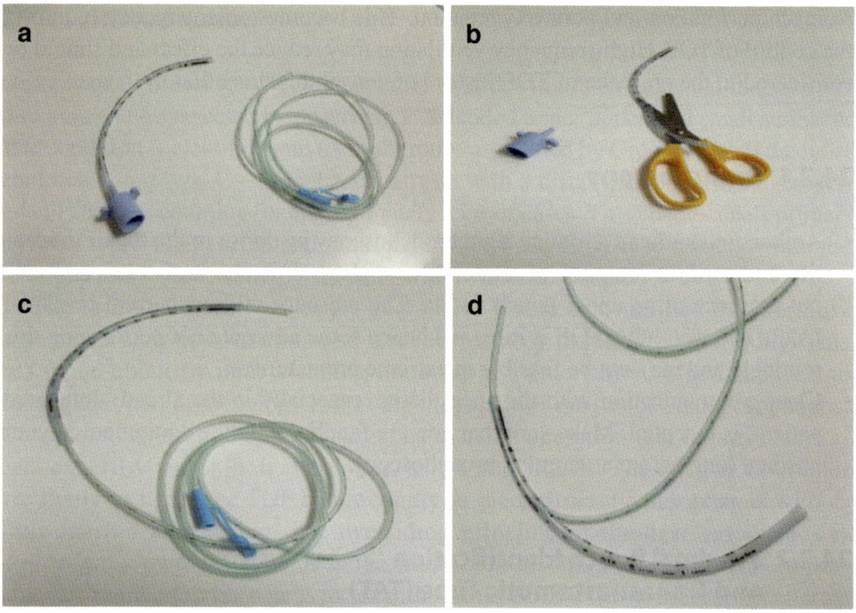

Fig. 24.1 (**a–d**) A longitudinal cut to open the lumen is created in the endotracheal tube (ETT) and a feeding tube passed through the lumen. This enables the more rigid ETT to be removed easily when required after passage of the TAT

Retraction of the pleura and lung with a malleable retractor avoids lung injury and allows adequate oxygenation during surgery. It helps to avoid hand bag ventilation during surgery and in keeping the baby warm.

- Azygous vein is ligated and divided by many to access the TOF ligation but is not necessary. Avoid ligating the azygous if it is found to be larger than expected, as it is possible there could be abnormalities of IVC, and is the only route of venous return from lower limbs and trunk.
- Careful identification of all the structures is paramount to prevent the disastrous situation of ligating an airway or major vessel. If in doubt, follow the vagus to locate the fistula. Minimise handling of the vagus to prevent injury.

24.2.4 TOF Division

- The fistula can be identified by incising the endothoracic fascia and by seeing its distension corresponding with ventilation and vagal nerve fibres coursing towards the lower oesophagus from trachea downwards.
- Always use a vascular sling to temporarily occlude the fistula prior to ligation—check with the anaesthetist to confirm easier ventilation and no change in circulation.

- Fistula ligation and division are performed (following control of proximal and distal ends with a stay suture) with interrupted non-absorbable suture preferably monofilament (authors use 5/0 or 6/0 Prolene).
- Always perform an air-leak test with saline after ligation of fistula.

24.2.5 Oesophageal Anastomosis

- Proximal pouch dissection—a stay suture can be passed through both the end of the pouch, and tubing passed earlier to facilitate easier dissection.
- A combination of bipolar and sharp dissection should be used to avoid thermal injury to the trachea.
- Proximal blood supply is robust, and significant dissection can be achieved if required.
- Distal pouch dissection is performed only to the extent required for repair, as the blood supply is segmental and not as robust as the proximal pouch. However, some dissection is feasible without damaging its blood supply if required and is still compatible with successful outcome.
- The posterior wall of the anastomosis is performed with interrupted absorbable sutures making sure to take full-thickness bites including both sides of the mucosa in the bites. If the two ends come together without tension, the suture does not cut through in a parachuted technique. Following passage of the TAT into the stomach, the anterior wall is repaired.
- Extrapleural drain placement is operator dependent. In reality there is no real evidence that a post-operative drain prevents complications. While saliva or air in the drain may indicate a leak, a small leak generally will resolve spontaneously without a drain, while a large leak will often require separate transpleural intercostal catheter placement or a second look with debridement of trapped lung [2].

24.2.6 Thoracoscopic OA Repair

The use of thoracoscopic repair has been increasing significantly in the last few years. Whereas initially attempted in selected cases, now the experience has broadened to encompass all types of atresia and patients' characteristics.

While requiring advanced minimally invasive skills, the advantages include much better vision (visualisation of the mucosa is much better with thoracoscopic surgery) and minimal scars.

- Position is via a semi-prone right side elevated to 30–45°. Initial 5 mm port is placed in the posterior axillary line in fifth intercostal space for a 30° scope. Two working ports are placed in mid- or between mid- and anterior axillary line. One port is placed two rib spaces above the camera port and second below the camera port in order to achieve triangulation. While 3 mm instruments are available for dissection and anastomosis, 5 mm ports are required for camera and clip application. Low pressure (5 mmHg) and flow rate (0.5–1 L) are good starting points and can be adjusted as tolerated.

- The repair is essentially the same as the open approach, though via a transpleural approach.
- Ligation of TOF is performed with 5 mm clips or suture transfixion, as is azygous ligation if required. Mackinlay uses sutures rather than clips due to the risk of the anastomotic suture looping on the clips and dislodging them [3] (Figs. 24.2 and 24.3).
- Mobilisation of upper pouch remaining close to the oesophagus avoids injury to the trachea (Fig. 24.4)

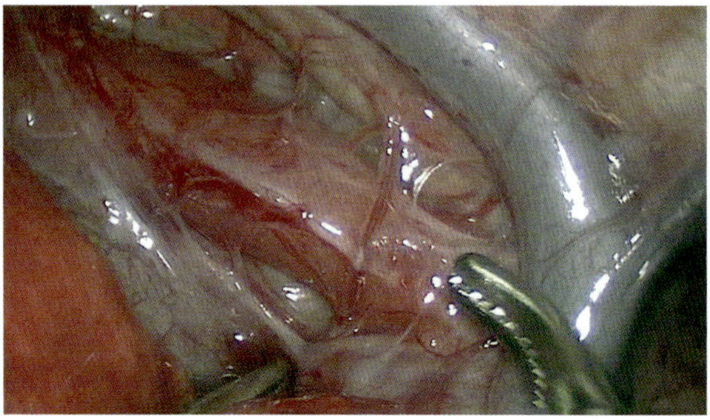

Fig. 24.2 Tracheo-oesophageal fistula—distal oesophagus connected to trachea—the pleura is divided carefully with minimal mobilisation of the fistula thus keeping as many vessels into the fistula intact to maintain excellent blood supply

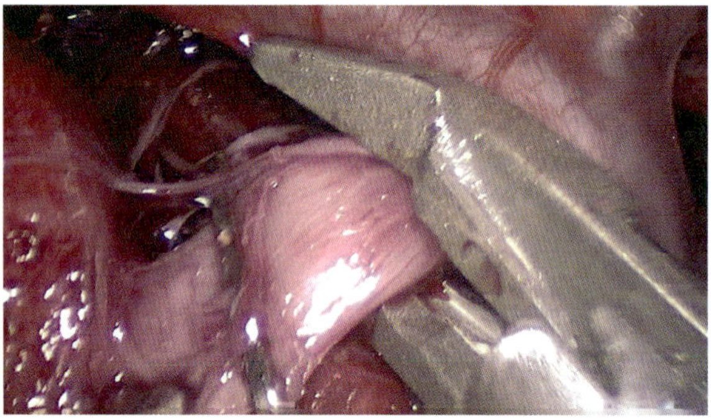

Fig. 24.3 TOF after mobilisation divided between two 5 mm endoclips. Azygous is preserved but can be divided if required. Some surgeons transfix the fistula with 4/0 suture near the trachea. Air leak is checked after division

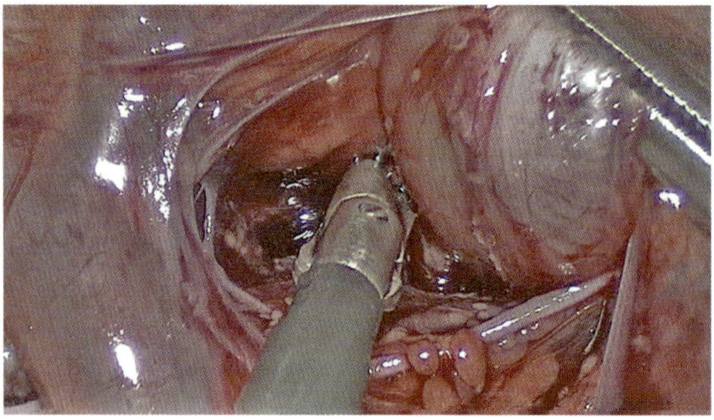

Fig. 24.4 Upper pouch mobilisation. Gentle rotation around the Yohan's forceps helps retraction and visualisation in a small space

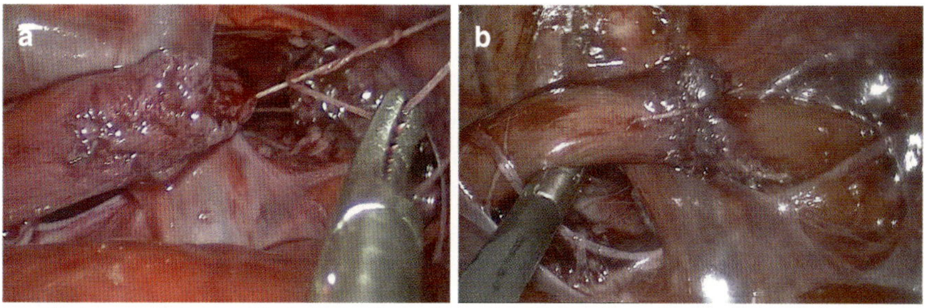

Fig. 24.5 (**a**) The anastomosis of the two ends of the oesophagus is performed with 5-0 Vicryl (RB-2 13 mm needle). The azygos vein is maintained intact. The first suture is a slip knot to bring two ends together. (**b**) Tension-free anastomosis. A transanastomotic 8Fr tube was passed beyond the anastomosis before its completion

- Anastomosis is performed using 4/0 or 5/0 absorbable interrupted sutures, using two 3 mm needle holders.
- If there is tension, then an approximation suture can be used first to relieve this and prevent tissue trauma during the initial anastomotic sutures (Fig. 24.5a, b).

24.2.7 H-Type Fistula

An uncommon diagnosis often suspected clinically via recurrent respiratory symptoms with an intact oesophagus, H-type fistula, is diagnosed via a tube oesophagram.

- Rigid bronchoscopy confirms the diagnosis and enables passage of either a guidewire or a ureteric stent through the fistula which can be retrieved via the oesophagus—this will act as a guide during dissection.
- Right transverse lower cervical approach; identify trachea and oesophagus and dissect distally till fistula identified, ligated and divided. Interrupted absorbable suture is commonly used.
- Ensure each end of the fistula is controlled with stay sutures prior to division as they can retract quickly. It is vital to divide the fistula as ligation by itself is associated with higher rates of recurrence
- The recurrent laryngeal nerve lies in the trachea/oesophageal groove. Beware this nerve on both sides and the possibility of vocal cord paralysis.

24.3 Difficult Situations

24.3.1 Long-Gap Type C Oesophageal Atresia

- While traditionally considered mainly as an issue for pure oesophageal atresia, Freidmacher showed that this problem is recognised in the more common variant. In a meta-analysis, 56% of long-gap patients were from the type C population [4].

- Delayed primary anastomosis at 8–12 weeks with gastrostomy feeds in the interim for growth was, until the last decade, the most common strategy. Muscle flaps and myotomies have been described, though rarely used in the author's experience. Over the last decade, internal and external traction sutures have gained increasing popularity.
- Gap assessments in theatre or interventional radiology are useful for assessing the deficiency and influencing timing of surgery (see long-gap chapter for more information).

24.3.2 Right-Sided Aortic Arch

Intraoperative right-sided aortic arch has been recorded in 1.8–13% of OA [5, 6]. Preoperative echocardiogram is used routinely to assess for concurrent cardiac abnormalities, but while it invariably comments on the location of the aorta (left- or right-sided), this should be regarded with caution if the surgeon uses this to influence surgery, as the accuracy of this is variable [5, 6]. Allen et al. found one third of right arches were incorrectly diagnosed preoperatively [7].

- Effective oesophageal anastomosis can be achieved via a right-sided thorax approach [5, 6, 8], and as this is the most familiar approach, then this should be continued with a suspected right-sided arch, with minimal complication rates recorded. The anatomy is slightly different, but the position of fistula and vagus coursing over it remains the constant phenomenon. The upper pouch dissection is slightly trickier in right aortic arch however not impossible. We do not advocate a conversion to left thoracotomy as the possibility of finding a double-sided arch is real (see below)
- Spitz believes that a right-sided aortic arch should be approached from the left thorax [2]. Babu et al. showed a high leak rate in right-sided approaches, though 25% of their series had a double aortic arch, so left side approach had to be abandoned [9]. Allen et al. also performed some via a left approach [7].
- Anastomosis can be performed either lateral to aortic arch [5] (preferable in short proximal pouch) or leaving the proximal oesophagus medial to the arch depending on the sightings of the upper pouch in the thorax during identification and dissection.

24.3.3 Respiratory Compromise

This situation is more common in the premature and *very-low-birth-weight* infant, with abdominal distension causing compromise of immature lungs.

- Transpleural approach can be used to quickly ligate the fistula if time does not allow an extrapleural dissection.
- If clinical status improves significantly enough, then primary anastomosis can be attempted, otherwise return to the intensive care setting and perform a delayed primary anastomosis when clinically improved.

24.3.4 Ruptured Stomach

With significant distension of the stomach, rupture and pneumoperitoneum may occur. The baby will typically show rapid respiratory decompensation with a distending abdomen.

- Urgent intervention required—needle abdominocentesis to decompress pneumoperitoneum—and then emergency operation.
- Operative intervention requires control and division of fistula and repair of stomach. Techniques have been described to control the fistula first via the stomach, e.g. using a Fogarty balloon via the distal oesophagus to occlude the fistula lumen [10], though this can be very difficult to achieve in an emergency situation. We would recommend decompressing the abdomen then turning expediently to the thorax and rapid transpleural fistula control and division, and then performing a laparotomy to repair the stomach with or without gastrostomy formation. Primary or delayed primary anastomosis would depend on the clinical setting.

24.3.5 Concurrent Duodenal Atresia and/or Anorectal Malformation

Duodenal atresia is usually diagnosed preoperatively by the presence of a double bubble on abdominal X-ray, while the anorectal malformation will be diagnosed on clinical examination.

- Top-down approach is recommended—deal firstly with fistula, then OA repair, then duodenal atresia and lastly the anorectal malformation (usually stoma formation).
- Do not feel pressure to perform all in one go—multiple operations is not a failure for this difficult constellation, while a long anaesthetic time may be detrimental to the patient.
- Strong consideration should be given for a gastrostomy for both initial decompression of stomach and feeding in the medium-long term, either gastrostomy or jejunal feeds.

24.4 Post-operative Care

The clinical setting for post-operative care will depend largely on concurrent comorbidities, difficulty of the operation and available resources. There is no routine requirement from a surgical point for mechanical ventilation, paralysis or intensive care, though these can be considered in extreme situations.

With a TAT feeds can be commenced the day after operation, while some wait for a normal oesophagram on day 5–7 before commencing feeds [11]. In those rare cases that required delayed closure, sham feeding can be commenced to encourage the suck reflex and minimise oral aversion.

Anti-reflux medication is routinely commenced post-operatively and continued for the medium-long term due to the high rates of gastro-oesophageal reflux.

24.5 Post-operative Complication

24.5.1 Large Anastomotic or Fistula Leak

A large post-operative leak often occurs within the first 3 days [2] and typically presents as a tension pneumothorax. Our experience in this population is that early intervention is beneficially as is usually represents an anastomotic defect which can be easily closed with interrupted sutures with good outcomes. Intercostal catheter placement may temporise the situation but will not avert reoperation and delay only makes this harder as the inflammatory response converts the operative field into a danger zone.

24.5.2 Small Anastomotic Leak

Small contained leaks can be conservatively managed, and 95% will close within the next few weeks [12]. Parenteral nutrition, drainage and antibiotics are treatments to consider while this resolves.

24.5.3 Recurrent Fistula

Recurrent fistula occurs in up to 8% of patients [2] and can be difficult to treat. Suspicion is usually raised following recurrent respiratory symptoms, is diagnosed by tube oesophagram and confirmed with bronchoscopy.

- Operative approach is via the neck or thorax depending on type and location.
- Repair is as previously described, though muscle flaps or pleura may be used to interpose between trachea and oesophagus.
- Be careful to exclude missed proximal fistula when performing the bronchoscopy
- Novel techniques via rigid bronchoscopy have been reported such as using fibrin glue.

24.5.4 Stricture

Anastomotic strictures are a common issue and occur in up to 35% [12]. Causes include GORD, gap >2.5 cm (and presumed tension on the anastomosis), significant

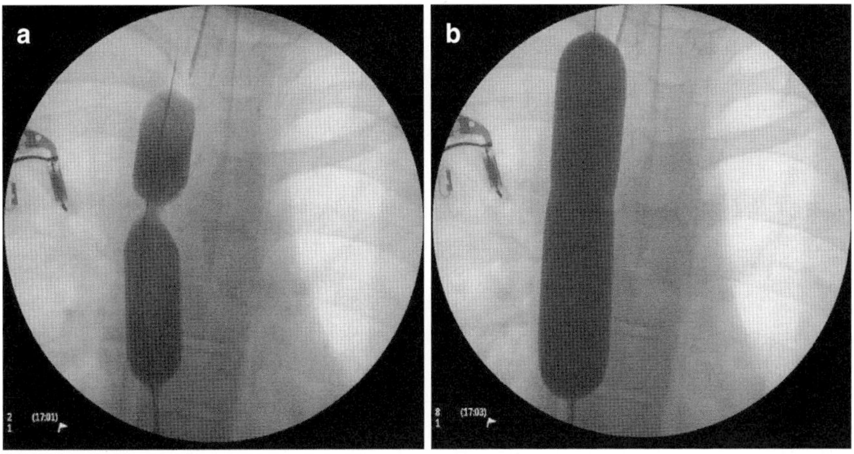

Fig. 24.6 (**a**) Anastomotic stricture shown by narrowing of balloon. (**b**) Following successful balloon dilatation

dissection of distal pouch, [12, 13] and anastomotic leak (up to 50% of anastomotic leaks complicated by stricture) [12].

- On contrast imaging, the anastomosis site will always appear narrower on imaging, but demonstration of a functional obstruction on contrast is diagnostic. Clinical symptoms such as food bolus obstruction and dysphagia are often enough to warrant endoscopy.
- Based on personal experience, the author considers that balloon dilatation under endoscopic and fluoroscopic control is superior to bouginage to dilate strictures. Gradual radial dilatation causes less shearing force than the bouginage [14]. Jayakrishnan reported lower rates of perforation and technical failures in the balloon dilatation group [15] (Fig. 24.6a, b).
- Risk factors include GORD, so ensure adequate anti-reflux treatment, and consider fundoplication in those with difficult to control disease. Engun et al. showed that in OA, up to 58% had reflux with 44% of these required an anti-reflux procedure [12].

24.5.5 Tracheomalacia

The occurrence of tracheomalacia in patients with OA/TOF is well recognised, and it is likely that this results from a field defect during embryology. Probably most if not all have some degree of tracheomalacia, though the assessment for this is not required unless clinically indicated. Ongoing respiratory compromise, e.g. inability to wean from ventilation, or acute life-threatening events (ALTE) will lead to the investigation for this using a flexible bronchoscope. While the majority of patients with tracheomalacia will improve with time and growth, occasionally intervention will be required.

- Aortopexy is one option that involves suturing the aortic wall to the posterior sternum, bringing the trachea (attached posteriorly to the aortic adventitia) forward, opening the airway lumen and preventing anterior wall collapse [16].
  - This can be performed either thoracoscopically or via an open approach (anterior or lateral thoracotomy) from right to left sides, using non-absorbable sutures.
  - The ascending aorta is used up to (and potentially including) the right innominate artery.
  - Care during suture placement must be taken, and a partial thickness suture is advocated. These can be pledgetted to reduce stress on the artery wall. The important point is to not remove a full-thickness suture, if placed, to avoid catastrophic haemorrhage.
  - Flexible bronchoscopy is required intraoperatively before, during and after the procedure to evaluate the results immediately. If inadequate results, then further sutures can be placed.
- In ALTE's, some will favour fundoplication primarily over aortopexy, as there is an association between GORD and spasm of the airway, which in the setting of tracheomalacia may be the stimulus for the ALTE. Laparoscopic or open fundoplication will resolve the majority of symptoms and in addition protect the oesophagus from reflux disease.

Conclusion

While requiring significant skill to perform an oesophageal atresia repair, it is often the recognition and management of the difficulties and complications that make a successful surgeon. The Pediatric surgeon needs to anticipate these both intra- and post-operatively. Preservation of the patient's own oesophagus remains the goal in all these patients.

References

1. Gross R. The surgery of infancy and childhood. Philadelphia: WB Saunders; 1953.
2. Spitz L. Esophageal atresia: lessons I have learned in a 40-year experience. J Pediatr Surg. 2006;41(10):1635–40.
3. MacKinlay GA. Esophageal atresia surgery in the 21st century. Semin Pediatr Surg. 2009;18(1):20–2.
4. Friedmacher F, Puri P. Delayed primary anastomosis for management of long gap esophageal atresia: a meta-analysis of complications and long-term outcome. Pediatr Surg Int. 2012;28(9):899–906.
5. Bowkett B, Beasley SW, Myers NA. The frequency, significance, and management of a right aortic arch in association with esophageal atresia. Pediatr Surg Int. 1999;15:28–31.
6. Bicakci U, Tander B, Ariturk E, Rizalar R, Ayyildiz SH, Bernay F. The right-sided aortic arch in children with esophageal atresia and tracheo-esophageal fistula: a repair through the right thoracotomy. Pediatr Surg Int. 2009;25(5):423–5.
7. Allen S, et al. The effect of a rightsided aortic arch on outcome in children with esophageal atresia and tracheoesophageal fistula. J Pediatr Surg. 2006;41(3):479–83.
8. Wood JA, Carachi R. The right-sided aortic arch in children with oesophageal atresia and tracheo-oesophageal fistula. Eur J Pediatr Surg. 2012;22(1):3–7.

9. Babu R, Pierro A, Spitz L, Drake DP, Kiely EM. The management of oesophageal atresia in neonates with right-sided aortic arch. J Pediatr Surg. 2000;35(1):56–8.
10. Conforti A, Morini F, Bagolan P. Difficult esophageal atresia: Trick and treat. Semin Pediatr Surg. 2014;23(5):261–69.
11. Slater BJ, Rothenberg SS. Tracheoesophageal atresia. Semin Pediatr Surg. 2016;25(3):176–8.
12. Engun SA, Grosfeld JL, West KW, et al. Analysis of morbidity and mortality in 227 cases of esophageal atresia and/or tracheoesophageal fistula over two decades. Arch Surg. 1995;130:502–8.
13. Chittmittrapap S, Spitz L, Kiely EM, et al. Anastomotic stricture following repair of esophageal atresia. J Pediatr Surg. 1990;25:508–11.
14. McLean GK, Leveen RF. Shear stress in the performance of oesophageal dilatation: comparison of balloon dilatation and bouginage. Radiology. 1989;172:983–6.
15. Jayakrishnan VK, Wilkinson AG. Treatment of oesophageal strictures in children: a comparison of fluroscopically guided balloon dilatation with surgical bouginage. Pediatr Radiol. 2001;31:98–101.
16. Fraga FC, Jennings RW, Kim PCW. Pediatric tracheomalacia. Semin Pediatr Surg. 2016;25(3):156–64.

Long-Gap Oesophageal Atresia

25

David C. van der Zee

Abstract

This chapter describes the evolution from delayed management of long-gap oesophageal atresia to thoracoscopic treatment directly after birth without the placement of a gastrostomy.

Long-gap oesophageal atresia remains a challenge for pediatric surgeons. Over the years several techniques have been described to manage long-gap oesophageal atresia. More recently a traction technique has been advocated. With the advent of minimal invasive surgery, the thoracoscopic elongation technique has been developed.

This chapter describes the single-center experience with the thoracoscopic treatment of patients with long-gap oesophageal atresia.

Initially all patients had a gastrostomy. During the course the technique evolved into delayed primary anastomosis directly after birth without the use of a gastrostomy.

It is shown that thoracoscopic elongation technique in long-gap oesophageal atresia is not only feasible; it can nowadays also be performed directly after birth without the use of a gastrostomy. With this development we have entered a new era in the management of long-gap oesophageal atresia.

Keywords

Oesophageal atresia · Long-gap · Thoracoscopic elongation · Traction technique

D.C. van der Zee, M.D., Ph.D.
Department of Pediatric Surgery, KE 04.140.5, University Medical Center Utrecht, Utrecht, The Netherlands
e-mail: d.c.vanderzee@umcutrecht.nl

D. Parikh, P.B. Rajesh (eds.), *Tips and Tricks in Thoracic Surgery*,
https://doi.org/10.1007/978-1-4471-7355-7_25

25.1 Introduction

The term long-gap oesophageal atresia is principally reserved for pure oesophageal atresia where there is no connection between oesophagus and trachea. In those cases the distance between the proximal and distal pouch is so long that a primary anastomosis is not possible. In practice the same accounts for in cases where there is a proximal fistula present, because this fistula usually withholds the oesophagus from migrating downward into the thorax. In cases where there is a distal tracheoesophageal fistula, there may be a long distance between the two pouches, but they are not called long-gap oesophageal atresia.

Long-gap oesophageal atresia remains a challenge for pediatric surgeons. Where in the past the problem was dealt with delayed management with colon interposition or gastric pull-up [1, 2]; in more recent years, jejunal interposition and oesophageal traction techniques have been described with satisfactory results [3, 4]. Nowadays long-gap oesophageal atresia can even be managed in the neonatal period with the thoracoscopic traction technique [5].

25.2 Technical Tips and Tricks of Thoracoscopic Elongation on Long-Gap Oesophageal Atresia

Today long-gap oesophageal atresia can be managed in the neonatal period. After the standard preoperative work-up with X-ray thorax/abdomen to determine the level of obstruction in the proximal pouch and the absence of air in the abdomen, ultrasound to detect cardiac malformations and the position of the aortic arch, abnormalities of the urinary tract and kidneys, and establishment of the anus or other gross external pathologies, a multidisciplinary meeting is arranged with neonatologists, ENT surgeons, and anesthesiologists to discuss the foreseen procedure. The further work-up with consultation of the medical geneticist and exclusion of other pathologies and VACTERL association can be executed at a later stage during admission.

All patients are monitored according to protocol with a central venous line, arterial line, urine catheter, and transcutaneous saturation device. Brain perfusion is continuously measured by near-infrared spectrometry (NIRS) and a-EEG pre-, during, and postoperatively.

The procedure is started with a rigid tracheobronchoscopy to determine or exclude a proximal tracheoesophageal fistula, tracheomalacia, and bronchial malformations. A proximal fistula can more easily be missed by flexible tracheoscopy. With the use of the rigid endoscope, the ENT specialist can "scrape" over the posterior wall and pars membranacae. By doing so, sometimes the aperture of a proximal fistula can be pulled open that otherwise would go undetermined. Afterward the child is intubated. Selective intubation is not warranted.

The child is then turned in a ¾ left-sided position with a little role under the left armpit to prevent the arm from being compressed too much. The right arm is fixed over the head of the patient over a gel pad. The plaster over the Replogle tube is detached and only lightly fixed against the nose, so it can be manipulated during the mobilization of the proximal pouch.

A first 5 mm trocar is placed approximately 1 cm below and anterior of the scapula tip by incision in the skin and blunt perforation of the muscles and pleura with a mosquito. Insufflation is started with 5 mmHg pressure and a flow of 1 L/min. Usually the anesthesiologist will have to increase the frequency of ventilation up to 40–60×/min with a constant breathing minute volume. If the insufflation is not tolerated initially, the insufflation tube can be disconnected temporarily and restarted at a lower initial pressure (2–3 mmHg) after restoration of 100% oxygenation. After anesthesiological stabilization, the pressure can be further increased to 5 mmHg. The right lung lobes should be slowly deflated by the CO_2 insufflation. If the ventilation is exerted at a too high PEEP, the lung will have difficulty to deflate. If this is necessary to keep the child sufficiently oxygenated, an additional 3 mm trocar can be inserted with a flexible lung retractor to carefully depress the lung so far that adequate view of the proximal and distal pouch can be obtained. The procedure should only be continued when the anesthesiologist is convinced of a stable anesthesiological situation.

Two additional 3 mm trocars are placed under direct vision in a triangle around the 5 mm optic but also in a manner that both the upper pouch and lower pouch can be dissected.

It is usually started with the determination of both pouches. Proximally the Replogle tube can be pushed forward by the anesthesiologist to identify proximal oesophageal pouch. The vagal nerve is proximally running over the course of the trachea. The tip of the upper oesophagus should be lying posterior to the trachea.

Distally the vagal nerve is running over the lower pouch. If the distal pouch is not visible at the level of the diaphragm, the pleura at the level of the hiatus can be opened and the vagal nerve followed downward until the distal pouch is identified (Fig. 25.1). At that point with the use of an Endoclose®, a Vicryl 4×0 suture can be introduced into the thoracic cavity as high as possible posterior from the scapula. The needle follows passively through the opening and can be picked up with an endoscopic needle holder. The distal pouch is hitched with the needle, preferably at

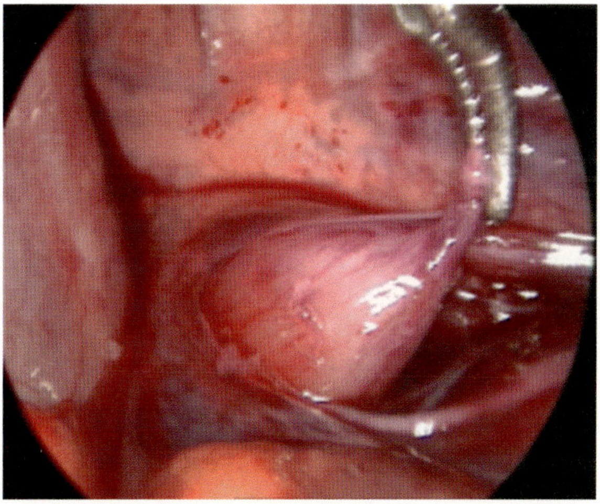

Fig. 25.1 Mobilization of distal oesophagus out of hiatus

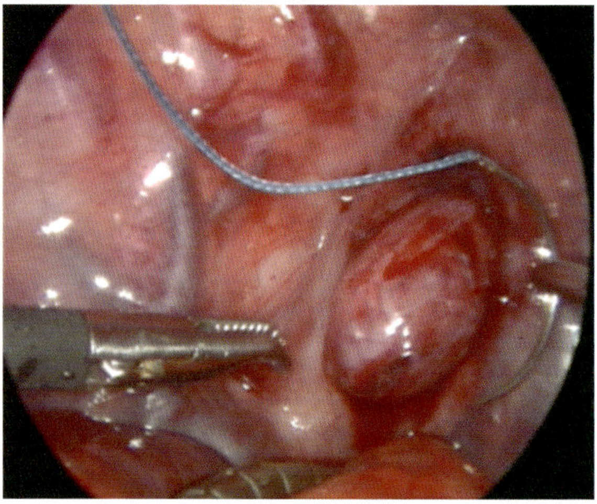

Fig. 25.2 Placement of sutures in proximal oesophagus

the posterior side, and the thread is guided back into the reintroduced Endoclose® and carefully pulled out and clamped with a mosquito. By carefully pulling on the thread, the distal pouch can be mobilized out of the hiatus. Additional stay sutures are placed at the four corners to exert symmetrical traction with the use of the Endoclose®, and the distal pouch is maximally dissected out of the hiatus. The same procedure is carried out at the proximal pouch, where the sutures are led out as low as possible on the thoracic wall (Fig. 25.2). In case a proximal fistula is present, this can be dealt with thoracoscopically by completely dissecting around the fistula with identification of the vagal nerve. A transfixing suture is placed through the fistula at the tracheal side after which the fistula can be transected. The oesophagus is closed with interrupted sutures. The location is usually somewhat higher up and does not interfere with the stay sutures that are placed in the proximal pouch for traction. In case the fistula is too high for a thoracoscopic approach, it will be closed through the neck. The preoperative tracheoscopy usually gives an idea on the level of the proximal fistula and if it can be closed thoracoscopically.

When all stay sutures are in place, the optic is replaced for a 3 mm optic to allow introduction of a 5 mm clip applier (Fig. 25.3). Two clips are applied on the sutures at the level of the tip of both pouches to allow observation of the progression of the two ends toward each other.

On the outside the threads are pulled through a piece of silicone tubing with the use of the Endoclose® to serve as a cushion at the skin level (Fig. 25.4). Maximum traction on the sutures is applied under direct vision of the endoscope. The silicone tubing is advanced against the skin, and a mini-mosquito is applied on the threads against the silicone tubing to maintain the traction.

The trocars are removed under direct vision, after which the defect from the 5 mm trocar is closed with a Vicryl 5×0 suture. All skin defects are closed using Steristrips®.

When the child is operated in the first days of life, a gastrostomy is not made. Instead the ventral gastric wall is fixed to the anterior abdominal wall using two

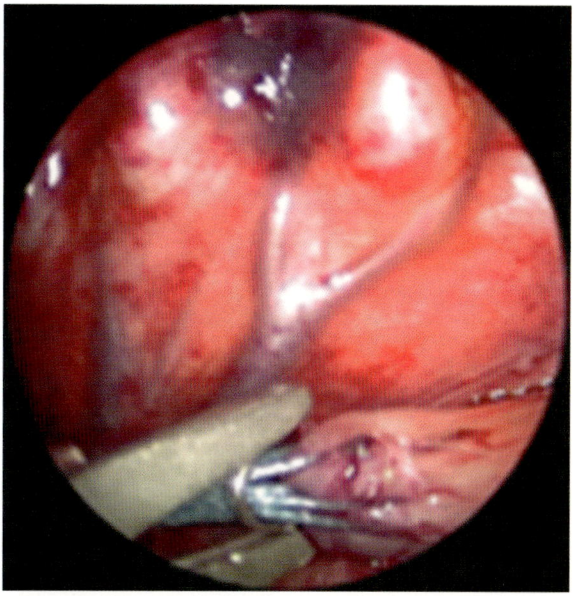

Fig. 25.3 Placement of clips at the ends of the oesophageal pouches

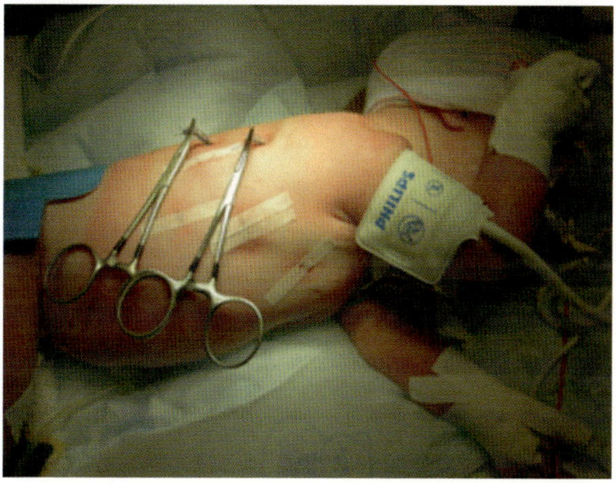

Fig. 25.4 Overview after placement of traction sutures

Ethibond® 5×0 sutures in a laparoscopic fashion to avoid migration of the stomach into the thorax (gastropexy).

The infant is sedated and appropriately given pain relief; the muscle paralysis is not indicated. Infant is nursed in a ¾ or left lateral or prone position.

Postoperatively an X-ray thorax is made to determine the start position for traction (Fig. 25.5). Thereafter once daily an X-ray thorax is made to measure the progress. Twice daily the sutures are tested for traction. It is important not to try to exert additional traction to avoid tearing of the sutures. Only when there is no more traction and the sutures can be moved freely, renewed traction may be applied on the sutures with the mini-mosquitos. An X-ray thorax should exclude that the sutures

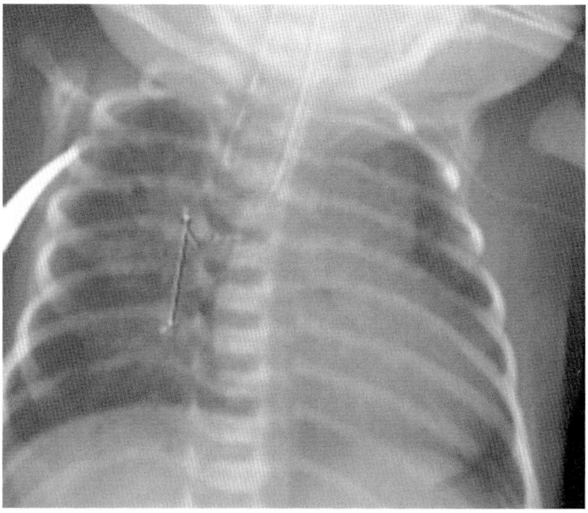

Fig. 25.5 X-ray after placement of traction sutures

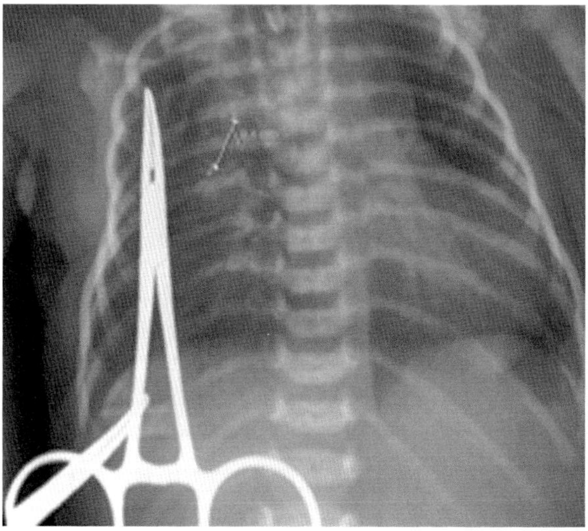

Fig. 25.6 Distance between clips after 3 days of traction

have come out of the pouch and the clip is against the thoracic wall. In that case renewed thoracoscopy is indicated. This is also the case when after 3–4 days there is no more progression of the elongation of the oesophagus (Fig. 25.6). During renewed thoracoscopy the adhesions between the oesophagus and lung tissue can be mobilized by gently sweeping an instrument between both tissues. In case a suture has come out and there is no perforation, the suture can be renewed.

If a perforation has occurred and there is contamination of the thoracic cavity, it is our policy to abandon the traction technique and convert to one of the other available techniques, in order to avoid complications.

When after 4–6 days (Fig. 25.7) the clips have approached each other, a renewed thoracoscopy is performed for a delayed primary anastomosis. For this anastomosis the proximal pouch is opened in a horizontal fashion and two Vicryl 5×0 are laid in

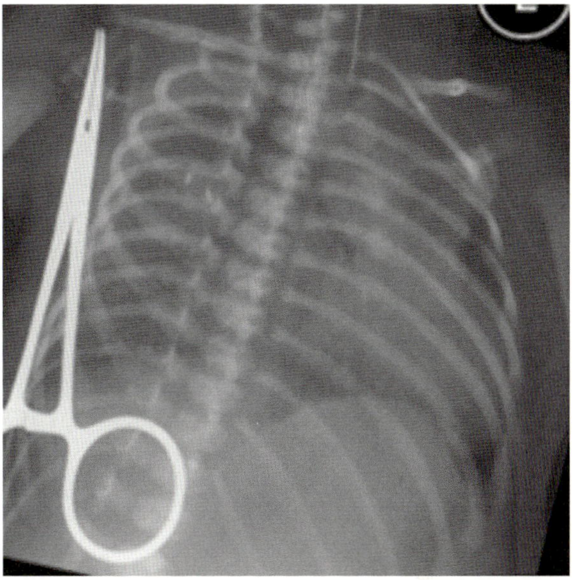

Fig. 25.7 X-ray on day 5: The clips have approached each other.

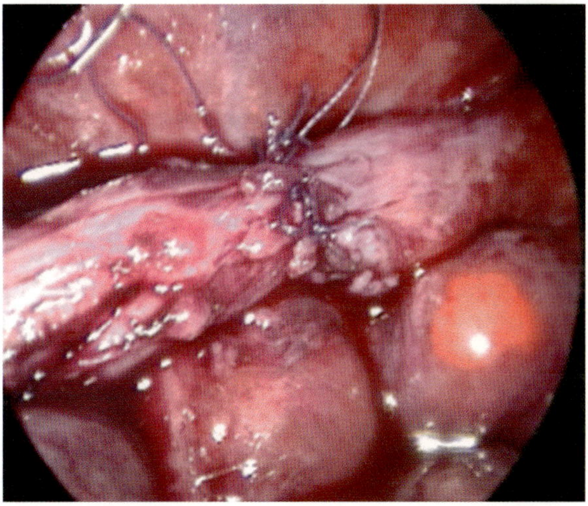

Fig. 25.8 Delayed primary anastomosis has been made

the corners with sliding knots to slowly approximate the two ends. The distal oesophagus is also opened in a horizontal way. Sometimes the mucosa is somewhat retracted, and the incision has to be opened further to identify and open the mucosa sufficiently for an adequate anastomosis. If a gastrostomy is in place, a bougie can be introduced to push up the mucosa during opening of the distal pouch.

A third suture is placed in the posterior wall after which a transanastomotic tube 6–8F is passed into the stomach. The anterior wall is closed with either interrupted or a running suture, including both the mucosa and muscle wall (Fig. 25.8). Depending on the quality of the anastomosis a postoperative chest drain is left in situ next to the anastomosis.

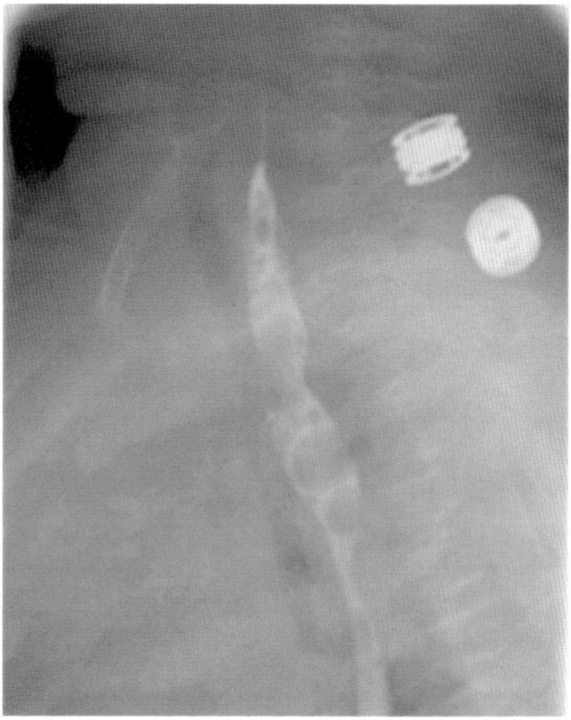

Fig. 25.9 Contrast study 5 days postoperatively. There is no leakage and the child can start drinking

After 5 days an oesophageal contrast study is performed to determine the patency of the anastomosis (Fig. 25.9). When no extravasation is present, oral feeds can be started. It should be noted that many of these patients have a small stomach and will need an adjusted feeding pattern with oral and tube feeding to ensure sufficient caloric intake.

All patients are administered antacids in the first postoperative month. From experience it is known that many of these children will need an antireflux procedure after 1–2 months, because during the traction period the oesophageal gastric junction is stretched to such an extent that gastroesophageal reflux is inevitable. Performing an antireflux operation in the same procedure as the delayed primary anastomosis is not wanted, as (1) considerable traction will be exerted on the newly made anastomosis, (2) the liver at this time is still very friable, and (3) the procedure will last longer, which is undesirable.

25.3 Other Procedures That May Be Considered in Variation of Presentation

Alternative techniques are the gastric pull-up, jejunal, and colon interposition.

Advantage of the gastric pull-up is that there will only be one anastomosis. The technique is straightforward. The disadvantage is transection of the vagal nerves with gastric emptying disturbances, superseding of the lung in the thorax, reduced feeding capabilities and reflux with concomitant pulmonary sequelae. Jejunal interposition has the advantage that it has similar to the oesophagus in size and growth. The disadvantage is that there will be two anastomoses with the risk of leakage or stenosis, the technique is technical demanding. There are less sequelae of reflux and pulmonary complications. Colon interposition is technically easier because of the arcade vascularization; it can easily be brought up into the neck, contrary to jejunal interponate. The disadvantage is the unequal growth during childhood with kinking and bulging in the neck, motility problems, and foetor ex ore.

25.4 Tips and Tricks That Will Avoid and Deal with Intraoperative Anticipated and Unanticipated Complications

1. Preoperative multidisciplinary deliberation will avoid unexpected actions to occur.
2. Close collaboration with the anesthesiologist on the positioning of the patient and during the insufflation is important to avoid deterioration of ventilation. Usually ventilation will have to be increased in minute frequency.
3. Careful exertion of pressure on the Replogle tube during dissection of the proximal oesophagus to avoid perforation.
4. Identification and sparing of the vagal nerve.
5. Blunt introduction of the trocars with a mosquito will avoid damage and bleeding of the intercostal vessels and lung.
6. Introduction of the traction sutures should be sufficiently high behind the scapula. This also holds for the distal entrée point of the traction sutures. Try to introduce the Endoclose® through the same hole every time a suture is introduced and retrieved to avoid postoperative air leakage and reduce the entry point for infection.
7. Guard the mini-mosquitos when transferring the child from operating table to incubation crib, and carefully instruct the nurses to be aware of inadvertent traction on the mini-mosquitos.
8. Upon starting the rethoracoscopy, beware of adhesion of the lung at the site of the 5 mm trocar. When reopening the skin and muscle defect, carefully swipe away the pleura in a horizontal direction parallel to the ribs. Use the optic to carefully detach the adhesions from pleura to the thoracic wall. Only when there is room, introduce the second and third trocar to avoid inadvertent injury to the lung with potential continuing air leakage.
9. In case the traction sutures have come out, make sure there is no leakage into the thoracic cavity with mediastinitis. It is our policy to abandon the technique with a low threshold to prevent future calamities. In case of small defects with no contamination, the leak can be over sewn with the application of new traction sutures away from the perforation.
10. In case during the delayed primary anastomosis, it remains difficult to bridge the distance between the pouches; it can be decided to take down the gastropexy

sutures or gastrostomy to gain more length to accomplish the anastomosis. A later antireflux procedure will need to restore the transition between the oesophagus and stomach.

25.5 Discussion of Uncommon Pathology and Operative Findings

25.5.1 Proximal Tracheoesophageal Fistula

Proximal tracheoesophageal fistulae apparently occur more often than described in the literature. Therefore a standard preoperative tracheoscopy is mandatory.

In case of a proximal tracheoesophageal fistula, this has to be dealt with during the first procedure, because the fistula will prevent the proximal oesophagus from coming down. It should be noticed that because of long-standing swallowing during pregnancy, the proximal pouch is already more or maximally stretched and will not descend very much more. When the proximal fistula is very high and the light of the tracheoscope can been seen in the neck when at the level of the fistula, it should be managed from the neck. If the fistula is situated at a lower level, it can be closed during the dissection of the proximal fistula.

25.5.2 Unusual Forms

Sometimes unusual forms of oesophageal atresia can be found where fibrous bands run from the proximal and/or distal oesophagus upward in the direction of the trachea or even thoracic wall. These strands often have a positive influence on the length of the pouch, and primary anastomosis with the use of two or three sliding knot sutures is possible.

25.5.3 Tips and Tricks to Deal with Postoperative Complications

1. Anastomotic leakage: when leakage is present on contrast study, a drain can be placed. If not a drain has already been placed at the level of the anastomosis; this can be performed through the 5 mm trocar incision and placed in the posterior mediastinum near the anastomosis. Principally the leaks will always fall dry in a few days to a weeks' time. Usually is suffices to leave the drain on a water slot. If the tissue around has sealed off the rest of the thorax, the drain can slowly be withdrawn.
2. Anastomotic stenosis: is a common problem after anastomosis under tension. The transanastomotic tube has secured a passage. Two to 3 weeks after surgery, dilatation can be performed for the first time. A supple guidewire is introduced through the anastomosis in to the stomach over which an 8 mm/4 cm balloon

catheter can been passed through the anastomosis. The anastomosis is carefully dilated. Be sure not to use shearing forces as this may break down the anastomosis (see also chapter on oesophageal stenosis). After 2 weeks the dilatation can be repeated with a larger size balloon catheter, followed by a laparoscopic antireflux procedure. This may be challenging, because usually the stomach is small and there is little tissue to create a valve.

3. Dysmotility of the oesophagus is a common problem in children with oesophageal atresia that is difficult to treat. Sometimes propulsitoria may have a beneficial effect.

25.6 Discussion

Long-gap oesophageal atresia is a seldom-occurring anomaly. Only 6% of all cases of oesophageal malformations concern a Gross type A atresia without fistula. This makes it difficult to acquire a large experience. There are some referral centers for long-gap oesophageal atresia, but mostly they deal with secondary referrals. In this era of high standard care and transportation facilities, it would be preferable to concentrate these patients in referral centers. The fact that several different techniques have been developed over time indicates that no technique is ideal. In all patients definitive treatment is delayed until a later stage when the children are older and better capable of enduring major surgery. Initial treatment consists of tube feeding through a gastrostomy. Sometimes even a cervical esophagostomy is made to allow for sham feeding and disposal of salivation. Children that have not been fed orally later have considerable difficulties in learning and willingness to eat. Cervical esophagostomies have also been used to try to elongate the proximal oesophagus (Kimura). However, quite often a proximal anastomosis has to be made in the neck, excluding some of the available techniques for replacement of the oesophagus, such as jejunal interposition and probably also traction elongation.

With the advent of minimal invasive surgery more recently, the thoracoscopic elongation technique has been described. Nowadays these children can be operated in the first week of life without a gastrostomy, and when the contrast study shows no leakage, they can start drinking after 2–3 weeks of life. This technique seems promising and makes these patients comparable to children with type C oesophageal atresia with much less secondary sequelae.

References

1. Stone MM, Fonkalsrud EW, Mahour GH, et al. Esophageal replacement with colon interposition in children. Ann Surg. 1986;203:346–51.
2. Spitz L. Gastric transposition for esophageal substitution in children. J Pediatr Surg. 1992;27:252–7; discussion 257–9. Review.
3. Bax KM. Jejunum for bridging long-gap esophageal atresia. Semin Pediatr Surg. 2009;18:34–9.

4. Foker JE, Linden BC, Boyle EM Jr, et al. Development of a true primary repair for the full spectrum of esophageal atresia. Ann Surg. 1997;226:533–41; discussion 541–3.
5. van der Zee DC, Vieirra-Travassos D, Kramer WL, et al. Thoracoscopic elongation of the esophagus in long gap esophageal atresia. J Pediatr Surg. 2007;42:1785–8.

Foregut Duplication Cysts

26

Michael Singh

Abstract
Foregut duplication cysts originate from the foetal foregut and can be oesophageal duplications or bronchogenic cyst. The majority of patients are diagnosed antenatally and are asymptomatic at birth. A postnatal CT scan will confirm the diagnosis. All foregut duplications should be removed as they will eventually cause symptoms. If the patient is asymptomatic, thoracic cysts are best excised thoracoscopically.

Keywords
Foregut duplications · Oesophageal duplication · Bronchogenic cyst · Neuroenteric cyst · Thoracoscopy

26.1 Introduction

Foregut duplication cysts are a spectrum of congenital malformations with origins from the foetal foregut [1]. They comprise oesophageal duplications and bronchogenic cysts. In the modern era, the majority of patients are diagnosed during antenatal scanning. They account for one third of all mediastinal cysts and are the main differential diagnosis for posterior mediastinal cysts. Oesophageal duplication cysts can account for up to 21% of all gastrointestinal duplications [2, 3]. The majority of children are asymptomatic at birth. Occasionally some may have acute respiratory distress, stridor, dysphagia, haematemesis, meningitis and sudden appearance of a cervical mass. They may be found incidentally on a chest X-ray. All foregut duplications should be removed as they will eventually cause symptoms.

M. Singh, M.B.B.S., F.R.C.S.Ed. (Ped Surg)
Department of Pediatric Surgery, Birmingham Children's Hospital NHS Foundation Trust, Birmingham, UK
e-mail: michael.singh@bch.nhs.uk

D. Parikh, P.B. Rajesh (eds.), *Tips and Tricks in Thoracic Surgery*,
https://doi.org/10.1007/978-1-4471-7355-7_26

26.2 Technical Tips and Tricks

Symptomatic neonates should undergo urgent investigations to confirm the diagnosis. A CT scan with intravenous contrast should be done. The typical appearance is of a low attenuation, homogenous cystic mass, with a smooth border adjacent to the oesophagus or trachea (Figs. 26.1a, b and 26.2). A contrast swallow may show communication with the oesophagus in an oesophageal duplication. The spine should also be assessed for vertebral anomalies in cases of a neurenteric cyst [4]. As the majority of patients are asymptomatic, these investigations can be done between 9 and 12 months of age. Elective thoracoscopic surgery should be performed at about 1 year of age.

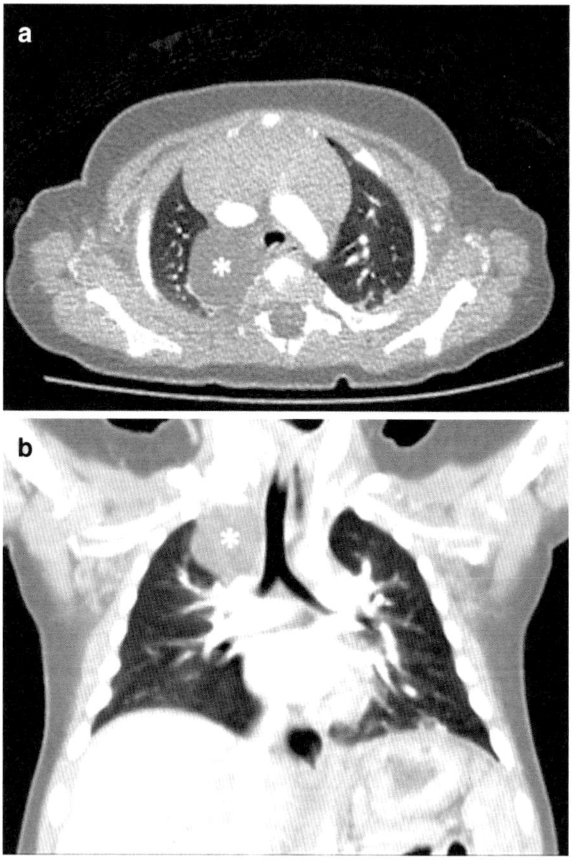

Fig. 26.1 (**a**, **b**) A CT scan of a right-sided and superior bronchogenic cyst. The typical appearance is of a low attenuation, homogenous cystic mass with a smooth border adjacent to the oesophagus (asterisk)

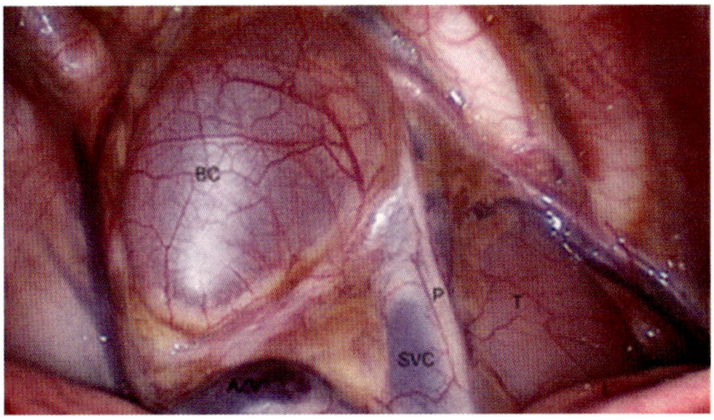

Fig. 26.2 This cyst is located in close proximity to the great vessels. Bronchogenic cyst (BC), azygos vein (AZV), superior vena cava (SVC), phrenic nerve (P), thymus (T), lung (L)

26.3 Thoracoscopic Surgery

The location of the lesion is confirmed and the chest is marked on that side. Blood loss is usually not significant; however there should be one unit of blood cross-matched. Central endotracheal intubation, with the use of a pneumothorax, is sufficient in most cases. In the older child, single-lung ventilation can be achieved by the use of bronchial blockers. A single dose of prophylactic antibiotics (co-amoxiclav) is administered.

1. 5 mm instruments are used in patients 7 kg or more. The instruments used include 0 degree scope, straight and curved graspers, needle holders, monopolar hook diathermy, suction irrigation and a sealing device such as the LigaSure© (Valley Lab, Boulder, CO, USA). A thoracotomy tray should be on standby if a thoracotomy is needed.
2. The patient is placed on an axillary roll, in the lateral position with the affected side up. For a superior lesion, the patient's hip is flexed, and the surgeon stands at the foot of the table. For an inferior lesion, the surgeon stands at the head end of the table. The monitor is positioned directly over the patient's head or pelvis.
3. The first port (optical) is inserted just anterior to the inferior angle of the scapula. A pneumothorax of 5–6 mmHg with flows of 1–2 L/min is created.
4. Following lung collapse, the two other working ports are inserted under direct vision in the same intercostal space, at the anterior axillary line and posteriorly. There should be adequate triangulation so as to create ergonomic and efficient working.
5. Large cysts can be aspirated by using a spinal needle. The cyst is grasped, and the mediastinal pleura at its base is incised with the monopolar hook (Figs. 26.3 and 26.4). Progressive dissection is continued with the hook by staying close to the surface of the cyst. The monopolar diathermy should be used sparingly so

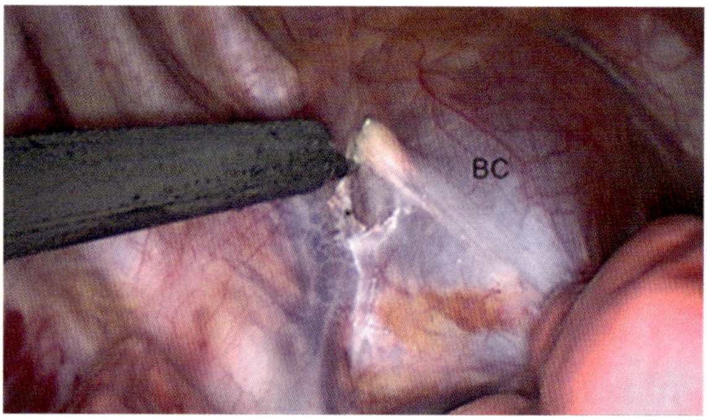

Fig. 26.3 The cyst (BC) is grasped, and the mediastinal pleura (asterisk) at its base is incised with a monopolar hook

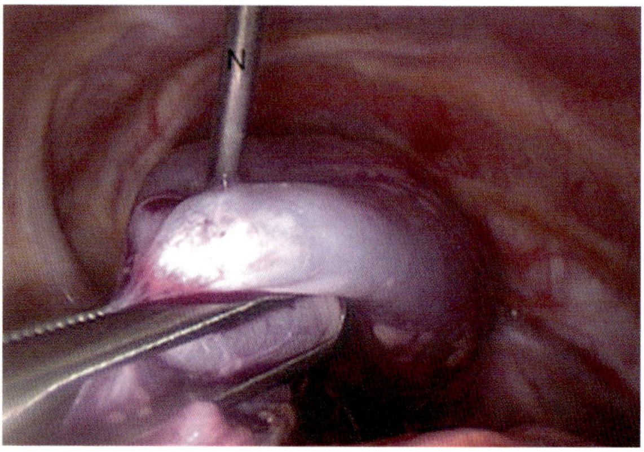

Fig. 26.4 The cyst can be aspirated with a spinal needle (N) to facilitate dissection and removal

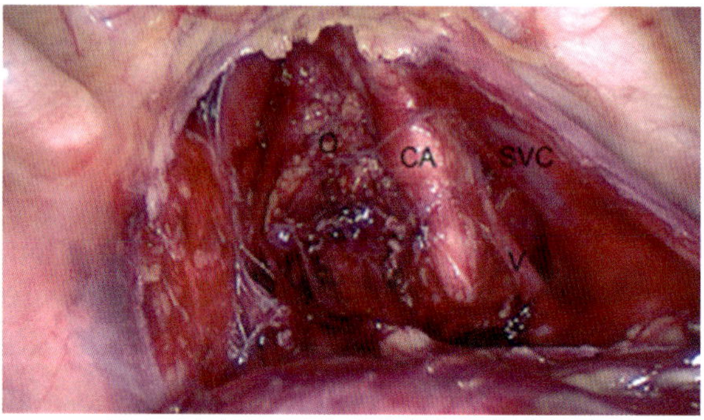

Fig. 26.5 The bed of the cyst after removal is shown: oesophagus (O), carotid artery (CA), vagus nerve (V), superior vena cava (SVC)

as to avoid inadvertent electrical or thermal injury to the phrenic and vagus nerves and the oesophagus.

6. Oesophageal duplication cysts can have a common wall with the native oesophagus. The cyst should be carefully excised and the oesophageal mucosa left intact (Fig. 26.5). The muscular defect is then sutured with absorbable sutures.
7. Marsupialisation of the cyst should be avoided as recurrence will occur.

8. The specimen is extracted via the anterior port site, and the pneumothorax is aspirated with a temporary under water seal. There is no need to insert a chest drain if the lung is re-expanded and the resection is straight forward.
9. If there is injury to the lung, trachea or oesophagus, a 16 Fr chest drain should be inserted via the anterior port.
10. A chest X-ray is done the following day. A contrast swallow can be performed to check for an oesophageal leak if necessary.

26.4 Thoracotomy

1. Thoracotomy and resection is indicated for the following reasons:
   - Thoracoscopic expertise is not available.
   - A large infected cyst.
   - Inability to clearly visualise the base of the cyst.
   - Complications during thoracoscopic resection.
2. The patient is positioned as for a thoracoscopic resection, and the surgeon stands towards the patient's back.
3. The posterolateral muscle-cutting thoracotomy is performed. Subperiosteal resection of the fourth or fifth rib is performed, and the pleura is opened.
4. The cyst is excised in a similar way as in a thoracoscopic resection.
5. The periosteum is closed with absorbable sutures, and the chest muscles are closed in layers.

26.5 Cervical Excision

1. This is indicated if the cyst is palpable at the base of the neck, in the anterior triangle.
2. A roll is placed under the patients shoulder to extend the neck.
3. The skin and platysma muscle are incised. Blunt dissection is then used until the surface of the cyst is reached.
4. The vagus and recurrent laryngeal nerves can be pushed onto the anterior surface of the cyst. Careful dissection by staying on the surface of the cyst is carried out with the minimal use of diathermy.
5. The cyst is excised and the oesophagus is repaired. The neck muscles are closed.

26.6 Intraoperative Anticipated and Unanticipated Complications

1. Bleeding
   (a) Careful dissection, staying close to the cyst wall, should not result in significant bleeding. Crossmatched blood should be available if there is a large infected oesophageal duplication or the cyst is adjacent to the large mediastinal vessels.

2. Injury to the phrenic and vagus nerves
   (a) The surgeon should aim to stay close to the surface of the cyst during its dissection. Minimal use of electrosurgical devices would reduce the risk of conduction and thermal injuries to the adjacent structures.
3. Oesophageal and thoracic duct injury
   (a) Both can present as a postoperative pleural effusion or increased output from the chest drain.
   (b) An oesophageal leak is suspected if frothy liquid (saliva) is draining from the chest drain. There may be associated sepsis. As small leak that is adequately draining via the chest drain can be managed conservatively. This includes: intravenous antibiotics, nil by mouth and total parenteral nutrition. A contrast swallow or tube oesophagogram is performed after 10 days. Oral diet can be started if no continued leakage is demonstrated. However, if an empyema develops than a thoracotomy, debridement and oesophageal repair are necessary.
   (c) If a thoracic duct injury is recognised intraoperatively, then it should be ligated or clipped. Fibrin glue can also be applied over the area. Postoperatively, it presents as the typical milky effusion, draining via the chest drain. Conservative management can include: nil by mouth and total parenteral nutrition, medium chain triglyceride feeds and subcutaneous octreotide. A persistent chylothorax can also be managed by thoracoscopic clipping of the injured duct or clipping as it comes through the right diaphragm.
4. Tracheal injury
   (a) This can occur if the bronchogenic cyst shares a common wall with the trachea. It requires rapid conversion to a thoracotomy for repair. The anaesthetist may have to advance the endotracheal tube beyond the defect in order to maintain ventilation. The trachea is sutured using a continuous polypropylene suture. A chest drain should be inserted.

Conclusions

The majority of patients with foregut duplications are diagnosed antenatally and are asymptomatic at birth. In asymptomatic patients, an elective CT scan should be done at 9–12 months of age. Elective thoracoscopic excision should be planned at about 1 year of age. Surgical complications can be avoided with careful dissection, staying close to the cyst surface and the minimal use of electrosurgical instruments.

References

1. Ponski TA, Rothenberg SS. Foregut duplication cysts. In: Parikh DH, Crabb D, Aldist A, Rothenberg SS, editors. Paediatric thoracic surgery. London: Springer; 2009. p. 383–90.
2. Stringer MD, Spitz L, Abel R, et al. Management of alimentary tract duplication in children. Br J Surg. 1995;82:74–8.
3. Holcomb GW III, Gheissari A, O'Neill JA Jr, et al. Surgical management of alimentary tract duplications. Ann Surg. 1989;209:167–74.
4. Weiss LM, Fagelman D, Warhit JM. CT demonstration of an esophageal duplication cyst. J Comput Assist Tomogr. 1983;7:716–8.

Oesophageal Tumours: Benign and Malignant

27

S. Michael Griffin, Barry Dent, and Shajahan Wahed

Abstract

Oesophageal tumours provide a challenge in management. Curative treatment for adenocarcinoma and squamous cancer invariably involve surgical resection. Small cell cancer is managed without surgical intervention. Benign lesions such as leiomyomas must be monitored but rarely require intervention unless they are causing obstruction. The staging investigations are often extensive and complex as there is no place for palliative surgery for metastatic disease. Surgery requires alymphadenectomy and feeding access. The procedures are high risk and complications are common. This chapter highlights practical ideas to make the procedure and the management of the complications more clear and straightforward.

Keywords

Oesophageal tumours • Oesophagectomy • Lymphadenectomy • Omentoplasty • Jenenostomy

27.1 Introduction

The most common malignant tumours of the oesophagus are adenocarcinoma and squamous cell carcinoma. Squamous cell carcinoma is the most predominant histological type worldwide. In the UK and western world, adenocarcinoma predominates and accounts for over half of all oesophageal cancers [1–3]. The incidence of

S. Michael Griffin, O.B.E., M.D., F.R.C.S.Ed (✉) • B. Dent, M.B. B.Chir., F.R.C.S.Ed
S. Wahed, B.Sc., M.D., F.R.C.S
Northern Oesophago-Gastric Unit, Royal Victoria Infirmary, Queen Victoria Infirmary, Newcastle upon Tyne, UK
e-mail: michael.griffin@nuth.nhs.uk

D. Parikh, P.B. Rajesh (eds.), *Tips and Tricks in Thoracic Surgery*,
https://doi.org/10.1007/978-1-4471-7355-7_27

adenocarcinoma continues to rise, and is strongly associated with reflux disease, obesity and Barrett's oesophagus [4, 5]. Rare malignant tumours of the oesophagus include primary melanoma, small cell carcinoma, leiomyosarcoma and adenoid cystic carcinomas.

Benign tumours of the oesophagus include leiomyomas and gastrointestinal stromal tumours (GIST). Leiomyomas are more common but in the majority of patients can be left alone. Surgery is rarely required but may be indicated if necrosis or obstructive symptoms occur. Endoscopic ultrasound and fine needle aspirate can be used if there is diagnostic uncertainty. The risk of malignancy with a leiomyoma is extremely low. Oesophageal GISTs are rare. Larger GISTs can demonstrate malignant behaviour so warrant full investigation and treatment. Rare granular cell tumours can be observed.

Patients with oesophageal cancers should undergo clinical staging and discussion at a specialist upper GI multidisciplinary meeting (MDT). Staging investigations will include endoscopy, endoscopic ultrasound and computed tomography of the chest, abdomen and pelvis. Most patients also will have a positron emission tomogram (PET-CT) to look for distant metastases [6]. Neck ultrasound and magnetic resonance imaging of the liver can clarify the nature of lymph nodes in the neck or lesions in the liver, respectively. Patients should undergo formal fitness assessment and review by an anaesthetist specialising in oesophageal surgery to risk stratify patients and identify any aspects of a patient's condition that can be optimised. Cardiopulmonary exercise testing has been adopted in recent years although its value in predicting morbidity and mortality is yet to be clarified. Nutritional assessment by a specialist dietician is equally as crucial.

Most patients with potentially curative oesophageal cancer present with locally advanced disease and will receive neoadjuvant chemotherapy or chemoradiotherapy prior to surgical resection [7–9]. It is important to recognise that resection should not be performed in the palliative setting. This includes cancers that have perforated, as the development of recurrent disease is inevitable [10]. Oesophagectomy is in most cases performed as a two-phase procedure with a radical en bloc two-field lymphadenectomy. The stomach is the most common conduit replacement for resected oesophagus [11]. The aims of surgical resection are to remove all cancerous tissue, provide the optimal chance of cure and optimal disease staging whilst maintaining as best possible the patient's quality of life.

27.2 Technical Tips and Tricks

Oesophagectomy is performed under general anaesthesia with a double lumen endotracheal tube, nasogastric tube insertion, intravenous antibiotic prophylaxis and mechanical venous thromboembolism prophylaxis. A thoracic epidural has traditionally been used although paravertebral and wound catheters offer an alternative approach to postoperative pain management.

1. Abdominal access and gastric mobilisation

   Excision of the xiphisternum will improve access from a long midline incision. A retractor anchored to the operating table such as the Omni-tract® is crucial

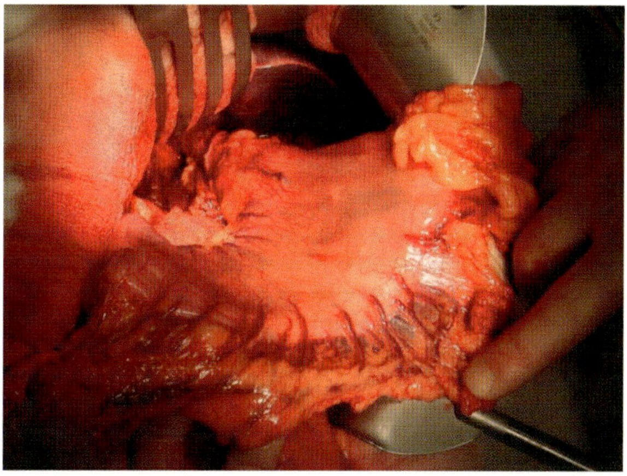

Fig. 27.1 Preservation of the right gastroepiploic vessels and arcade

to provide the required exposure, with more traction required for the left side of the abdominal wall. The left triangular ligament attaching the left lobe of the liver to the diaphragm can be divided to aid hiatal exposure but ensuring the dissection does not injure the diaphragm, liver, phrenic vein or inferior vena cava. Use of a headlight significantly enhances visualisation of the operative field.

Palpating and tracing the route of the gastroepiploic vessels is the first step before commencing gastric mobilisation. Variations in the anatomy need to be appreciated as the arcade can sometimes take a course much further away from the greater curve than expected [12, 13]. Some of the omentum from the greater curve should be preserved to wrap the oesophagogastric anastomosis and conduit staple line in the thorax. Bipolar scissors and an energy-sealing device are used for the dissection (Fig. 27.1).

The duodenum should be kocherised and the tissue within the 'C' of the duodenum dissected to free any attachments to the colon and allow the pylorus to reach the hiatus. Failure to achieve sufficient mobility and leaving the pylorus or distal stomach in the abdominal cavity can result in significant postoperative gastric emptying problems.

2. En bloc lymph node dissection

   Diathermy forceps or bipolar scissors are a good instrument for the abdominal nodal dissection in order to coagulate the small surrounding vessels. The easiest starting point is around the anterior common hepatic node, using atraumatic grasping forceps to lift the lymph node and continuing the dissection back to the junction with the splenic artery. The proximal splenic nodes are dissected in a similar way. The left gastric vein will be encountered and needs to be ligated in continuity before being divided. The dissection is continued onto the left gastric lymph nodes, left gastric artery (ligated and divided in continuity) and coeliac vessels before progressing up to the hiatus. This part of the dissection is often best approached with the stomach retracted in the cranial direction, although the view through the pars flaccida window can also be utilised (Fig. 27.2).

3. Hiatal dissection

   This part of the dissection proceeds along the pre-aortic plane, resecting pleura and the pericardial fat en bloc. A renal vein retractor provides good retraction to

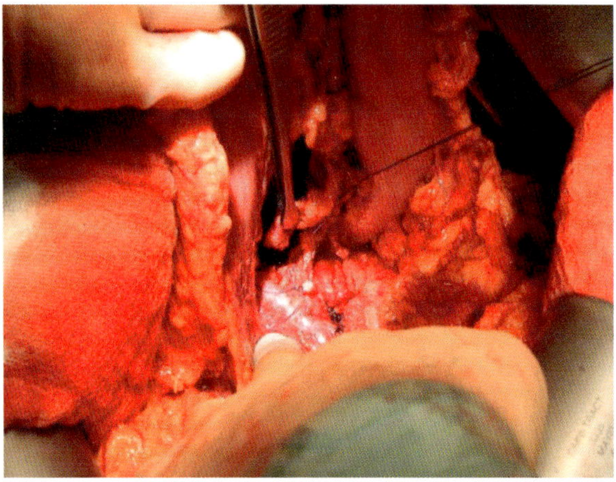

Fig. 27.2 En bloc abdominal lymphadenectomy

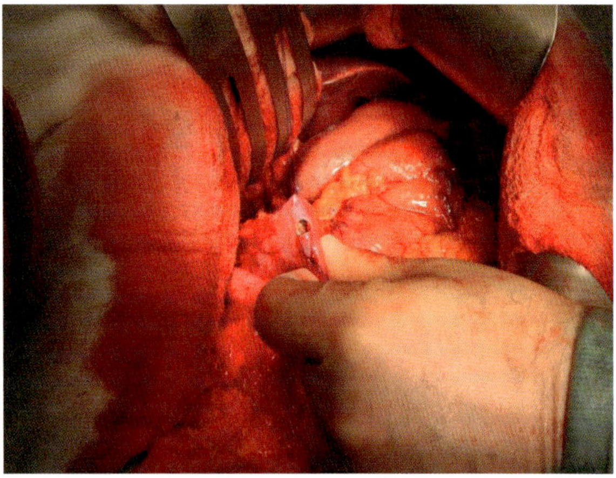

Fig. 27.3 Performing a pyloroplasty

allow exposure for the dissection. Part of each crus is resected en bloc, and this will allow tension-free delivery of the gastric conduit during the thoracotomy. Complete mobilisation can be checked by running a hand freely from above the hiatus behind the stomach to the duodenum without any obstructing tissue.

4. Pyloroplasty

   A pyloroplasty is used to prevent postoperative gastric drainage problems. Diathermy is used to divide the muscle between stay sutures. Forceps or the sucker tip can be used to open up the anterior wall. A Gambee-type suture at either end can reduce bleeding from submucosal vessels. It is crucial to confirm that a small amount of mucosa is incorporated in the sutures whilst checking that no sutures catch the posterior wall (Fig. 27.3).

5. Feeding jejunostomy

   This is routinely performed to provide nutritional support in the postoperative period. It becomes especially important in the event of any postoperative complications that delay resumption of oral intake or necessitate additional nutritional requirements [14]. It is however a potential source of morbidity in itself, so the technique to insert it should be meticulous.

The authors use a 14Fr MIC feeding tube. The flushed tube is drawn through the abdominal wall after making a stab incision and cut to the appropriate length (approximately 30 cm from the balloon). This is inserted through a 2.0 Vicryl™ purse-string into the proximal jejunum, leaving a 1 cm gap from the balloon to the entry point. The purse-string is tied and the two ends wrapped back around the tube and retied to prevent the tube from slipping back out. The tube is covered with a Witzel tunnel created with interrupted 2.0 Vicryl™ and then anchored to the abdominal wall with three or four anchor sutures. It is easier to insert the lateral sutures first before pulling the balloon back into the abdominal wall and tying. The medial sutures are inserted next. A split is created in a suitable part of the omentum that is attached to the transverse colon. This is placed around the jejunostomy before tying proximal and distal anchor sutures that incorporate peritoneum, omentum, jejunum and omentum. These sutures prevent twisting at the jejunostomy site whilst the omental wrap reduces the possibility of infracolic contents herniating through the hiatus. The balloon is inflated with 2–4 mL of sterile water within the preperitoneal abdominal wall. The jejunostomy should be flushed at this point to ensure there is free flow.

6. Thoracic access

   The ideal space for the right posterolateral thoracotomy is the fourth intercostal space. The neck of the rib should be excised to allow the rib space to open up fully without fracturing further ribs. It is the authors' experience that post-thoracotomy wound pain is reduced if a length of intercostal nerve is excised at the level of rib resection. The Omni-tract® or a finochietto retractor is used for retraction and exposure.

7. Ligation of azygos vein

   When mobilising the arch of the azygos vein, it is important to identify branches of the bronchial vessels that can cause nuisance bleeding. The knots from the ligatures on the azygos arch need to be tied squarely to avoid twisting of the vein and slippage of the ties that could result in catastrophic bleeding.

8. Dissection and ligation of thoracic duct

   The dissection should follow the line of the azygos vein caudally. Bipolar scissors are the authors' instrument of choice for this. The dissection is deepened onto the pre-aortic plane. At the level of the hiatus, the thoracic duct should be clearly identified and ligated in the groove between the azygos vein and aorta. It is vital that no traction is placed on the thoracic duct to avoid avulsing small branches off the main duct (Fig. 27.4).

9. Para-aortic dissection

   The dissection in the pre-aortic plane takes the dissection back in the cranial direction and onto the infracarinal tissue. The fingers of the retracting left hand are crucial in elevating and stretching the tissue to allow dissection with the bipolar scissors taking everything away from the aorta. Any vessels branching directly off the aorta need to be identified and controlled before division. It is important not to retract tissue from the left side of the aorta, because bleeding

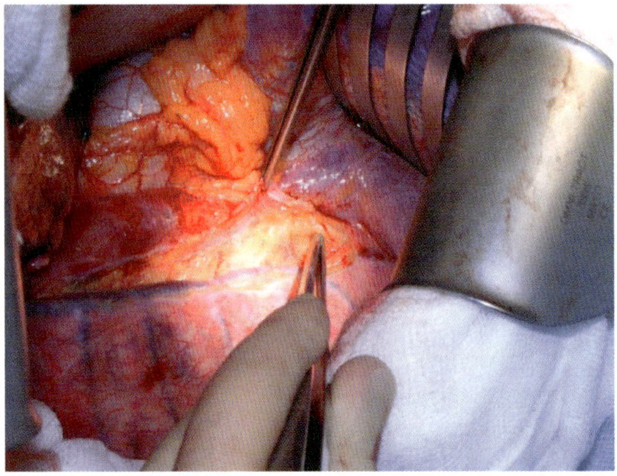

Fig. 27.4 Identification of the thoracic duct at the level of the hiatus

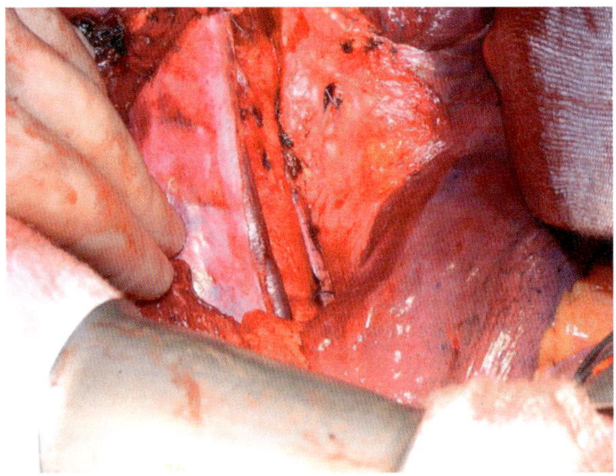

Fig. 27.5 Appearance after mediastinal dissection including en bloc lymphadenectomy around the bronchi

from any divided tissue on that side will be extremely difficult to control. Once a window has been created in this plane, a Nylon tape can be used to sling the oesophagus up and open the plane cranially for further dissection.

10. Tracheobronchial lymphadenectomy

    The optimal approach for this part of the dissection is to continue the dissection up from the back of the pericardium. The upper and lower edges of the cartilaginous rings of both bronchi need to be identified before dissecting into this region to avoid injury. The balloon on the endotracheal cuff should be palpable in the left main bronchus. Traction (consider Wangensteens or Babcock forceps) can help pull these infracarinal lymph nodes away from the pericardium and allow a clean dissection. There will be vessels supplying the lymph nodes at the apex within the carina and at the edge of each bronchial node that should be ligated to prevent bleeding (Fig. 27.5).

    The dissection continues onto the right paratracheal tissue. The vagus nerve should be divided without diathermy to avoid conduction of energy damaging the recurrent laryngeal nerve. The stay sutures are inserted into the proximal oesophagus once the mobilisation is complete. Interrupted full-thickness 2-0

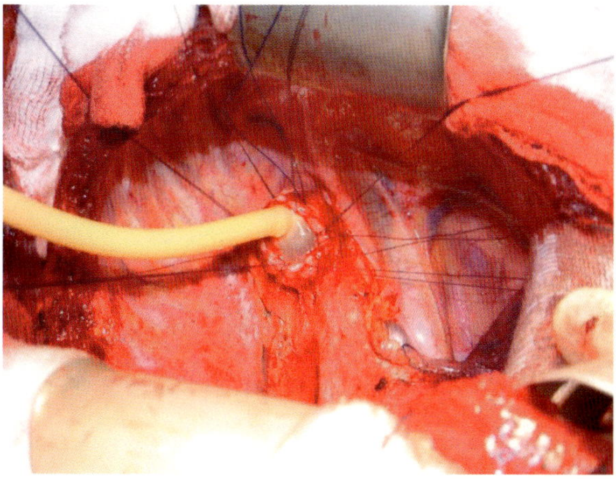

Fig. 27.6 Using a Foley catheter to dilate the proximal oesophagus after the purse-string suture has been inserted

Monocryl sutures are inserted before a 0 Prolene purse-string suture that is used to tie in the anvil of an appropriately sized anvil. The proximal oesophagus is dilated with the balloon of a Foley catheter prior to the anvil insertion (25 or 28 mm). It is important to take the tension off the interrupted sutures when tying the purse-string (Fig. 27.6).

11. Delivery and formation of conduit

Completion of the hiatal dissection is left until the end of the oesophageal mobilisation to avoid abdominal fluid spilling into the thorax and obscuring the operative field. Once the dissection has been completed, the gastric conduit should be delivered by gentle traction along the greater curve of the stomach. The pyloroplasty should lie at or above the level of the hiatus with the sutures palpable anteriorly. It is crucial to ensure that the stomach has not twisted during delivery.

12. Anastomosis and drainage

The conduit should be prepared by dividing the lesser curve fat at the junction between the left and right gastric arteries. The high point of the stomach needs to be identified and checked so that it will reach the proximal oesophagus. The anastomosis should lie above the level of the divided azygos arch. A long oesophageal clamp is used to mark the level of transection from the point on the lesser curve and the stomach divided with diathermy below this. Babcock forceps are used to pick up the gastric conduit edges. It is imperative to ensure that the distance between the chosen anastomosis site and gastrotomy edge is not too short. The conduit itself should not be narrowed too much (the authors' minimum recommendation is 5 cm) as this will damage intramural vascular arcades and put the conduit at risk of ischaemic necrosis [15].

When the circular stapler is inserted, the distance to the edge of the gastrotomy should again be checked to ensure it is not too short (minimum 2 cm). The stapler point should be advanced through the gastric wall whilst two fingers press either side of the exit point. A purse-string suture is inserted around the exit point of the anvil to prevent a split in the gastric wall. After engaging the stapler and anvil, a check is made to ensure no other tissue is caught in between. The doughnuts should be inspected for complete circumferential integrity after the stapler has been fired and the staple gun removed. The nasogastric tube

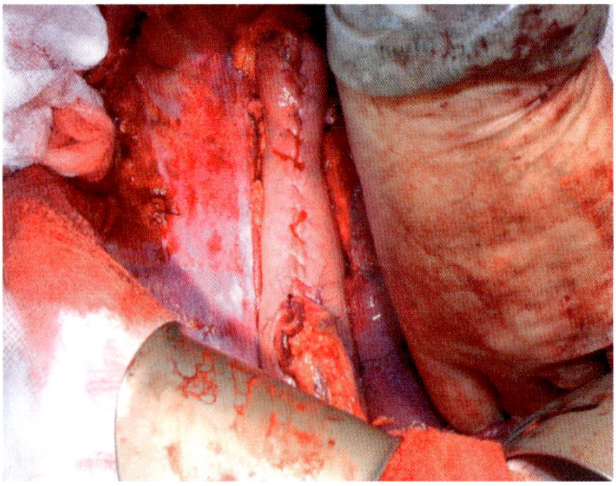

Fig. 27.7 The gastric conduit after inversion of the gastrotomy staple line

should be sited in the distal stomach and secured to a nasal bridle. Although the gastrotomy is closed with a stapler, the authors invert the staple line with a continuous suture.

The greater curve fat/omentum is placed alongside the airways and wrapped over the anastomosis and gastrotomy with interrupted sutures. The parietal pleura at the apex of the thoracic cavity is used to provide additional cover over the fat at the anastomosis.

The authors use two soft 24Fr chest drains to drain the apex and base of the right thoracic cavity (Fig. 27.7).

27.3 Tips and Tricks that Will Avoid and Deal with Intraoperative Anticipated and Unanticipated Complications

27.3.1 Splenic Injury

The first manoeuvre in the abdominal dissection should be to identify and release any adhesions from the gastrosplenic ligament to the lower pole of the spleen to prevent inadvertent traction injury and bleeding. Placing the patient head up and right side down helps with the exposure for this step.

Control of bleeding from small tears on the spleen can be achieved by using ball diathermy or haemostatic tissue glues in order to preserve the spleen.

27.3.2 Bleeding

Ensure the short gastric vessels are clearly defined before ligation and division or before application of an energy device to seal the vessels. Inadequate exposure can lead to troublesome bleeding if vessels are only partially sealed before division. Use of energy devices is not a substitute for adequate dissection.

The small vessels branching directly off the aorta are encountered during the pre-aortic dissection and oesophagus mobilisation. These can cause significant bleeding. Prevention is the best course of action, so firm retraction with the fingers of the left hand will stretch the para-aortic tissue and allow identification of these branches before they are inadvertently cut. The dissection should take one layer of the pre-aortic tissue at a time with the bipolar scissors. The safest option for the aortic branches is ligation, although controlled bipolar diathermy is suitable for the smallest branches. The dissection should ensure that a small stump of the vessel is left on the aortic wall to facilitate ligation in continuity. The branch that appears near the start of the arch of the aorta is a particularly sizeable vessel and in most cases can be avoided. If it enters the plane of dissection, it should be ligated and then divided.

27.3.3 Chyle Leaks

A double (or rarely triple) thoracic duct is sometimes encountered, more commonly in females. In these cases both ducts need to be ligated and divided. There are often large side branches from the main thoracic duct particularly in its distal part that need to be ligated separately.

During the hiatal dissection of the abdominal phase, the cisterna chyli is at risk of injury, particularly in thin patients. The dissection of the pre-aortic plane at this level needs to avoid damaging this structure.

The small lymphatics around the abdominal lymph nodes rarely cause significant chyle leak, but they can be ligated during the lymphadenectomy to prevent small pools of chyle.

27.3.4 Lymph Node Fracture

It is best practice to avoid holding lymph nodes if at all possible as they fracture easily. If there is no other option, then use of atraumatic forceps such as Wangensteens is least likely to cause disruption. Babcock forceps to completely encircle the lymph node are the other instruments that are useful during lymphadenectomy. The posterior common hepatic node often needs to be ligated at an appropriate level to avoid injury to the portal vein.

27.3.5 Airway Injury

The membranous part of the trachea and bronchi are fragile and particularly susceptible to injury. The edges of these structures should be clearly identified by vision and palpation. Avoiding the use of diathermy in close proximity to these structures is recommended. If diathermy is necessary, it should be with bipolar scissors. Dissection in the direction of the airways is made safer by placing the fingers of the retracting hand flat against the airways to protect them.

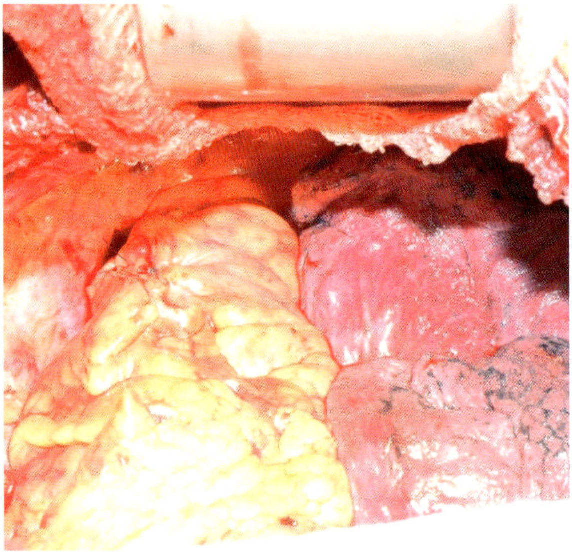

Fig. 27.8 Omentoplasty covering the anastomosis and gastrotomy and acting as a barrier between the conduit and the airways

The omentum should be placed between the airways and conduit and then onto cover the gastrotomy and anastomosis. This offers additional protection should there be any leak from either part of the staple line (Fig. 27.8).

27.4 Alternative Methods

Endoscopic resection is a potentially curative option in patients with T1a (mucosal) cancer [16]. These cases should still be fully staged as with any other oesophageal cancer and be discussed in the MDT prior to endoscopic resection. Endoscopic mucosal resection is performed under sedation and intravenous analgesia in the endoscopy department by a specialist endoscopist. Mucosal lesions with histologically clear vertical and circumferential margins (including biopsies from the edge of the resection site) can be followed up with endoscopic surveillance. Endoscopic resection is not suitable for cancers that have reached the submucosal layer because of the risk of lymph node metastases [17].

The use of minimally invasive techniques for oesophagectomy has increased in the UK [18]. The same resection as in open surgery should be performed if minimally invasive techniques are chosen. Appropriate placement of the ports is crucial in making the dissection less onerous, particularly of mobilising the distal stomach and performing the pyloroplasty. Using the Nathanson retractor to lift up the whole stomach once the left gastric vessels have been divided helps with mobilising the duodenum free from hepatic flexure attachments and with kocherisation. The feeding jejunostomy can be performed more easily by extending the left side supraumbilical port and placing the sutures under direct vision in the same way as described above.

One major pitfall when performing laparoscopic mobilisation is failure to identify the route of the gastroepiploic arcade particularly in obese patients. This can be inadvertently damaged, rendering the stomach unsuitable as the conduit and, if not recognised at the time of operation, resulting in gastric necrosis [19]. Creation of a too narrow conduit will also significantly increase the risk of conduit necrosis [12, 15].

Thoracoscopic mobilisation can be helped by appropriate port placement, with the arm abducted and rotated above the patient's head.

27.5 Uncommon Pathology

A duplicate or even triplicate thoracic duct is sometimes encountered. Failure to appreciate that this variant exists can result in a postoperative chyle leak.

27.6 Postoperative Management

Patients should be prepared in advance for the postoperative period. Enhanced recovery programmes have been demonstrated to improve outcomes and reduce hospital stay in patients undergoing oesophagectomy [20]. Early, regular physiotherapy and mobilisation is crucial to reduce the risk of atelectasis, respiratory tract infections and venous thromboembolism. It also helps gut function return quicker. Enteral nutrition can be provided via the feeding jejunostomy according to local dietetic protocols. It is important to build up enteral jejunostomy feeds gradually to prevent nausea, bloating and pain. Routine use of laxatives can also help expedite the return of gut function.

27.7 Tips and Tricks to Deal with Postoperative Complications

Patients who have had an oesophagectomy can deteriorate rapidly in the event of postoperative complications. Prevention is the best strategy and involves preoperative optimisation, meticulous surgical technique and postoperative mobilisation and physiotherapy. A high index of suspicion must be adopted when reviewing patients with a low threshold for prompt investigation.

In the majority of patients, anastomotic leaks can be successfully managed with intensive conservative management [21]. This includes intravenous antibiotics and antifungals, intravenous proton pump inhibitor, enteral feeding, targeted chest drainage and stopping any oral intake. A radiological nasogastric tube should be placed. Patients should be endoscoped to identify the degree of disruption. A return to theatre is infrequently required in these cases. Surgical options in patients requiring intervention include closure of defects over a T-tube and the use of intercostal muscle flaps. Formation of an oesophagostomy with take down of the anastomosis is rarely required. The routine use of oesophageal stents to treat anastomotic leaks is unnecessary. Stents are associated with significant complications including mortality [22].

Chyle leaks can result in immunosuppression and malnutrition. It is usually due to damage to the main thoracic duct or a large side branch, although occasionally can arise from damage to the cisterna chyli. Chyle can be confirmed by sending drain fluid for chylomicrons or triglycerides. The differential serum lymphocyte count should be checked. Management involves reducing the flow of chyle, draining any chylothorax, maintaining nutritional status and preventing opportunistic infection. Enteral feeds should be switched to medium chain triglyceride types. Intravenous co-trimoxazole is given to prevent opportunistic infections. Fluid and electrolyte balance should be strictly monitored. Indications for a return to theatre for thoracotomy would be a persistent leak of >1000 mL/24 h persistent for 48 h. Radiological insertion of a pleuroperitoneal shunt is an option for persistent leaks where there is no identifiable duct or branch to ligate surgically.

27.8 Conclusions and the Future

Oesophageal cancer is a condition requiring specialist and complex management. Oesophagectomy requires meticulous attention to detail. This chapter has highlighted some techniques that can be adopted into practice to prevent intraoperative and postoperative difficulties.

References

1. Cancer Research UK oesophageal cancer incidence statistics. http://www.cancerresearchuk.org/cancer-info/cancerstats/types/oesophagus/incidence/.
2. Coupland VH, Allum W, Blazeby JM, Mendall MA, Hardwick RH, Linklater KM, Moller H, Davies EA. Incidence and survival of oesophageal and gastric cancer in England between 1998 and 2007, a population-based study. BMC Cancer. 2012;12:10.
3. Pennathur A, Gibson MK, Jobe BA, Luketich JD. Oesophageal carcinoma. Lancet. 2013;381(9864):400–12.
4. Lagergren J, Bergstrom R, Lindgren A, Nyren O. Symptomatic gastroesophageal reflux as a risk factor for esophageal adenocarcinoma. N Engl J Med. 1999;340(11):825–31.
5. Rubenstein JH, Taylor JB. Meta-analysis: the association of oesophageal adenocarcinoma with symptoms of gastro-oesophageal reflux. Aliment Pharmacol Ther. 2010;32(10):1222–7.
6. Allum WH, Blazeby JM, Griffin SM, Cunningham D, Jankowski JA, Wong R, British Assoc Surgical O. Guidelines for the management of oesophageal and gastric cancer. Gut. 2011;60(11):1449–72.
7. Shapiro J, Van Lanschot JJB, Hulshof MCCM, van Hagen P, van Berge Henegouwen MI, Wijnhoven BPL, van Laarhoven HWM, Nieuwenhuijzen GAP, Hospers GAP, Bonenkamp JJ, Cuesta MA, Blaisse RJB, Busch ORC, ten Kate FJW, Creemers G-JM, Punt CJA, Plukker JTM, Verheul HMW, Bilgen EJS, van Dekken H, van der Sangen MJC, Rozema T, Biermann K, Beukema JC, Piet AHM, van Rij CM, Reinders JG, Tilanus HW, Steyerberg EW, van der Gaast A, CROSS Study Group. Neoadjuvant chemoradiotherapy plus surgery versus surgery alone for oesophageal or junctional cancer (CROSS): long-term results of a randomised controlled trial. Lancet Oncol. 2015;16(9):1090–8.

8. Allum WH, Stenning SP, Bancewicz J, Clark PI, Langley RE. Long-term results of a randomized trial of surgery with or without preoperative chemotherapy in esophageal cancer. J Clin Oncol. 2009;27(30):5062–7.
9. Cunningham D, Allum WH, Stenning SP, Thompson JN, Van de Velde CJH, Nicolson M, Scarffe JH, Lofts FJ, Falk SJ, Iveson TJ, Smith DB, Langley RE, Verma M, Weeden S, Chua YJ, Participants MT. Perioperative chemotherapy versus surgery alone for resectable gastroesophageal cancer. N Engl J Med. 2006;355(1):11–20.
10. Di Franco F, Lamb PJ, Karat D, Hayes N, Griffin SM. Iatrogenic perforation of localized oesophageal cancer. Br J Surg. 2008;95(7):837–9.
11. Griffin SM, Raimes SA, Shenfine J. Oesophagogastric surgery: a companion to specialist surgical practice. 5th ed. Philadelphia: Saunders; 2013.
12. Ndoye JM, Dia A, Ndiaye A, Fall B, Diop M, Ndiaye A, Sow ML. Arteriography of three models of gastric oesophagoplasty: the whole stomach, a wide gastric tube and a narrow gastric tube. Surg Radiol Anat. 2006;28(5):429–37.
13. Takeda FR, Cecconello I, Szachnowicz S, Tacconi MR, Gama-Rodriguez J. Anatomic study of gastric vascularization and its relationship to cervical gastroplasty. J Gastrointest Surg. 2005;9(1):132–7.
14. Couper G. Jejunostomy after oesophagectomy: a review of evidence and current practice. Proc Nutr Soc. 2011;70(3):316–20.
15. Luketich JD, Alvelo-Rivera M, Buenaventura PO, Christie NA, McCaughan JS, Litle VR, Schauer PR, Close JM, Fernando HC. Minimally invasive esophagectomy – outcomes in 222 patients. Ann Surg. 2003;238(4):486–94.
16. Pech O, May A, Manner H, Behrens A, Pohl J, Weferling M, Hartmann U, Manner N, Huijsmans J, Gossner L, Rabenstein T, Vieth M, Stolte M, Ell C. Long-term efficacy and safety of endoscopic resection for patients with mucosal adenocarcinoma of the esophagus. Gastroenterology. 2014;146(3):652.
17. Griffin SM, Burt AD, Jennings NA. Lymph node metastasis in early esophageal adenocarcinoma. Ann Surg. 2011;254(5):731–7.
18. National Oesophago-Gastric Cancer Audit - 2013. http://www.hscic.gov.uk/catalogue/PUB11093.
19. Berrisford RG, Wajed SA, Sanders D, Rucklidge MWM. Short-term outcomes following total minimally invasive oesophagectomy. Br J Surg. 2008;95(5):602–10.
20. Markar SR, Karthikesalingam A, Low DE. Enhanced recovery pathways lead to an improvement in postoperative outcomes following esophagectomy: systematic review and pooled analysis. Dis Esophagus. 2015;28(5):468–75.
21. Dent BM, Wahed S, Jones R, Immanuel A, Hayes N, Griffin SM. Outcomes following anastomotic leak in patients undergoing oesophagectomy. Br J Surg. 2016;103(8):1033–8.
22. Schweigert M, Dubecz A, Stadlhuber RJ, Muschweck H, Stein HJ. Risk of stent-related aortic erosion after endoscopic stent insertion for intrathoracic anastomotic leaks after esophagectomy. Ann Thorac Surg. 2011;92(2):513–9.

Oesophageal Strictures

28

David C. van der Zee

Abstract

Congenital oesophageal strictures are rare and are commonly associated with cartilaginous rings. Surgical intervention in congenital stenosis in shown to be beneficial with very good outcome. Acquired oesophageal strictures in children are related to severe gastro-oesophageal reflux, anastomosis and accidental ingestion of corrosive bleach or button batteries. Most oesophageal anastomotic surgery are actively followed up and monitored for stricture and gastro-oesophageal reflux. Early diagnosis and management is advocated. Only the resistant stricture may require surgical intervention. The outcome of acquired strictures is demanding and requires dedication to improve its long-term outcome. We advocate that after initial forced dilatation leaving an indwelling balloon is left at the site of stricture and the balloon is inflated three times daily with 15-20 cc of air. This may be easily taught to the parents, so they can do this at home. The dilatation is continued until the stricture has healed completely. Our experience with this management strategy has produced very good outcome of the difficult corrosive and resistant strictures and has avoided oesophageal replacement surgery.

Keywords

Oesophageal stenosis · Balloon dilatation · Oesophageal atresia · Lye burns · Reflux esophagitis

D.C. van der Zee, M.D., Ph.D.
Department of Pediatric Surgery, University Medical Center Utrecht, Utrecht, The Netherlands
e-mail: d.c.vanderzee@umcutrecht.nl

D. Parikh, P.B. Rajesh (eds.), *Tips and Tricks in Thoracic Surgery*,
https://doi.org/10.1007/978-1-4471-7355-7_28

28.1 Introduction

Oesophageal strictures may be divided into congenital or acquired in origin. Congenital strictures can be caused by muscular hypertrophy, cartilaginous ring, or oesophageal web. Acquired strictures may be due to gastroesophageal reflux, corrosive ingestion, eosinophilic esophagitis, post-oesophageal atresia repair, achalasia, and others [1].

Management varies from dilatation to resection in case of persistent stenosis.

28.2 Diagnosis and General Management

Diagnosis of oesophageal stricture usually is determined by oesophageal contrast studies and endoscopy. Congenital muscular hypertrophy or oesophageal web can be principally managed with balloon dilatation. In case of cartilaginous rings, dilatation will not be successful and surgery is warranted. When oesophageal reflux is suspected, further determination by reflux questionnaires, pH/impedance and manometry, and 13-C breath test is protocol in our institution. The stricture can usually be managed by balloon dilatation and (laparoscopic) antireflux surgery. This will solve the problem in most cases. Special attention should be directed toward eosinophilic esophagitis that may look similar to reflux esophagitis. Biopsies taken from the lower, middle, and upper oesophagus will lead to the diagnosis. Apart from dilatation medical treatment is required.

Strictures occurring after oesophageal atresia repair are usually due to gastroesophageal reflux after pulling up the distal pouch for anastomosis, compromised circulation, leakage, or a combination of all. Simple reflux can usually be managed by dilatation and antireflux medication. If the stricture persists (laparoscopic), antireflux procedure principally cures the problem. In case the stricture persists, forced dilatation followed by indwelling balloon dilatation until the defect has healed solves the problem [2].

In corrosive strictures it is important to prevent strictures from occurring. Therefore prophylactic indwelling balloon(s) are used for the duration of the healing process. This management is started within 24 h after the lye ingestion. At renewed endoscopy 1 week later, the extent of burn is evaluated, and continuation of indwelling balloon treatment is determined. In case of late management of corrosive strictures at first, forceful bouginage of the stricture is necessary. When an adequate diameter has been achieved, treatment is continued with indwelling balloons to keep the oesophagus at the desired diameter until complete healing has taken place. This may take several months. During the time of indwelling balloon treatment, feeding can be achieved both through the balloon catheter as tube feeding and when the acute symptoms of the lye burn have subsided by eating (semi-)solid food along the (not inflated) balloon. There are several lengths of balloon catheters available, and even the placement of two balloons is possible.

In children with achalasia, Heller myotomy is the first choice. In case of recurrence, positive results have been obtained with balloon dilatation. Injections with mitomycin or botulinum toxin have been described in the treatment of achalasia or recurrent strictures. It should be noted however that morbidity and mortality has been described after injection due to sepsis and mediastinitis.

28.3 Technical Tips and Tricks of Indwelling Balloon Catheter Treatment for Persistent Oesophageal Strictures

In case of persistent stricture of the oesophagus, the use of an indwelling balloon catheter has been described before [2]. The principle is that, either with a balloon catheter or a bougie, a forceful dilatation takes place under general anesthesia. When the desired diameter cannot be reached in one session, the forceful dilatation may be spread out over more than one procedure. Otherwise or meanwhile a balloon catheter is left behind to maintain the acquired diameter. This may be done by inflating the balloon three times daily with 15–20 cm^3 of air. This may be easily learned to the parents, so they can do this at home. The dilatation is continued until the stricture has healed completely.

28.3.1 Technique

Under general anesthesia esophagoscopy is performed. When the diagnosis is confirmed, a guidewire can be advanced orally through the stricture over which a balloon catheter is introduced. Usually a 4 cm/10 mm balloon is used. The balloon is placed with the upper marker well above the stricture. Under endoscopic vision the balloon is inflated with 20 cm^3 of air, and the effect on the stricture can be observed. If the stricture is not too solid, the stricture will tear. After retrieving the balloon, somewhat the endoscope can be advanced past the stricture and the distal oesophagus and stomach can be inspected for pathology. If the stricture is too solid, a forceful dilatation should be carried out. We usually use a Savary-Gilliard bougie that can be introduced over the guidewire and carries little risk of making a fausse route. The guidewire is stabilized at a fixed level to avoid the guidewire either from coming out or going in too deep. Because the tip is rather long, attention should be taken that the tip cannot perforate the stomach. By holding one hand on the abdomen, the tip of the bougie can usually be felt. After the desired diameter has been acquired, the guidewire is introduced through the nose and into the oesophagus under endoscopic control. The balloon catheter is taken, and the distal part, where the balloon is, is being bent every 2–3 mm in order to make it more supple. Instillagel® can be applied to the balloon to make it pass the nose more easily. Again under direct vision, the balloon is placed at the level of the stricture and inflated to keep it stable at the level of the stricture while retrieving the guidewire and subsequently bending the catheter at the level where it exits the nostril, so it does not pull on the nostril. The catheter is then fixed against the cheek up to under the level of the ear. First a strip of thin DuoDERM is fixed on the cheek to protect the skin, and then plaster is applied over the catheter to fix it on the DuoDERM. In case the catheter still pulls on the ala of

When a perforation occurs, treatment depends on the extent of the perforation. In case of a small lesion, it can be sustained to put in a nasogastric tube and refrain from further oral intake. Give antibiotics for 5 days, and perform a contrast study after 5 days to determine if the perforation has healed spontaneously. In somewhat bigger perforations with leakage into the thoracic cavity, a thoracic drain is placed to evacuate fluids and treat the pneumothorax. When there is no more production through the drain, a contrast study can confirm closure of the leak and oral feeds can be resumed.

In large perforations it may be advantageous to suture the perforation in the acute phase to avoid longtime sequelae.

28.7 Tips and Tricks to Deal with Postoperative Complications

1. In case of dislodgement, the balloon catheter can easily be replaced under fluoroscopy over a guidewire (Fig. 28.2). It is not necessary to replace the catheter under anesthesia.
2. In case the balloon brakes, the parents will report that they don't feel any resistance when inflating the balloon and also they cannot withdraw any air anymore from the balloon. Replacement is carried out as in point 1.
3. When giving tube feeding through the second channel, it is important to flush the channel after use to prevent clotting of the channel. Sometimes it helps to use sparkling water for flushing.

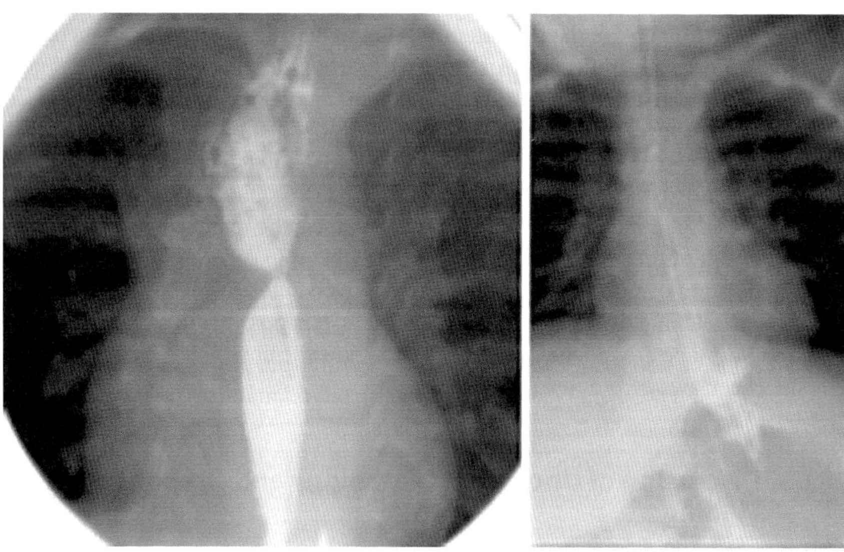

Fig. 28.2 Contrast study of oesophageal stricture (left). An indwelling balloon catheter is left behind to keep the oesophagus at the right diameter

28.8 Discussion

Oesophageal stenosis is a common occurring complication that can usually be managed by dilatation. If the stenosis is persistent or in case of caustic injury of the oesophagus, long-lasting therapy is warranted. The indwelling balloon catheter technique is an elegant way to avoid major surgery in persistent oesophageal stenosis. In a retrospective study, it was demonstrated that since the use of the indwelling balloon catheter, it has not been necessary anymore to resect the stenosis or replace the oesophagus with stomach, jejunum, or colon.

References

1. Ade-Ajayi N. Esophageal dilatation. In: Spitz L, Coran AG, editors. Operative pediatric surgery. New York: CRC Press; 2013. p. 90–6.
2. van der Zee D, Hulsker C. Indwelling esophageal balloon catheter for benign esophageal stenosis in infants and children. Surg Endosc. 2014;28(4):1126–30.

Oesophageal Replacement by Gastric Transposition

29

Emma L. Sidebotham and David C.G. Crabbe

Abstract

The oesophagus is usually the best conduit to convey food from the mouth to the GI tract. When the native oesophagus is absent or badly diseased, oesophageal replacement may be required. Gastric transposition has been used successfully to re-establish GI continuity in children since the 1980s. Several long-term follow-up studies report excellent outcomes and quality of life for these patients, superior to other procedures, especially colon interposition. Experience has highlighted a variety of intraoperative and post-operative problems and challenges for which we offer various technical tips and tricks.

Keywords

Long-gap oesophageal atresia · Caustic injury · Failed oesophageal atresia repair Stricture · Gastric transposition · Quality of life

29.1 Introduction

The oesophagus is the ideal conduit to propel food from the mouth to the stomach. However, if the oesophagus has failed to form or become irreparably damaged by injury or disease, then oesophageal replacement is necessary. In developed countries the commonest indication for oesophageal replacement is either long-gap oesophageal atresia or following failed attempts to repair oesophageal atresia. Injuries to the oesophagus by caustic ingestion or impaction of foreign bodies can cause such extensive damage that oesophagectomy is required. Rarely tumours or failed achalasia surgery necessitate removal of the oesophagus (Table 29.1). Whilst a

E.L. Sidebotham, M.D., F.R.C.S. (✉) • D.C.G. Crabbe, M.B. Ch.B., M.D., F.R.C.S.
Department of Pediatric Surgery, Leeds General Infirmary, Leeds, UK
e-mail: emma.sidebotham@nhs.net; david.crabbe@nhs.net

D. Parikh, P.B. Rajesh (eds.), *Tips and Tricks in Thoracic Surgery*,
https://doi.org/10.1007/978-1-4471-7355-7_29

Table 29.1 Indications for oesophageal replacement

Indications for oesophageal replacement
Long-gap oesophageal atresia
Failed primary repair of oesophageal atresia
Failed previous oesophageal substitution procedure
Caustic injuries
Foreign body impaction: especially batteries or prolonged impaction
Tumours, e.g. diffuse leiomyoma
Achalasia
Reflux-associated strictures

well-functioning native oesophagus is the ideal conduit, a poorly functioning scarred oesophagus requiring recurrent dilatations is usually better replaced [1–3].

In 1948 Sweet first proposed gastric transposition as a treatment for oesophageal atresia where primary anastomosis had proved unsuccessful based on his experience treating adults with oesophageal tumours [4]. However, it was 30 years later before the technique was introduced by Spitz and his colleagues as an alternative to colonic interposition for oesophageal replacement [5]. Thirty years on from this report of four children with long-gap oesophageal atresia, gastric transposition has become widely used for oesophageal replacement. Short- and long-term follow-up studies have confirmed the technique to be safe and effective [6, 7].

Colonic interposition is probably the most popular technique for oesophageal replacement in children worldwide. This procedure carries substantial morbidity in the short term because of graft infarction, anastomotic leak and stricture and gastro-oesophageal reflux. In the long term, the colon graft tends to become tortuous and redundant, often requiring revision because of progressive dysphagia. Jejunal interposition has the theoretical advantages of appropriate graft calibre to replace the oesophagus and active peristalsis, but the procedure is technically challenging because of the tenuous pedicle blood supply. Gastric tube interposition carries a high incidence of leak from the long suture lines in the chest and abdomen and problems with gastro-oesophageal reflux and anastomotic stricture. Tissue engineering offers hope for constructing a replacement oesophagus in the laboratory, but viable clinical application is still many years away.

29.2 Procedure of Gastric Transposition: Technical Tips and Tricks

29.2.1 Preoperative Planning

The details of preoperative planning will vary according to the indication for oesophageal replacement. Our practice, when using gastric transposition to treat oesophageal atresia, once it is apparent that primary repair has failed or is impossible, is to form an oesophagostomy and establish sham oral feeding. Bronchoscopy is mandatory in these infants to rule out an upper pouch tracheo-oesophageal fistula. We prefer to perform the gastric transposition when the baby is 6–8 kg in weight, although management of other co-morbidities (e.g. congenital heart disease, chronic lung disease) may necessitate the transposition being deferred. For other indications, such as caustic injuries, multiply recurrent tracheo-oesophageal fistulae, tumours, resection of the diseased oesophagus and oesophageal replacement may be simultaneous. There are reports of gastric transpositions in neonates less than 3 kg, partly to address problems with oesophagostomy and gastrostomy management outside hospital in developing countries. Perioperative mortality in one series was very high (15%), partly reflecting the general condition of the infants at the time of surgery [8].

Gastric transposition should be an elective procedure and every attempt made to optimise nutrition and cardiorespiratory function prior to surgery. Some authors have suggested that gastric transposition should be deferred until the child is walking, as the conduit may empty more efficiently in an upright posture [9]. We consider this unnecessarily prolongs the period of gastrostomy feeding and delays establishing normal oral feeding.

29.2.2 Operative Technique

The technique of gastric transposition varies somewhat depending on the indication for oesophageal replacement and previous surgery. The procedure is performed under general anaesthesia with endotracheal intubation, preferably via the nasal route. Central venous access and invasive arterial blood pressure monitoring are essential, ideally via the femoral vessels. A urethral catheter should be inserted.

The patient is positioned supine with a roll under the shoulders and the head turned away from the side of the cervical oesophagostomy, if present. The stomach is mobilised through an upper midline laparotomy extending caudally as necessary. Many patients will have a gastrostomy which should be taken down and closed in two layers. The left gastric artery is divided close to its origin. It is important to preserve the vascular arcade along the lesser curve of the stomach and the right gastric artery. The short gastric vessels are then divided leaving a narrow fringe of omentum on the greater curve of the stomach to ensure the gastroepiploic arcade is intact (Fig. 29.1). The remainder of the greater omentum is removed. The duodenum may be kocherised to allow mobilisation of the stomach such that the pylorus will sit at the level of the oesophageal hiatus in the diaphragm.

The distal oesophagus must be mobilised and removed. Both vagus nerves are divided. In long-gap oesophageal atresia or failed primary anastomosis where an oesophagostomy has been formed, the distal oesophagus can usually be mobilised safely by blunt dissection through the oesophageal hiatus in the diaphragm. Where there has been a severe transmural caustic injury, previous failed oesophageal replacement or extensive scarring from an anastomotic leak, thoracotomy may be required to mobilise the oesophagus safely because of adherence to the trachea or major vessels in the mediastinum. Where this has proved necessary, we have typically repositioned the patient and mobilised the thoracic oesophagus via a right lateral thoracotomy. Other authors use a thoracoabdominal incision: this needs to be planned from the outset with the patient in a semi lateral rather than supine position and the midline incision not extending cranially to the xiphisternum but deviating out to the costal margin.

Once freed the distal oesophagus is amputated at the level of the stomach. We use a stapling device (GIA™ or Endo GIA™ [Covidien]) to excise the oesophageal stump and close the stomach (Fig. 29.2). The adequacy of graft mobilisation can then be demonstrated by lifting the fundus of the stomach out of the wound over the front of the thorax. The fundus will easily reach to the base of the neck (Fig. 29.3).

Mobilisation of the stomach in this way divides the vagal nerve supply to the pylorus. Consequently a gastric drainage procedure is mandatory. We perform a Heineke-Mikulicz pyloroplasty (Fig. 29.4). Other authors perform a pyloromyotomy: this is technically difficult in the normal pylorus and may not continue to function long term. Radionuclide gastric emptying studies after gastric transposition have shown prolonged gastric emptying times after pyloromyotomy compared to relatively rapid emptying after pyloroplasty [10].

After the graft has been prepared, the proximal oesophagus needs to be mobilised in the neck. Most frequently we are performing a gastric transposition in a patient with oesophageal atresia where an oesophagostomy has already been established. The oesophagostomy is circumscribed to mobilise it from the skin margin,

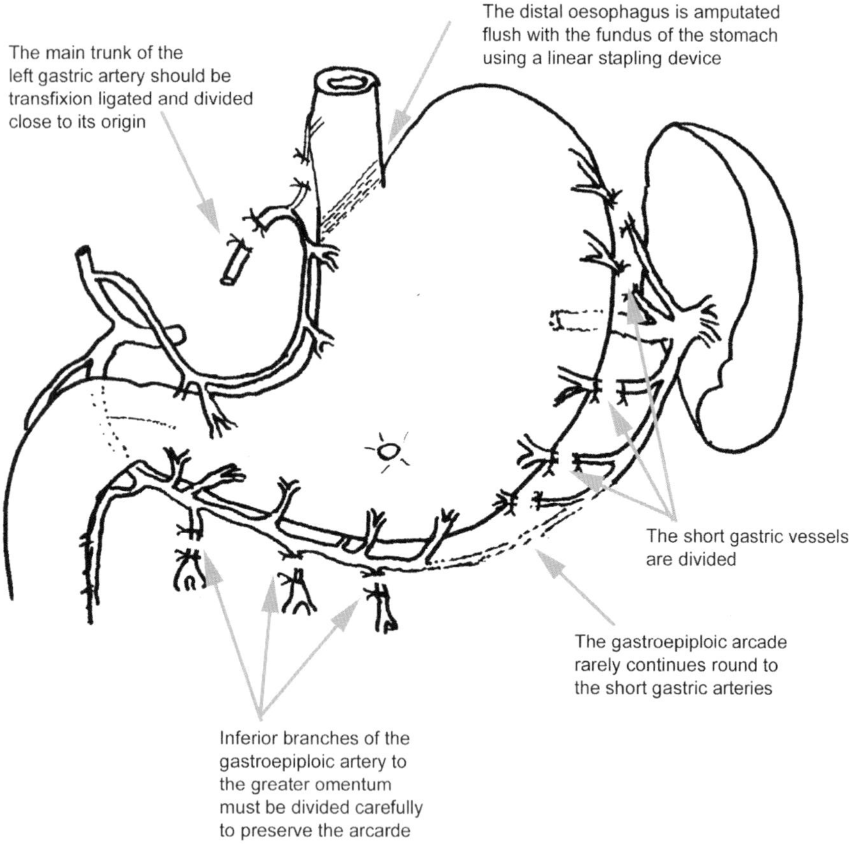

Fig. 29.1 The blood supply to the stomach

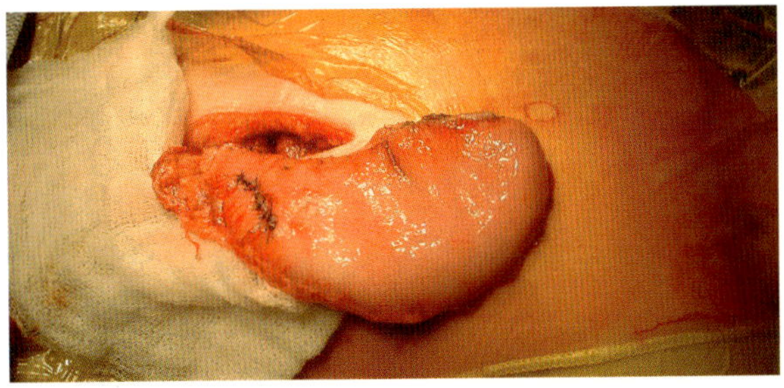

Fig. 29.2 The stomach mobilised, the old gastrostomy site closed and the stump of the distal oesophagus resected

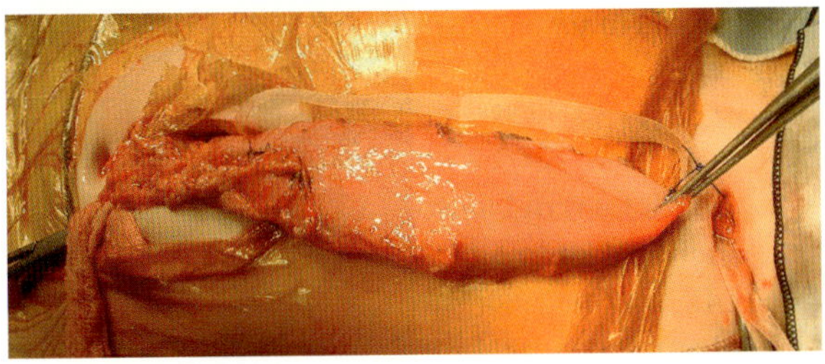

Fig. 29.3 The stomach mobilised on the right gastric and gastroepiploic pedicles easily reaches the neck

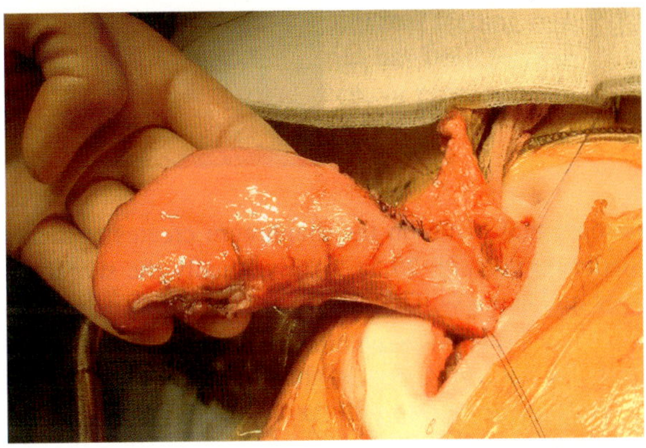

Fig. 29.4 Stay sutures placed for the pyloroplasty

and then a path is dissected to the thoracic inlet and down into the posterior mediastinum. Extreme care must be taken during the dissection to avoid damage to the recurrent laryngeal nerves whose position may be obscured or distorted by scarring from previous surgery. If the patient does not have an oesophagostomy, a skin crease incision is made in the lower neck. The sternomastoid is retracted laterally, and dissection proceeds medially to the carotid sheath down the cervical oesophagus behind the trachea.

We prefer to site an oesophagostomy on the left side of the neck, and consequently we approach the upper mediastinal dissection through the left side of the neck. Other authors report mobilising the cervical oesophagus from the right side [11].

The superior mediastinum is entered by blunt digital dissection following the posterior wall of the trachea. In this way a space is created in the posterior mediastinum down to the carina. Similarly, blunt digital dissection through the

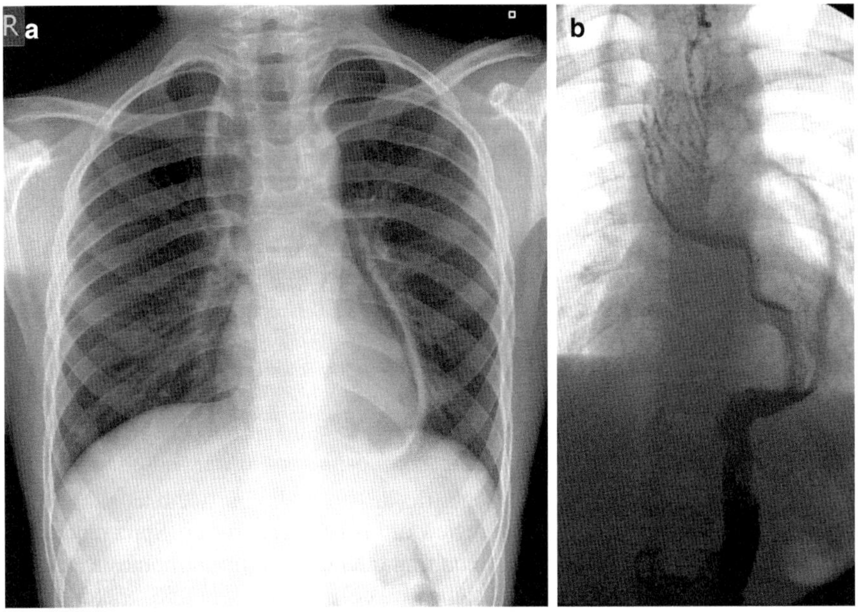

Fig. 29.7 (**a**, **b**) Chest X-ray and contrast swallow on a teenage boy who underwent oesophageal replacement by gastric transposition in infancy for long-gap OA

drawn up through the posterior mediastinum. Ensuring the posterior mediastinal dissection stays confined in the midline is probably important to prevent the stomach distending in the upper chest and kinking over the aortic arch and left main bronchus.

Whilst dumping can be induced by hypertonic glucose ingestion after gastric transposition, most children do not show clinical symptoms [10, 18]. If dumping is symptomatic, this can usually be managed by dietary modification in favour of complex carbohydrates.

29.4.5 Achlorhydria/Gastro-oesophageal Reflux

Vagotomy should result in achlorhydria although Jain et al. performed pH monitoring and found a mean pH of 1.7 and median pH of 1.4 over a 24 h testing period [14]. Studies in adults after gastric transposition have shown conflicting results. On the basis of these finding, acid suppression may be of benefit to symptomatic patients or in the case of a recurrent anastomotic stricture. Bile reflux into the stomach is common after pyloroplasty, but the significance of this is unclear [14, 18]. Achlorhydria can result in atrophic gastritis in the long term, and this is a common finding in adult patients. The long-term significance of this to the health of the gastric conduit is uncertain, but long-term follow-up is essential, and surveillance endoscopy should be considered.

A minority of patients report reflux symptoms after gastric transposition. The relative infrequency of this problem is attributed to the cervical oesophagogastric anastomosis in comparison to the often severe problems that follow an intrathoracic oesophagogastric anastomosis.

29.4.6 Barrett's Oesophagus

Chronic acid reflux oesophagitis is thought to be the cause of Barrett's metaplasia which is associated with a 40-fold increase in the frequency of adenocarcinoma of the oesophagus [23]. This is a source of concern for adult survivors of oesophageal atresia surgery where Barrett's metaplasia is found much earlier than the typical age 50+ years in the general population [24]. Lindahl et al. reported an 8.5% incidence of Barrett's change at a mean follow-up of 6.3 years following primary repair of oesophageal atresia, and this has been corroborated in many subsequent studies [19–21]. Whilst there are case reports of both adenocarcinoma and squamous carcinoma in adult survivors following correction of oesophageal atresia in infancy, there is no systematic evidence of an increased risk of oesophageal malignancy [22, 23].

It has long been argued that gastric transposition cervical oesophagogastric anastomosis offers freedom from gastro-oesophageal reflux but this may be optimistic. D'Journo and colleagues looked for Barrett's change in the residual oesophagus in 84 adults after oesophageal replacement surgery for various benign and malignant conditions. They compared 48 patients who had a cervical anastomosis with 36 who had an intrathoracic anastomosis. The incidence of columnar metaplasia was high in both groups (37% cervical anastomosis, 66% intrathoracic anastomosis) [24]. Lindahl et al. reported Barrett's metaplasia in the proximal oesophageal remnant following oesophageal replacement by gastric tube interposition in infancy, considering acid production in the gastric tube causative [25]. The situation after gastric transposition oesophageal replacement in infancy is unclear. There is anecdotal evidence that Barrett's change may occur [26] and it is certainly naive to think that the cervical oesophageal remnant in these patients is protected from columnar metaplasia. What is clear is that the importance of long-term follow-up in all oesophageal patients cannot be stressed highly enough.

29.4.7 Respiratory Function

Functional studies and quality of life assessments suggest that up to 50% of children experience chronic respiratory problems after oesophageal replacement. Formal lung function testing performed in patients after gastric transposition demonstrated parameters such as FEV_1 are significantly reduced in comparison to normal controls [10, 14]. There are several potential causes for respiratory symptoms including gastric distension affecting lung expansion, pressure on a malacic airway and recurrent minor aspiration secondary to reflux from the intrathoracic stomach. Of note in these studies, patients who underwent a primary transposition procedure had significantly better lung function than patients who had oesophageal replacement as a rescue procedure after a failed primary repair or anastomotic leak suggesting that scarring in the pleural cavity is an important contributory factor [14].

29.4.8 Quality of Life

Studies looking objectively at quality of life after gastric transposition in childhood report good overall results [10, 14, 15]. Whilst gastric transposition may not be ideal compared to a normal healthy oesophagus, determined attempts to retain a poorly functioning oesophagus are almost certainly not in the patient's best interests [2].

29.5 Conclusions and Future

Gastric transposition has been widely used as a technique for oesophageal replacement in children for over 30 years, predominantly long-gap oesophageal atresia, failed primary repair of oesophageal atresia and caustic strictures. There is now sufficient evidence from follow-up studies into adulthood to confirm good outcomes and good quality of life for this approach. Outcome studies demonstrate superiority of gastric transposition over colon interposition and gastric tube interposition as a strategy for oesophageal replacement. Comparison with jejunal interposition is less clear as the follow-up of these patients is much shorter.

There are many reports in the literature of heroic efforts to anastomose even the longest-gap oesophageal atresia. Some centres insist that alternative strategies are never necessary. Whilst it is reasonable to assume that the native oesophagus is best, it is important to not lose sight of the morbidity associated with a poorly functioning oesophagus. Oesophageal replacement would undoubtedly improve the quality of life of some of these children.

References

1. Conforti A, Bagolan P. Re: Which is better for esophageal substitution in children, esophagocoloplasty or gastric transposition? A 27-year experience of a single center. J Pediatr Surg. 2007;42(9):1633–4; author reply 4.
2. Hunter CJ, Petrosyan M, Connelly ME, Ford HR, Nguyen NX. Repair of long-gap esophageal atresia: gastric conduits may improve outcome-a 20-year single center experience. Pediatr Surg Int. 2009;25:1087.
3. Tannuri U, Maksoud-Filho JG, Tannuri AC, Andrade W, Maksoud JG. Which is better for esophageal substitution in children, esophagocoloplasty or gastric transposition? A 27-year experience of a single center. J Pediatr Surg. 2007;42(3):500–4.
4. Sweet RH. A new method of restoring continuity of the alimentary canal in cases of congenital atresia of the esophagus with tracheo-esophageal fistula not treated by immediate primary anastomosis. Ann Surg. 1948;127(4):757–68.

5. Spitz L. Gastric transposition via the mediastinal route for infants with long-gap esophageal atresia. J Pediatr Surg. 1984;19(2):149–54.
6. Cowles RA, Coran AG. Gastric transposition in infants and children. Pediatr Surg Int. 2010;26(12):1129–34.
7. Spitz L. Gastric transposition in children. Semin Pediatr Surg. 2009;18(1):30–3.
8. Gupta DK, Sharma S, Arora MK, Agarwal G, Gupta M, Grover VP. Esophageal replacement in the neonatal period in infants with esophageal atresia and tracheoesophageal fistula. J Pediatr Surg. 2007;42(9):1471–7.
9. Tannuri U, Tannuri AC. Should patients with esophageal atresia be submitted to esophageal substitution before they start walking? Dis Esophagus. 2011;24(1):25–9.
10. Davenport M, Hosie GP, Tasker RC, Gordon I, Kiely EM, Spitz L. Long-term effects of gastric transposition in children: a physiological study. J Pediatr Surg. 1996;31(4):588–93.
11. Ure BM, Jesch NK, Sumpelmann R, Nustede R. Laparoscopically assisted gastric pull-up for long gap esophageal atresia. J Pediatr Surg. 2003;38(11):1661–2.
12. Spitz L, Kiely E, Pierro A. Gastric transposition in children—a 21-year experience. J Pediatr Surg. 2004;39(3):276–81; discussion –81.
13. Ng J, Loukogeorgakis SP, Pierro A, Kiely EM, De Coppi P, Cross K, et al. Comparison of minimally invasive and open gastric transposition in children. J Laparoendosc Adv Surg Tech A. 2014;24(10):742–9.
14. Jain V, Sharma S, Kumar R, Kabra SK, Bhatia V, Gupta DK. Transposed intrathoracic stomach: functional evaluation. Afr J Paediatr Surg. 2012;9(3):210–6.
15. Ludman L, Spitz L. Quality of life after gastric transposition for oesophageal atresia. J Pediatr Surg. 2003;38(1):53–7; discussion –7.
16. Dunn JC, Fonkalsrud EW, Applebaum H, Shaw WW, Atkinson JB. Reoperation after esophageal replacement in childhood. J Pediatr Surg. 1999;34(11):1630–2.
17. Gupta DK, Charles AR, Srinivas M. Manometric evaluation of the intrathoracic stomach after gastric transposition in children. Pediatr Surg Int. 2004;20(6):415–8.
18. Ravelli AM, Spitz L, Milla PJ. Gastric emptying in children with gastric transposition. J Pediatr Gastroenterol Nutr. 1994;19(4):403–9.
19. Lindahl H, Rintala R, Louhimo I. Failure of the Nissen fundoplication to control gastroesophageal reflux in esophageal atresia patients. J Pediatr Surg. 1989;24(10):985–7.
20. Ijsselstijn H, van Beelen NW, Wijnen RM. Esophageal atresia: long-term morbidities in adolescence and adulthood. Dis Esophagus. 2013;26(4):417–21.
21. Sistonen SJ, Koivusalo A, Nieminen U, Lindahl H, Lohi J, Kero M, et al. Esophageal morbidity and function in adults with repaired esophageal atresia with tracheoesophageal fistula: a population-based long-term follow-up. Ann Surg. 2010;251(6):1167–73.
22. Jayasekera CS, Desmond PV, Holmes JA, Kitson M, Taylor AC. Cluster of 4 cases of esophageal squamous cell cancer developing in adults with surgically corrected esophageal atresia—time for screening to start. J Pediatr Surg. 2012;47(4):646–51.
23. Sistonen SJ, Koivusalo A, Lindahl H, Pukkala E, Rintala RJ, Pakarinen MP. Cancer after repair of esophageal atresia: population-based long-term follow-up. J Pediatr Surg. 2008;43(4):602–5.
24. D'Journo XB, Martin J, Rakovich G, Brigand C, Gaboury L, Ferraro P, et al. Mucosal damage in the esophageal remnant after esophagectomy and gastric transposition. Ann Surg. 2009;249(2):262–8.
25. Lindahl H, Rintala R, Sariola H, Louhimo I. Cervical Barrett's esophagus: a common complication of gastric tube reconstruction. J Pediatr Surg. 1990;25(4):446–8.
26. Hamza AF, Abdelhay S, Sherif H, Hasan T, Soliman H, Kabesh A, et al. Caustic esophageal strictures in children: 30 years' experience. J Pediatr Surg. 2003;38(6):828–33.

Oesophageal Replacement: Jejunal Interposition

30

Janet McNally and Eleri L. Cusick

Abstract

The jejunum has been utilized as an oesophageal replacement since the early 1900s. Decades of refinements and adjustments to the surgical techniques, in addition to improvements in both preoperative assessment and postoperative care, have resulted in the jejunum now being a reliable choice as an oesophageal substitute in both children and adults. It is widely utilized as either a free or pedicled graft or a combination of these as in the supercharged pedicled jejunal interposition. The most common indication for oesophageal replacement in infants is the management of long-gap oesophageal atresia and less frequently severe caustic strictures or resistant reflux strictures in older children. The benefits of the jejunum are it has a similar calibre to oesophagus, maintains intrinsic peristalsis, is much less likely than colon to develop redundant loops over time, is relatively abundant and is typically disease-free. Further benefits of the orthotopic pedicled jejunal interposition are retention of the native distal oesophageal pouch, including the oesophagogastric junction, thereby eliminating the long-term risks of reflux oesophagitis, an important consideration in the Pediatric population.

Keywords

Oesophageal atresia · Long-gap · Jejunal interposition · Oesophageal replacement
Oesophageal substitution · Ileal interposition

J. McNally (✉) • E.L. Cusick
Department of Pediatric Surgery, Bristol Royal Hospital for Children, Bristol, UK
e-mail: janet.mcnally@uhbristol.nhs.uk; eleri.cusick@uhbristol.nhs.uk

D. Parikh, P.B. Rajesh (eds.), *Tips and Tricks in Thoracic Surgery*,
https://doi.org/10.1007/978-1-4471-7355-7_30

Excluding malrotation is important as it may preclude the use of the jejunum as an oesophageal substitute. We found malrotation in one patient but were able to proceed by fixing the caecum with a temporary caecostomy to prevent volvulus developing later.

30.3.2 Orthotopic Pedicled Jejunal Interposition

The pedicled jejunal interposition starts with a right posterolateral muscle sparing (serratus anterior) thoracotomy via the sixth rib space to assess whether or not the two blind oesophageal ends can be brought together. Taking the midsection of the rib in the subperiosteal space improves access to the thoracic cavity, and the rib grows back within months.

Identifying the proximal or distal oesophageal pouches can be difficult if they are short, and using Hegar or Bakes dilators or a neonatal endoscope can help facilitate their identification. The vagus nerve can also be a useful pointer to the position of the distal pouch and should be preserved wherever possible. There is no need to mobilize the oesophageal pouches extensively if it is clear that primary anastomosis is unfeasible and to do so may contribute to postoperative oesophageal dysmotility.

The gap is measured between the two blind oesophageal ends to assess the length of graft required to bridge the gap. Ensure the distal oesophageal pouch is patent before measuring the gap otherwise the graft will be too short. It is also useful at this stage to open the pleura at the oesophageal hiatus behind the distal oesophagus, slinging the oesophagus with a coloured vascular loop as this will facilitate in identifying the right thoracic cavity from the abdomen and the passage of the graft from the abdomen into the chest later on in the procedure.

The chest is then closed temporarily and an upper midline laparotomy performed. Inspect the mesenteric vessels to the proximal jejunum carefully by transillumination of the mesentery. The first jejunal branch distal to the duodenojejunal flexure is spared to ensure adequate perfusion of the proximal jejunum. The jejunal pedicle is then developed by taking the second and third jejunal branches of artery and accompanying veins as close to the superior mesenteric vessels as possible. The fourth, or in some cases fifth (if a longer pedicle is anticipated) jejunal branch is preserved and will form the base of the vascular pedicle to the jejunal graft. It is reassuring to temporarily occlude the vessels with a vascular microclamp prior to ligation to ensure that the proximal jejunum remains adequately perfused. Some surgeons prefer to do the first part of a two-stage procedure at the time of gastrostomy formation, coming back to continue with the procedure a couple of months later, anticipating hyperplasia of the proposed pedicle vessels. Careful incision of the peritoneum overlying the mesentery can help with identification of the jejunal vascular arcades (Fig. 30.2).

When the vessels have been addressed, the proximal jejunum is transected between the first and second jejunal branches, approximately 10 cm from the duodenojejunal flexure. At this stage lifting the jejunal graft on to the chest can be useful to assess whether the length of the pedicle is adequate. The graft should reach the base of the neck. If not, a further jejunal branch may be taken. Once there is a pedicle that reaches as high as the proximal oesophageal pouch, the jejunum is transected for a second time, distal to the jejunal branch that forms the base of the vascular pedicle resulting in a jejunal graft that is usually about 20–30 cm long.

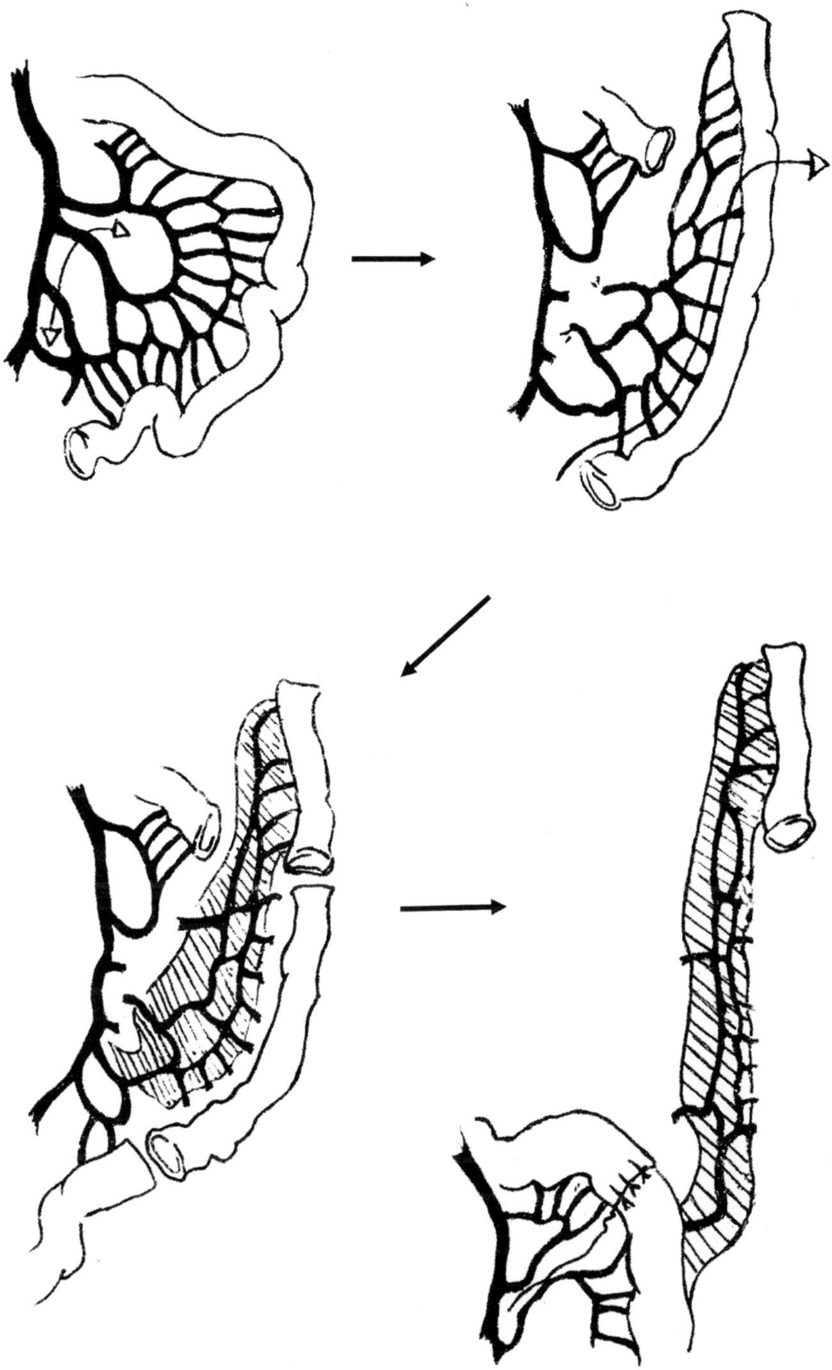

Fig. 30.2 Developing the pedicle and bowel graft for the orthotopic pedicle jejunal interposition graft

The full length of bowel that has been mobilized is not required, and a distal segment of the jejunum is sacrificed by cauterizing the vessels directly on the bowel wall starting distally and proceeding proximally to achieve a straight jejunal graft of the correct length to bridge the gap. The vascular pedicle is supported by a leash of mesenteric fat covered by peritoneum that is approximately 2 cm wide, with the graft at the proximal end. It is advisable to mark the proximal end of the graft with a small suture as once pushed into the chest, it can be difficult to identify the proximal and distal ends of the graft and it is important to ensure isoperistaltic graft placement. The graft should be kept moist at all times, the bowel should not be clamped, and handling of the graft and pedicle should be kept to a minimum to avoid desiccation and reduce the risk of ischaemia.

Bowel continuity of the jejunum is restored by a jejunojejunostomy anterior to the base of the pedicle, closing the mesenteric defect. A pathway is then created for the graft through the transverse mesocolon to the left of the middle colic vessels, into the lesser sac, behind the stomach, the oesophagogastric junction and the distal oesophagus and through the oesophageal hiatus into the chest. Once the peritoneum at the oesophageal hiatus has been incised, it is necessary to dilate the hiatus with an index finger or a large Hegar dilator. The graft can then be advanced atraumatically behind the stomach and on into the right hemi-thorax without compromising either the graft or the pedicle. Particular care must be taken to pass the proximal part of the graft first and to avoid twisting the pedicle during this manoeuvre. The abdomen is closed after refashioning the gastrostomy.

The patient is turned laterally once more to allow reopening of the thoracotomy. Adjustments to the length of the jejunal graft may be necessary to avoid redundant loops. The proximal anastomosis is usually performed first, and the graft finally trimmed before completing the distal anastomosis. Single-layer interrupted proximal and distal oesophago-jejunostomies over a nasogastric transanastomotic tube may be either end to end or end to side, whichever lies comfortably without tension or kinking. An intercostal drain is placed and the chest closed in the standard fashion. Postoperative contrast study is performed to delineate continuity (Fig. 30.3).

30.3.3 Alternative Operative Techniques

The jejunum has on occasion received a bad press. There are a number of different techniques described utilizing the jejunum as an oesophageal substitute. The different procedures are not all comparable when it comes to technical ease, complications or surgical outcomes [6, 7]. The pedicled jejunal graft described by Cusick et al. [8] and free jejunal grafts described by Cauchi et al. [9] both with microvascular anastomoses and distal jejunogastric anastomoses had a much higher rate of graft failure, reflux-associated morbidity and postoperative deaths. The reasons for this are multifactorial with postoperative fluid management, anaesthetic agents, the distal jejunogastric anastomosis bypassing the native oesophagogastric junction and the route utilized for the graft all being implicated. Reflux secondary to bypassing the oesophagogastric junction and lower oesophageal sphincter and leaving the blind distal pouch in situ has been implicated in the development of Barrett's

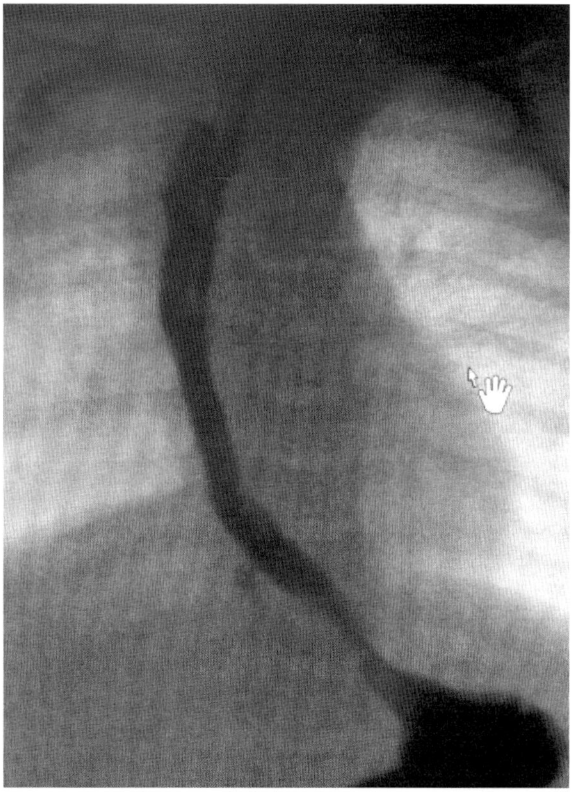

Fig. 30.3 A postoperative contrast study after an orthotopic jejunal interposition graft

oesophagitis and metaplasia predisposing these children to a risk of malignancy in later life [10]. The small size of the vessels in infants and children may also be a factor when performing a microvascular anastomosis. There is no advantage to this procedure over the pedicled jejunal interposition graft.

On rare occasions, when the distal oesophagus is diseased or absent and the distal graft has to be anastomosed onto the stomach, inversion of the jejunum into the gastric fundus creating a type of Thal fundoplication may protect against vomiting, reflux, ulceration and respiratory complications [11].

Saeki et al. routinely performed a pyloroplasty as part of their jejunal interpositions; however, we feel this predisposes the patients to dumping and have not found it necessary as we aim to preserve the vagus during the procedure [2].

We have had 15 patients over the last 10 years with long-gap oesophageal atresia (Fig. 30.4).

30.3.4 Uncommon Pathology

A very high proximal oesophageal pouch may require an anastomosis in the neck approached via a transverse cervical incision as in repair of an H-type tracheoesophageal fistula. A similar situation may arise in a child with caustic stricture affecting a long segment of the native oesophagus. In this situation a longer graft and pedicle

Achalasia of the Cardia

31

Oscar Crespin and Carlos A. Pellegrini

Abstract

The understanding of achalasia has evolved over time, and today the disease is defined manometrically by a non-relaxing lower oesophageal sphincter (LES) in association with aperistalsis of the oesophageal body.

We believe that there are two very important aspects in the surgical management of achalasia that are vital to obtaining excellent outcomes: patient selection and operative technique.

Thus, this chapter will describe a series of "tips" and "tricks" that we have used in those two domains. Because the chapter is directed to the practicing surgeon, we will follow the order in which a potential patient moves through the system starting with all aspects of diagnosis (or patient selection) and then continuing on through surgery.

The operation initially described by Heller has undergone numerous modifications in the last two decades as we learned the importance of a laparoscopic (rather than thoracoscopic) approach, the wisdom of an "extended myotomy" (more than 3 cm below the cardia), and the advantages associated with a partial anti-reflux procedure.

We will also address the treatment of "megaesophagus" and the role that myotomy plays vs. that of esophagectomy, and lastly we will examine the new endoscopic procedures that have been described.

Keywords

Achalasia · Laparoscopic · Standard · Extended · Heller · Myotomy · Tips · Tricks Surgical · Treatment

O. Crespin, M.D. • C.A. Pellegrini, M.D., F.A.C.S. (✉)
Department of Surgery, University of Washington, Seattle, WA, USA
e-mail: pellegri@uw.edu

D. Parikh, P.B. Rajesh (eds.), *Tips and Tricks in Thoracic Surgery*,
https://doi.org/10.1007/978-1-4471-7355-7_31

31.1 Introduction

Achalasia was first recognized more than 300 years ago as a disease that impaired the ability to swallow because of delayed transit of the food through the oesophagus. At that time it was proposed that a dilation of the gastroesophageal junction using whalebone might be effective [1]. Multiple theories involving viral, inflammatory, and autoimmune processes targeting oesophageal ganglion cells have been proposed, but the etiology remains unknown. The understanding of achalasia has evolved over time, and today the disease is defined manometrically by a non-relaxing lower oesophageal sphincter (LES) in association with aperistalsis of the oesophageal body. Thus, current treatment is directed at reducing the pressure gradient across the LES with the aim of relieving the patient's symptoms, particularly dysphagia. For many years the primary treatment for achalasia has been either endoscopic dilation or surgical myotomy. The first successful operation for achalasia was performed in 1913 by Ernest Heller who described an anterior and posterior lower oesophageal myotomy through a laparotomy [2]. Subsequently, the technique evolved to a single anterior myotomy, usually through a left posterior thoracotomy with a success rate of 60–94% in terms of relieving symptoms. However, the relatively high morbidity of this approach made it less attractive than dilation techniques until the advent of the minimally invasive surgical approach in the early 1990s [3, 4].

Today, laparoscopic Heller myotomy (LHM) is considered the gold standard for the treatment of achalasia in most centers in United States.

Given the importance that an accurate diagnosis plays in terms of patient selection and given that selection of patients is vital to a good outcome, we will first describe the diagnostic aspects that the surgeon must consider.

31.1.1 Clinics Visit

Patients that consult for the first time usually have been experiencing symptoms for a long period of time, occasionally years. In most instances, this is caused by the insidious and slowly progressive nature of the disease. In other instances, the initial symptoms are considered to be secondary to abnormal gastroesophageal reflux—a much more common problem—and the patient is mislabeled and continues with anti-reflux therapy for long periods of time [5].

31.2 Symptoms

Dysphagia: Represents the cardinal symptom. First typically to solids, then patients avoid meat but continue to report difficulty with leafy vegetables, bread, pastas, and frequently liquids. Anxiety while eating or emotional upset is common. "Washing foods down" to relieve a sensation of retrosternal fullness after meals with liquids is often ineffective, and relief is only obtained by belching and regurgitation of undigested food. The process may become so embarrassing that patients avoid eating in public.

Tip: Patients learn to eat using certain maneuvers, such as arching the back, raising the arms, lifting the neck, or throwing the shoulders back to ease progression of the food bolus. One has to be careful on how the issue of dysphagia is elicited. Frequently, the patients will say, "I can swallow OK" (when asked) only to recognize that "things get stuck down here" pointing to the retrosternal area.

Regurgitation: Regurgitation of bland undigested food or saliva is seen in 76–91% of patients with achalasia [6, 7]. The food particles are undigested and may be brought up several hours after ingestion. Patients also often complain of waking up in the mornings with remnants of the previous night's supper in their mouth.

Chest pain: It is found in 40% of patients with achalasia. There are at least two different types of chest pain experienced by patients with achalasia. The obstructive type is associated with swallowing a food bolus and resolves with passage of food into the stomach. The second type is unrelated to eating and is more often seen in patients with vigorous achalasia. The etiology is unclear as it does not correlate with radiographic or manometric findings [6]. It is more common in younger patients and often fails to respond to surgical treatment but tends to diminish over the course of several years.

Tip: Be careful when creating expectations of cure or relief of pain with a Heller myotomy. We advise our patients that "while they can expect substantial improvement in dysphagia, pain is unlikely to be resolved."

Heartburn: Patients frequently report retrosternal burning. This may be due to gastroesophageal reflux disease or more likely to direct irritation of the oesophageal lining by food, pills, or lactate production by bacterial fermentation of retained carbohydrates [8].

Tip: Many patients are treated for gastroesophageal reflux disease before the diagnosis of achalasia is made. In someone who does not respond to the usual medical therapy for reflux, one ought to measure oesophageal acid exposure and oesophageal function by manometry to rule out achalasia and other motor disorders.

Other symptoms: Patients may have hiccups due to obstruction of the distal oesophagus.

In rare cases, patients may present with a globus sensation.

Weight loss: Usually mild in patients with achalasia, but it can be substantial if the disease has gone on for some time. Weight loss should be very well evaluated since (a) it could be misdiagnosed with anorexia nervosa or psychiatric symptoms and (b) malignant tumors near or at the esophagogastric junction may mimic achalasia symptoms.

Tip: In an adolescent girl with weight loss and regurgitation, achalasia must be ruled out.

Tip: Young patient with recent-onset dysphagia and weight loss, endoscopy and biopsy of any suspicious lesion should be performed before definitive treatment is entertained.

31.3 Preoperative Workup

Manometry: Is required to establish the diagnosis of achalasia and characterized by the absence of peristaltic contractions and incomplete relaxation of the lower oesophageal sphincter. Manometry is the gold standard in the diagnosis of this disease and should be performed in every patient prior to planning an operative procedure.

Chest radiograph: A plain radiograph of the chest may reveal widening of the mediastinum due to the dilated oesophagus. The normal gastric air bubble may be absent due to the failure of LES relaxation that prevents air from entering the stomach. This is usually not a test that yields useful information and should be avoided in most patients suspected of having achalasia.

Barium esophagram: Findings that are suggestive of achalasia include the following.

The most common finding in over 90% of patients with achalasia is the presence of an air-fluid level indicative of poor emptying. Dilation of the oesophagus, narrow esophagogastric junction with "bird-beak" appearance caused by the persistently contracted LES, and aperistalsis are also seen and can be very helpful in the diagnosis.

In patients with late- or end-stage achalasia, the oesophagus may appear significantly dilated (megaesophagus), angulated, and tortuous giving it a sigmoid shape.

Tip: Epiphrenic diverticula may accompany this picture. In most cases of achalasia, the GE junction is smoothly narrowed, giving rise to the classic bird's beak and allowing only very small amounts of contrast to pass through to the stomach.

Endoscopy: Findings suggestive of achalasia—oesophageal dilation with food material or secretions, lack of contractions or multiple simultaneous contractions, oesophageal mucosa with erythema, erosions, or even ulceration.

Tip: A tight but relatively elastic feel as the endoscope passes (or pops) through the GE junction is characteristic of achalasia but may be easily overlooked if the diagnosis is not specifically searched.

Tip: The inability to pass the scope despite moderate amounts of pressure is highly suggestive of an inflammatory or a neoplastic stricture.

Differential diagnosis: The diagnosis of achalasia is established by all the above-mentioned tests having in mind that some recognized diseases can cause oesophageal motor abnormalities similar or identical to those of primary (idiopathic) achalasia: gastric carcinoma, Chagas disease, amyloidosis, sarcoidosis, neurofibromatosis, eosinophilic gastroenteritis, multiple endocrine neoplasia, type 2B juvenile Sjögren's syndrome with achalasia and gastric hypersecretion, chronic idiopathic intestinal pseudo-obstruction, and Anderson-Fabry disease.

Occasionally achalasia may result from a parasitic infection, Chagas disease. This is endemic in some areas of South America. Pseudoachalasia is a syndrome that has the manometric and the clinical characteristics of achalasia and is caused by an infiltrative (usually neoplastic) process that involves the GE junction but does not manifest intraluminally.

Primary achalasia can be distinguished from most other causes of an achalasia-like motility disorder based on the clinical, manometric, and radiologic features and upper endoscopy with biopsies. However, pseudoachalasia due to a malignancy may be more difficult to differentiate from primary achalasia with the usual tests.

Tip: Short duration of symptoms (less than 6 months), presentation after age 60, excessive weight loss in relation to the duration of symptoms, and difficult passage of the endoscope through the gastroesophageal junction should raise the suspicion of pseudoachalasia. In these situations, a CT scan or/and endoscopic ultrasound may show evidence of the disease and prevent an unnecessary myotomy.

31.3.1 Patient Preparation

The patient is prepared for surgery in the standard fashion, with orders to be NPO after midnight.

Tip: If the oesophageal dilatation is greater than 4 cm and/or with a long or tortuous oesophagus, we recommend patients discontinue solid food 4–5 days prior to the procedure and utilize a high-energy liquid diet. The idea is to clear the oesophagus of solid debris as much as possible to prevent aspiration during induction and decrease contamination in case of a mucosal laceration.

31.3.2 Operative Technique

Patient position: Patients are placed in lithotomy position with padding, such as a surgical beanbag. This position provides optimal ergonomics and access to the hiatus. The patient is positioned in a steep reverse Trendelenburg position, which allows the stomach and other organs to fall away from the oesophageal hiatus.

Access to the oesophagus: The lower oesophagus and the gastroesophageal junction can be accessed via laparoscopy or via thoracoscopy. Laparoscopic approach yields better results than the thoracoscopic approach for the average patient. Thoracoscopy requires collapse of the lung and makes access to the proximal stomach more difficult. By contrast, laparoscopy is better tolerated, allows access to the critical area (GE junction and upper stomach), and provides excellent exposure of the distal oesophagus. In a study involving 168 patients with achalasia who underwent myotomy with minimally invasive techniques, we found that the laparoscopic approach was (a) more effective in relieving dysphagia, (b) associated with a shorter hospital stay, and (c) resulted in lower incidence of postoperative reflux [9].

Tip: We reserve thoracoscopic access for patients who, for one reason or another, cannot be safely done via laparoscopy.

Abdominal access and port placement: Abdominal access is obtained at the left upper quadrant just inferior to the costal margin. Pneumoperitoneum is established according to standard laparoscopic techniques. Four operative ports (two of 5 mm for the surgeon (S), one of 5 mm for the assistant (A), and one of 10 mm for the scope (SC)) are then placed under direct visualization, and liver retraction (R) is then achieved by any number of such devices on the market via an abdominal port site (Fig. 31.1).

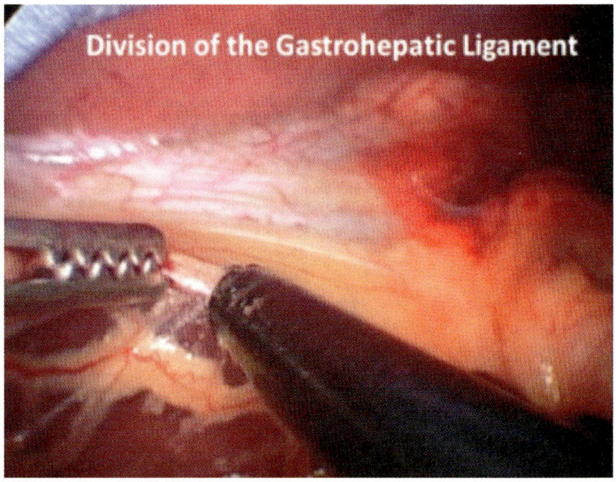

Fig. 31.5 Gastrohepatic ligament division

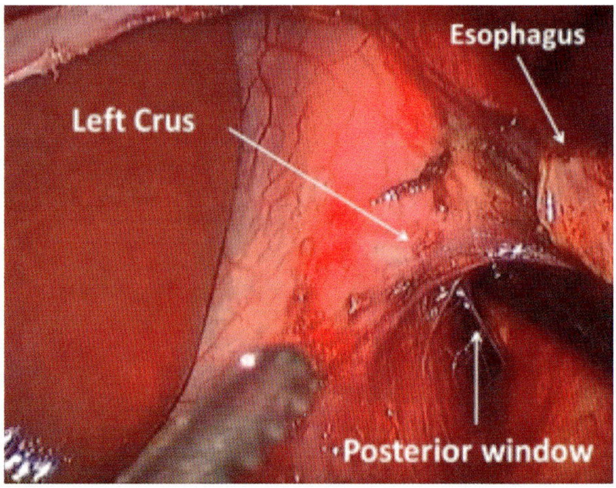

Fig. 31.6 Creation of a posterior oesophageal window

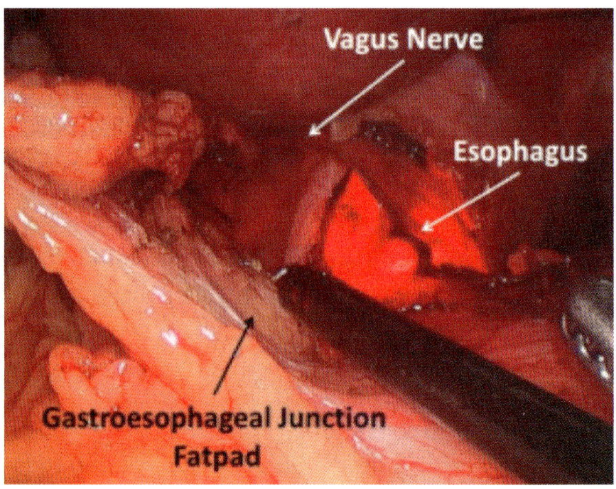

Fig. 31.7 Dissection of the GEJ fat pad

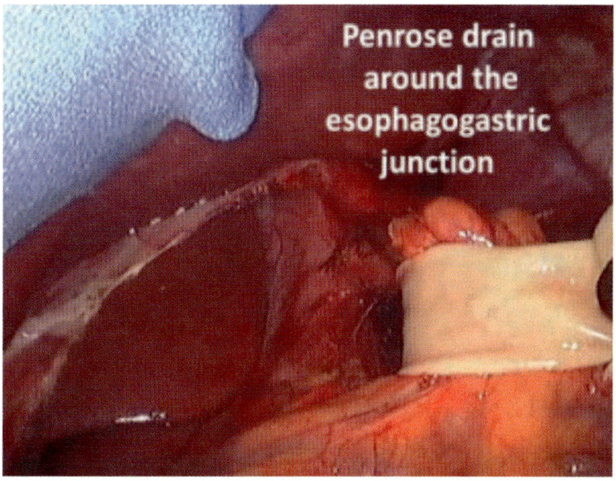

Fig. 31.8 Penrose drain for oesophageal retraction

Trick: Although in the majority of the patients, the maneuvers described above can be done with relative ease, in some patients mobilization of the distal oesophagus may be difficult. Retraction downwards with a sling around the gastroesophageal junction may be helpful in these situations. A 1/2 in. Penrose drain placed around the esophagogastric junction is helpful to retract the GE junction and to complete the oesophageal dissection and to bring the distal oesophagus more easily into the operative field (Fig. 31.8).

Myotomy: There is general consensus that a Heller myotomy should extend 6–7 cm above the gastroesophageal junction. The standard myotomy (SM) extends only 1.5–2 cm below the GEJ. In 2003 we proposed that an extended gastric myotomy (3 cm below the GE junction) would eliminate in a more complete way the oblique fibers of the angle and facilitate oesophageal emptying. We found a significant improvement in dysphagia scores postoperatively [10, 11].

Tip: Extending the myotomy 3 cm onto the gastric cardia is the key to obtain reproducible results in terms of relief of dysphagia.

Trick: We use a 50 FR lighted bougie as a platform to perform a gastric myotomy. It is placed by the anaesthesiologist transorally and advanced all the way into the stomach close to the lesser curvature. The bougie serves as a nice platform over which to perform the myotomy which extends 3 cm distal to the GE junction and as high as it is safe above it, usually 5–6 cm.

Tip: It is essential to have an anesthesiologist who is familiar with this surgical procedure and thus experienced and comfortable with placement of the bougie, to best avoid oesophageal perforation. Otherwise, it is beneficial for a member of the surgical team to perform this important step.

Trick: The anterior surface of the oesophagus is completely exposed, and slight tension is created by retracting caudally with an open grasper or Babcock over the bougie (Fig. 31.9).

We prefer to start on the stomach; while this is a more difficult submucosal plane to identify, we find it easier to proceed in a cephalad than caudal direction.

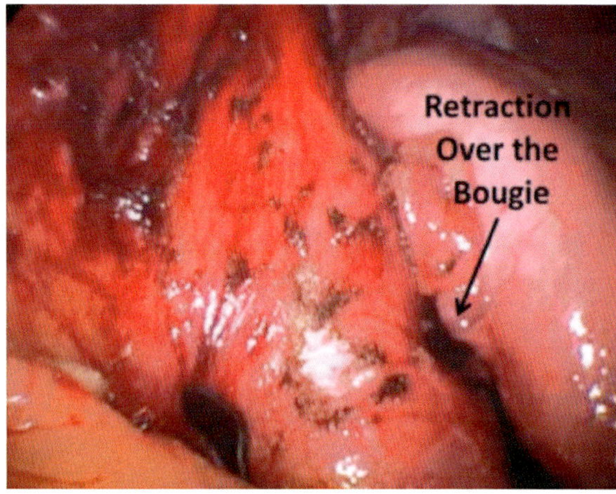

Fig. 31.9 Gastric retraction over a bougie

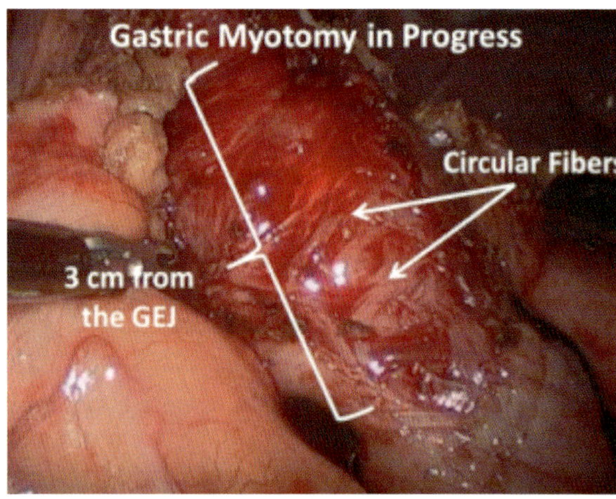

Fig. 31.10 Myotomy in progress

If bleeding is encountered, it should be controlled with pressure and patience since thermal injury can lead to an unrecognized injury and/or perforation of the oesophagus. The myotomy is performed by individually dividing the oesophageal and gastric muscle fibers until reaching the submucosa in the stomach and the mucosa in the oesophagus. The longitudinal muscles are divided first, which exposes the underlying circular muscles (Fig. 31.10). Division of the circular layer reveals a bulging mucosal plane that should appear smooth and slightly pink. Both the outer longitudinal and inner circular muscle layers must be identified and divided (Fig. 31.11).

Fundoplication: A laparoscopic myotomy alone is associated with a high incidence of reflux. On the other hand, a total fundoplication may cause too much resistance at the level of the gastroesophageal junction, impeding the emptying of food from the aperistaltic oesophagus into the stomach by gravity and eventually causing persistent or recurrent dysphagia. The addition of a partial anti-reflux procedure, whether Dor anterior or Toupet posterior fundoplication, leads to a relatively low incidence of reflux-related complaints while providing good to excellent relief of dysphagia in the majority of patients.

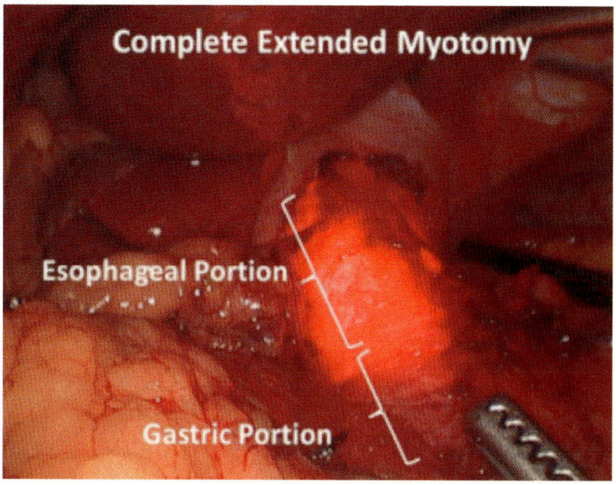

Fig. 31.11 Complete myotomy

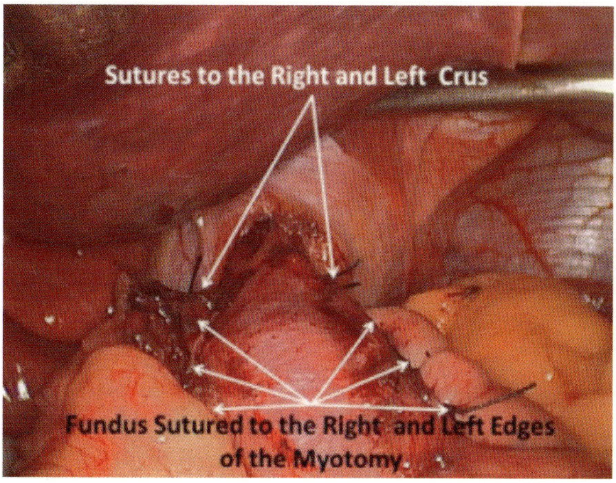

Fig. 31.12 Toupet fundoplication and myotomy

In a recent multicenter, prospective, randomized, controlled trial, we found no significant difference in the acid exposure of the distal oesophagus among of 60 patients who underwent Dor (36) or Toupet (24) fundoplications after Heller myotomy at 6–12 months. Abnormal acid reflux was present in 10 of 24 patients in the Dor group (41.7%) and in 4 of 19 patients in the Toupet (21.0%) ($p = 0.152$). Similarly, dysphagia, regurgitation, and quality of life measures improved significantly in both groups compared to preoperative scores. Therefore, LHM provides significant improvement in dysphagia and regurgitation symptoms in achalasia patients regardless of the type of partial fundoplication [12].

We prefer to perform a 270° posterior fundoplication by passing the tip of the gastric fundus posterior to the esophagogastric junction and securing it with interrupted sutures of 2–0 silk to the right crus of the diaphragm. The fundic tip is then sutured to the right edge of the myotomy, using three sutures. Similarly, the proximal aspect of the fundus is sutured to the left edge of the myotomy and also to the left crus (Fig. 31.12).

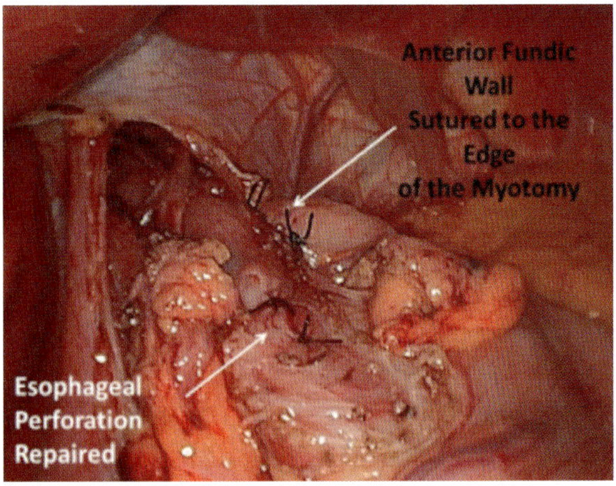

Fig. 31.13 Oesophageal perforation and Dor fundoplication in progress

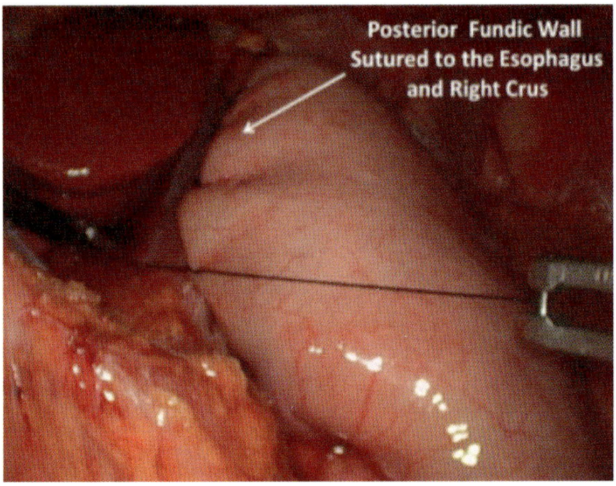

Fig. 31.14 Dor fundoplication to buttress an oesophageal perforation

Trick: A Dor fundoplication is routinely chosen in patients in whom there has been a perforation of the mucosa so as to buttress the mucosal closure (Figs. 31.13 and 31.14) [13].

31.4 Other Technical Considerations

Bleeding: ***Tip***—The vessels that tend to be more worrisome are always within the wall of the oesophagus and start bleeding as the muscularis, or the adventitia is divided (the latter is more common in large esophagi, and the vessels are superficial to the muscularis).

These vessels can and should be controlled either with electrocautery, making sure that the electrocautery is pressed against the muscle and not in contact with the mucosa, or, should the bleeding be more substantial, with an ultrasonic coagulator, a clip (with a tiny piece of muscle attached) or a suture.

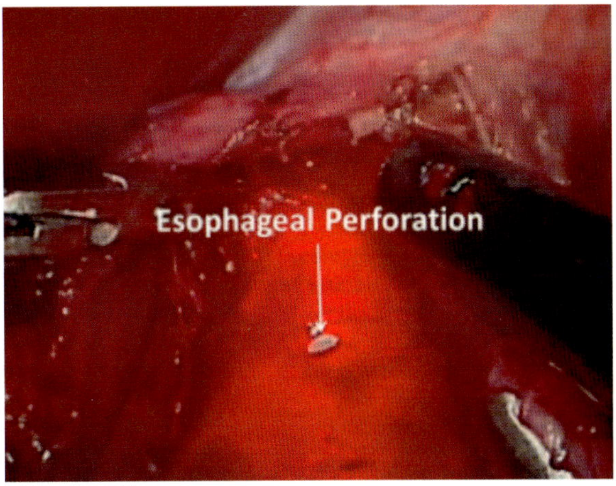

Fig. 31.15 Oesophageal perforation repair

Perforation: During the performance of a myotomy the mucosa may be lacerated. Laceration/injury to the mucosa is usually obvious. It should be treated by primary closure (we prefer a nonabsorbable suture such as fine silk) and use a small curved needle with a four or five zero size silk. One stitch is all that is needed in most instances (Fig. 31.15).

Tip: Always remove the bougie before suturing the laceration because its presence tends to stretch the tissue making placement and tying of the suture difficult *and* it is easy to incorporate the outer layer of the bougie with the suture if the bougie is still present. Always perform a Dor in these situations to bring a well-vascularized tissue flap over the suture line.

Several authors have reported that Heller myotomy generates less favorable results when preceded by endoscopic dilation [14, 15]. We reported on 57 patients treated with esophagomyotomy, 15 had received one or more injections of botulinum toxin preoperatively and 42 had not. Difficulties in dissection of the submucosal plane were encountered in 8 (53.3%) of the 15 patients and resulted in a mucosal laceration in 2 patients. By contrast, similar difficulties were present in only 3 (7%) of patients without previous treatment. All mucosal injuries were repaired laparoscopically, and the patients recovered without obvious sequel [16].

Tip: When performing a myotomy after Botox injection, one must be extra careful with the mucosa since the submucosal plane is usually obliterated.

Tip: Another useful tool to identify a perforation is to turn on the lighted bougie to review the myotomy immediately after finishing the myotomy (Fig. 31.16).

Stage of the disease: With time, the oesophagus of patients with achalasia widens and eventually elongates. Elongation leads to the formation of a "sigmoid" curve at the bottom of the oesophagus which provides a reservoir for food and fluid and impairs emptying. Contrary to what one would expect, we have seen excellent results in patients with advanced disease after a Heller myotomy and "straightening" of the distal oesophagus which is fixed at the crura. Food retention is a common event in such patients, even in those reporting an improvement in symptoms after myotomy [17].

21. Patti MG, Feo CV, Arcerito M, De Pinto M, Tamburini A, Diener U, Gantert W, Way LW. Effects of previous treatment on results of laparoscopic Heller myotomy for achalasia. Dig Dis Sci. 1999;44(11):2270–6.
22. Stefanidis D, Richardson W, Farrell TM, Kohn GP, Augenstein V, Fanelli RD, Society of American Gastrointestinal and Endoscopic Surgeons. SAGES guidelines for the surgical treatment of esophageal achalasia. Surg Endosc. 2012;26(2):296–311. https://doi.org/10.1007/s00464-011-2017-2. Epub 2011 Nov 2.
23. Boeckxstaens GE, Annese V, des Varannes SB, Chaussade S, Costantini M, Cuttitta A, Elizalde JI, Fumagalli U, Gaudric M, Rohof WO, Smout AJ, Tack J, Zwinderman AH, Zaninotto G, Busch OR, European Achalasia Trial Investigators. Pneumatic dilation versus laparoscopic Heller's myotomy for idiopathic achalasia. N Engl J Med. 2011;364(19):1807–16. https://doi.org/10.1056/NEJMoa1010502.
24. West RL, Hirsch DP, Bartelsman JF, de Borst J, Ferwerda G, Tytgat GN, Boeckxstaens GE. Long term results of pneumatic dilation in achalasia followed for more than 5 years. Am J Gastroenterol. 2002;97(6):1346–51.
25. Inoue H, Minami H, Kobayashi Y, Sato Y, Kaga M, Suzuki M, Satodate H, Odaka N, Itoh H, Kudo S. Peroral endoscopic myotomy (POEM) for esophageal achalasia. Endoscopy. 2010;42(4):265–71. https://doi.org/10.1055/s-0029-1244080. Epub 2010 Mar 30.
26. Swanstrom LL, Kurian A, Dunst CM, Sharata A, Bhayani N, Rieder E. Long-term outcomes of an endoscopic myotomy for achalasia: the POEM procedure. Ann Surg. 2012;256(4):659–67. https://doi.org/10.1097/SLA.0b013e31826b5212.
27. Hungness ES, Teitelbaum EN, Santos BF, Arafat FO, Pandolfino JE, Kahrilas PJ, Soper NJ. Comparison of perioperative outcomes between peroral esophageal myotomy (POEM) and laparoscopic Heller myotomy. J Gastrointest Surg. 2013;17(2):228–35. https://doi.org/10.1007/s11605-012-2030-3. Epub 2012 Sep 28.

Anti-Reflux Surgery

32

Simon Paterson-Brown, Graeme W. Couper, and Peter J. Lamb

Abstract

The surgical management of gastro-oesophageal reflux involves a variety of techniques and is associated with many different approaches depending on the underlying problem. As a result the associated complications which arise require to be managed according to the initial underlying condition. The key areas which will be addressed here relate to the decision for surgery and the type of surgery required; the different underlying problems for which surgery is indicated; and the identification and management of the potential complications.

Keywords

Gastro-oesophageal reflux · Surgery · Post-operative complications

32.1 Introduction

Over the last 20 years, there has been a seismic shift of antireflux surgery from open to laparoscopic, which in turn has made the thoracic approach, at least for primary procedures, almost extinct. Patients can now undergo fundoplication as a day case, or at least within a 23-h stay, without the need for several days in hospital and a painful and often protracted recovery. Not surprisingly this has resulted in more patients being considered for surgery and more being referred from medical gastroenterologists. However the risks remain [1], and one must never forget the

S. Paterson-Brown, M.S., M.Phil., F.R.C.S(Ed) (✉) • G.W. Couper, M.B.Ch.B., M.D., F.R.C.S(Ed)
P.J. Lamb, M.B.B.S., M.D., F.R.C.S(Ed)
Department of General and Upper GI Surgery,
Royal Infirmary of Edinburgh, Edinburgh, UK
e-mail: spb@doctors.org.uk; graeme.couper@nhslothian.scot.nhs.uk;
Peter.lamb@nhslothian.scot.nhs.uk

D. Parikh, P.B. Rajesh (eds.), *Tips and Tricks in Thoracic Surgery*,
https://doi.org/10.1007/978-1-4471-7355-7_32

disastrous consequences of oesophageal or gastric perforation, especially if such injuries go unnoticed at the first operation. Meticulous attention to detail, gentle and careful dissection at all times and careful inspection of the result at the end of the procedure, is essential if the risks are to be kept to a minimum and patients to gain the most benefit from what is still a 'major' procedure.

32.2 Selection for Surgery

32.2.1 Gastro-Oesophageal Reflux Disease (GORD)

Careful assessment includes a good history to make sure the symptoms are actually reflux and not a possible underlying motility disorder or malignant dysphagia. Particular caution should be exercised in patients who might have gastric emptying problems and those with primarily extra-oesophageal symptoms. It is vital to ensure that the priorities and expectations of the patient match those of the surgeon; reflux is a common symptom and if other functional symptoms predominate, these might well be exacerbated by fundoplication.

Examination should assess potential difficulties of surgery (such as scars from previous surgery, obesity, etc.). A high-quality gastroscopy is essential—to exclude Barrett's oesophagus, to assess the size of any underlying hiatus hernia, to observe any oesophagitis/strictures and to make sure there is no other pathology which might take precedence (such malignancy or gastro-duodenal ulceration). If Barrett's is present, multiple biopsies are required to assess for underlying dysplasia, and this must be treated before a decision can be taken to proceed with antireflux surgery [2]. All patients being considered for antireflux surgery should undergo manometry studies to exclude other motility disorders such as achalasia (for which fundoplication is a disaster!). Although not essential in those with erosive oesophagitis, pH and increasingly impedance studies are useful to confirm the underlying diagnosis and severity of the reflux, particularly in patients with atypical symptoms. They are also useful in the postoperative period in patients who develop recurrent symptoms or have a less than an excellent result after surgery. If there is a history of previous peptic ulcer surgery, in particular vagotomy and pyloroplasty, a history of reflux, oesophagitis and elevated acid exposure time may all be due to decreased gastric motility. In these patients gastric emptying studies may be required.

As in all areas of surgery, the best results are achieved by selecting the right patient for the right operation at the right time.

32.2.2 Giant Hiatus Hernia/Intrathoracic Stomach with Gastric Volvulus

A large para-oesophageal hiatus hernia is relatively common, particularly in the elderly, and is increasingly being identified on imaging for other cardiorespiratory problems (Fig. 32.1). Patients with troublesome mechanical symptoms (chest pain, dysphagia and regurgitation) or acute attacks of volvulus should be considered for surgery [3]. Although shortness of breath will often improve following

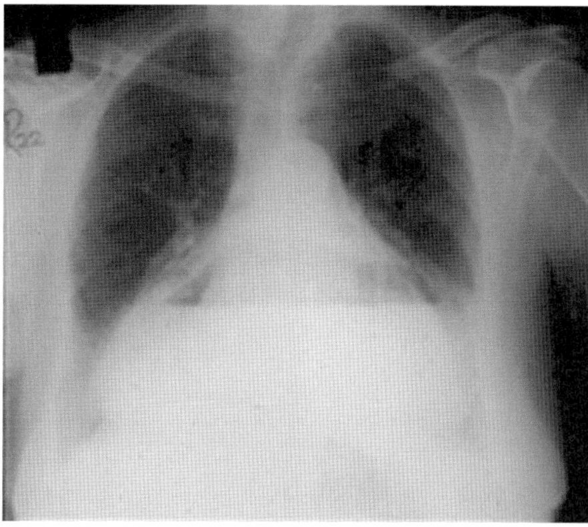

Fig. 32.1 Routine chest X-ray demonstrating a large retrocardiac air fluid level from an intrathoracic stomach

surgery, care should be taken to exclude other cardiorespiratory diagnoses, particularly in those patients without other symptoms warranting surgery. Iron deficiency anaemia is not uncommon secondary to Cameron's lesions at the hiatus and is another factor that needs to be considered when making a decision for surgery. Despite the small potential risk of life-threatening gastric volvulus with ischaemia, the authors would not recommend routine repair of totally asymptomatic radiological findings in elderly patients, and this would be supported by the literature and long-term observational studies [4]. Our experience is that patients who have required an emergency admission with an obstructed stomach and have settled with nasogastric decompression nearly always represent with identical symptoms if surgery is not undertaken. If this is to be performed during the acute admission, it is advisable to decompress the stomach with a nasogastric tube for a period of 48 h to reduce the resulting gastric oedema and increase the chance of a successful laparoscopic repair.

Assessment in the elective setting includes gastroscopy and either a CT (Fig. 32.2) or contrast swallow (Fig. 32.3) to delineate the anatomy. For patients with associated symptoms of shortness of breath or weight loss, CT is preferred to exclude other significant pathology. Oesophageal manometry or pH studies are not required.

32.3 Primary Laparoscopic Fundoplication

(a) Port placement and position of surgeon

There are basically two positions for a laparoscopic fundoplication: the surgeon on the left with the camera assistant on the right or the surgeon between the legs and the camera person either on the right or left. Port positions vary, but the majority of surgeons prefer the camera port to be on the left of the midline about half way from the costal margin and the umbilicus, depending on whether the patient is large or small. The authors all use different port positions!

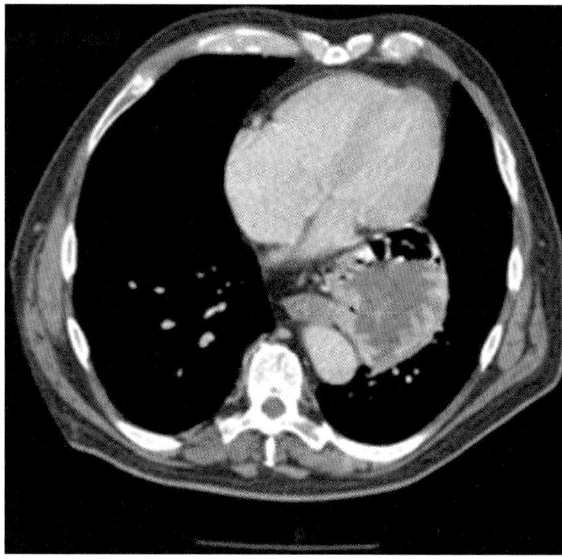

Fig. 32.2 CT showing large intrathoracic stomach with volvulus

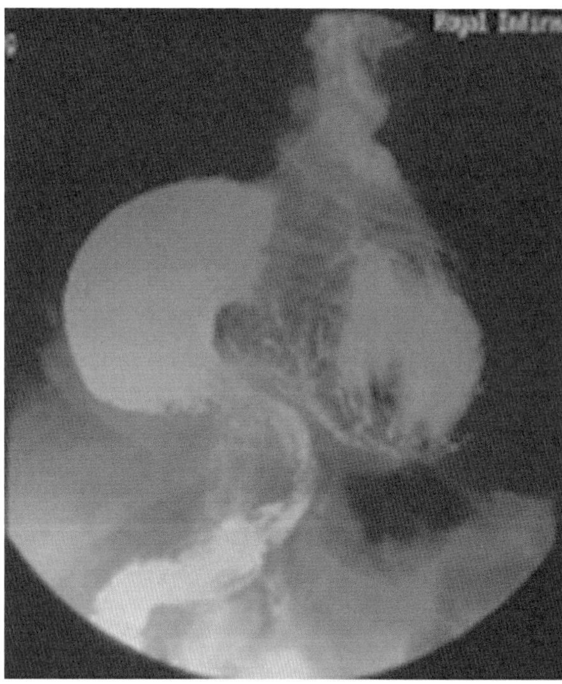

Fig. 32.3 Barium meal demonstrating a gastric volvulus within the hiatus

(b) Liver retraction

It is an essential manoeuvre, and the authors all use the Nathanson retractor which comes in a number of sizes and is anchored to a rigid structure attached to the right side of the operating table (Fig. 32.4).

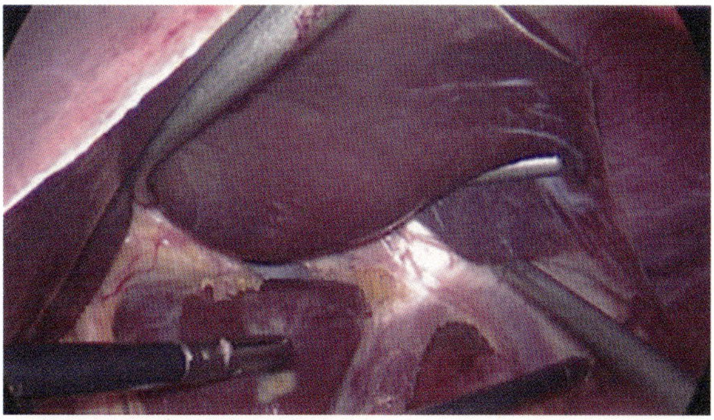

Fig. 32.4 Nathanson liver retractor

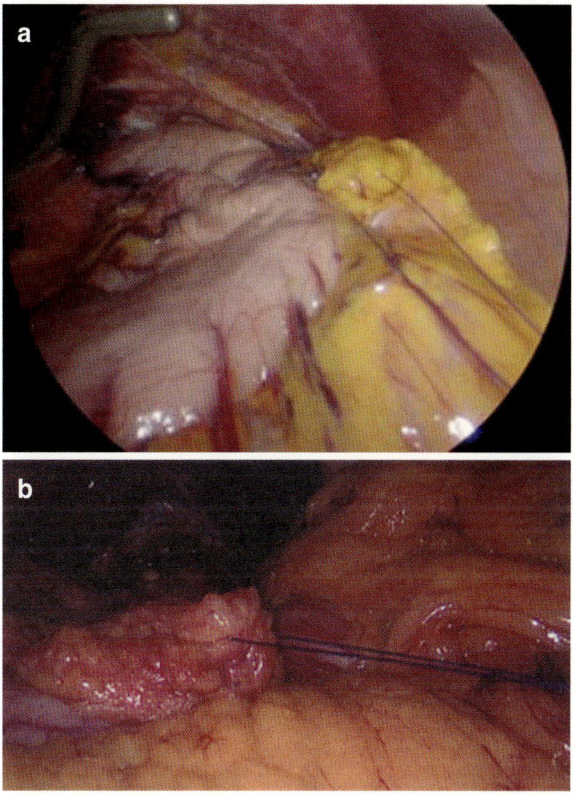

Fig. 32.5 Fat stitch retracting (**a**) the greater omentum and (**b**) the lesser omentum

(c) Fat stitches to greater and lesser omentum
They are very useful, particularly in patients with significant amounts of intra-abdominal fat. In very large patients, as many as three or four may be required (Fig. 32.5). They are generally brought out through the furthest left port and clipped at the skin edge.

(d) Dissection of hiatus
The key to the dissection of the hiatus is identifying either crus and then working round to the other. Identifying the phreno-oesophageal ligaments is a very useful technique to help avoid oesophageal injury and allow entry into the

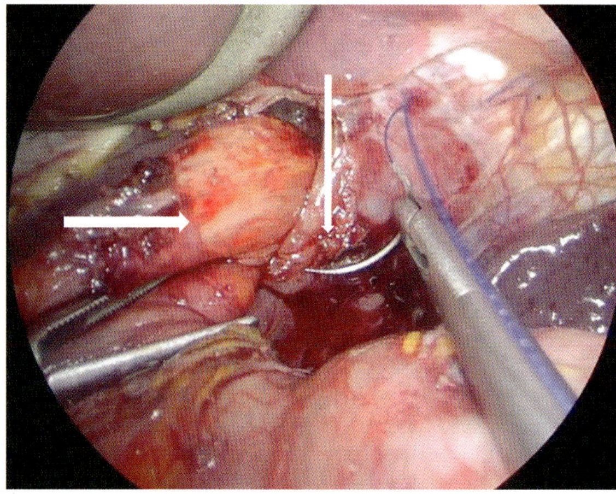

Fig. 32.6 Left phreno-oesophageal ligament (arrowed) being sutured closed before the fundoplication

avascular plane within the hiatus. There appears to be some evidence emerging that closure/repair of the left phreno-oesophageal ligament reduces the chance of revisional surgery. This can be performed with a continuous non-absorbable suture (Fig. 32.6). The authors are cautious with diathermy and preserve both vagi, incorporating the posterior vagus with the oesophagus during the mobilisation. The posterior part of the oesophagus must be dissected under direct vision, following which a retractor or sling can be passed behind to draw the oesophagus forward. This is facilitated by first mobilising the angle of His on the left side. Where possible the hepatic branch of the vagus nerve should also be preserved. If a posterior wrap is going to be used, preserving this structure helps to prevent distal slippage.

(e) Position of wrap: posterior/anterior and partial/full

There are many varieties of fundoplication, and there remains controversy regarding the best type, anterior or posterior, total or partial. Two recent meta-analyses from the same first author reached different conclusions [5, 6], but most of the problem relates to grouping all posterior and all anterior fundoplications together [7]. Overall it seems that long-term acid control is better with a Nissen than an anterior fundoplication but at the expense of more problems with dysphagia and gas bloat. What is perhaps of more importance is the expertise of the surgeon; choose your procedure and then become good at it!

(f) Management of short gastric vessels

A Nissen requires division of the short gastric vessels (SGV). A 360° wrap can be performed without division of the SGV, as in the Nissen-Rossetti procedure, although in such cases, the wrap involves the anterior part of the gastric fundus and not the greater curve, as in a Nissen. A fat stitch retracting the greater omentum greatly facilitates dissection and division of the SGV. A good tip to ensure that there is an adequate wrap with no tension when forming a posterior fundoplication is to make a good posterior window behind the oesophagus (Fig. 32.7) and then make sure that the wrap lies free after bringing it round (Fig. 32.8).

(g) Crural repair

This is most commonly carried out posteriorly, but a few anterior sutures can be useful, particularly in larger defects and where the posterior crura might start to

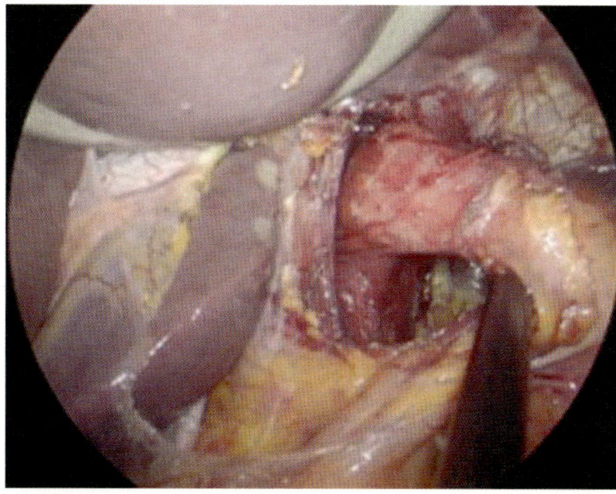

Fig. 32.7 Good posterior window behind the oesophagus

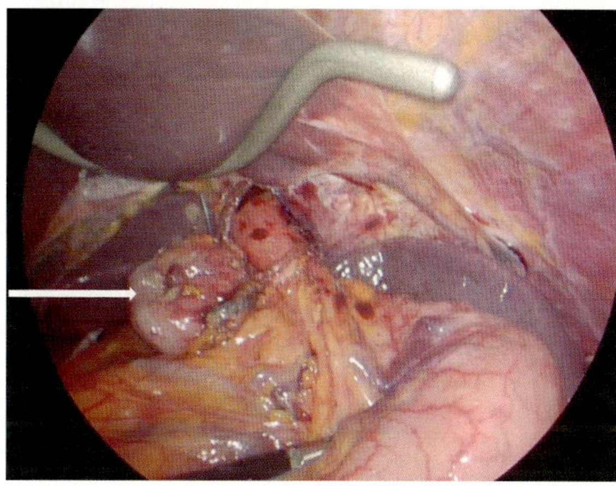

Fig. 32.8 Posterior wrap (arrow) lying with no tension behind oesophagus

'tear'. The authors recommend large bites using zero gauge non-absorbable sutures (either monofilament or braided). The hiatus should be calibrated so there is about 1 cm gap around the oesophagus. This can be measured using an instrument or over a bougie. Although some report that a bougie provides better consistency particularly with a Nissen, this must be balanced against the very small risk of iatrogenic oesophageal injury. The role of meshes (or not) is discussed in the section on giant hiatus hernia repair.

32.4 Revision Fundoplication

32.4.1 Assessment for Revisional Surgery

These patients require careful assessment as the risks of revisional surgery are higher and the results are less certain (around 70% good outcomes compared to 90% for primary fundoplication). It is important to determine whether patient's recurrent symptoms are related to recurrent reflux and whether there is an anatomical abnormality to correct. Endoscopy should be performed by the operating surgeon and combined with contrast studies, pH and manometry and if indicated gastric emptying studies. Outcome is variable, but good results can be obtained both laparoscopically and after open surgery. Results are better for recurrent reflux than dysphagia [8].

The basic principle is to take down the existing fundoplication, repair any hiatal defect and reconstitute a new wrap, but in certain situations a more tailored approach can be used.

(a) After previous open abdominal fundoplication
Key tips—The left lobe of the liver is often adherent to the stomach or wrap and should be fully mobilised before commencing dissection. Both the right crus and left crus must be identified to delineate anatomy and reduce the risk of oesophageal injury. A soft flexible bougie or endoscope inserted across the OGJ can help identify the oesophagus in difficult cases but must be inserted carefully. Conversion to open surgery is often required.

(b) After previous thoracotomy
Difficulties here are found within the hiatus and the trans-abdominal approach can usually be carried out relatively easily laparoscopically. The decision on what type of wrap will obviously depend on the previous thoracic procedure which will have often been one of the many varieties of 'Belsey' operations.

(c) After previous laparoscopic Nissen (i.e. with Division of SGV) or other types of posterior wrap
The underlying problem here is often either a slipped wrap, which must then be dissected free from its position within the hiatus, or disruption of the wrap, which will require to be taken down, re-formed or converted to some other wraps. Previous division of the SGV can make revisional surgery difficult as the right side of the wrap will usually be densely adherent to the left lobe of the liver and the right crus. In such cases if the anatomy cannot be identified with careful dissection, the surgeon can either convert to open surgery (when dissection is often not much easier) or leave the right side of the wrap in situ, mobilising the left side and refashion it as it lies on the assumption that the OGJ and right crus are likely to be fixed. If the two edges of the wrap are difficult to identify, an endoscopic stapler can be used to divide the wrap anteriorly if a safe window can be created between the oesophagus and wrap.

(d) After previous anterior fundoplication
The defect is often a para-oesophageal hernia on the left side or anteriorly. It is usually reasonably straightforward to take the wrap down, reduce the hernia sac and then repair the defect in the diaphragmatic hiatus. Biological meshes again may have a role here to help improve healing but remain controversial. Again synthetic non-absorbable meshes have no role to play anywhere around the oesophagus.

(e) After failed revisional surgery
In a few patients hiatal breakdown and troublesome reflux will develop despite revisional surgery. These are few and far between, and if further surgery is required, a further attempt can be made at revising the fundoplication and repairing any recurrent hiatus hernia. However this is often extremely difficult and as a

result hazardous. However if symptoms justify a further operation and some form of revision looks to be too difficult or dangerous, a subtotal gastrectomy with Roux-en-Y reconstruction is one solution. In these revisional patients, adhesions around the hiatus have essentially ‘fixed’ the OGJ within the hiatus and reducing the gastric reservoir and hence the volume of refluxate, by a subtotal gastrectomy Roux-en-Y usually solves the problem. In many of these patients, the SGVs will have previously been divided. It is therefore important not to ligate the left gastric artery in order to ensure adequate blood supply to the stomach remnant; otherwise a near total gastrectomy will be required.

(f) The short oesophagus
The authors believe that with adequate dissection, it is extremely rare to encounter a true ‘short oesophagus’ and do not believe in the practice of Collis gastroplasty. In the unusual situation where adequate oesophageal length cannot be obtained, such as a patient who has undergone multiple procedures for reflux as a child, then the option lies between creating a wrap that could lie above the diaphragm or performing a more definitive procedure such as a subtotal gastrectomy.

32.5 Giant Hiatus Hernia and Gastric Volvulus

(a) It is important to fully dissect the entire peritoneal sac, ignoring the contents. Multiple fat stitches may be required to help expose the hiatus and contents. Care must be taken where possible to preserve both vagus nerves, although damage to either is not uncommon. The fat pad is a good guide to the gastro-oesophageal junction at the base of the right crus. It is important to fully reduce the posterior sac, which is also present.
(b) Approximation of crura usually requires several sutures both anteriorly and posteriorly. A biological mesh can be used to help support the sutures but should not be used to ‘bridge’ any defect. Such a policy is doomed to failure. In such occasions when the crura cannot be adequately approximated, some form of fixation of the fundoplication around the hiatus will help prevent recurrence. Buttressing of the sutures with Teflon pledgets can help when the quality of the crus is poor. In difficult cases conversion to open surgery may be required, but access and closure may not be any easier. The main objective in such patients is the reduction of the stomach from the mediastinum and prevention of it returning. Controlling reflux is very much a secondary aim. The authors routinely perform either an anterior or posterior fundoplication, and in these cases the fundus is usually very mobile. In our experience, some patients never regain normal gastric function and retain a degree of gastric stasis. It is unclear whether this results from chronic twisting/stretching of the stomach within the chest or from vagal damage during what is often a very extensive dissection.
(c) Use of biological meshes
There is increasing interest in using biological meshes to help encourage fibrosis formation around the crural repair and reduce recurrent defects. They are

In many patients these investigations do not confirm recurrent reflux, and the 'recurrent' symptoms are related to some form of motility problem. In most patients symptoms can be relatively well controlled with medical therapy, and only a few (around 5% in most studies [5]) will require revisional surgery. As mentioned earlier, recurrence does seem to be higher in those patients undergoing an anterior fundoplication, but their longer-term complications are perhaps slightly lower than for those with a posterior wrap.

(b) Dysphagia—migration of the wrap up into the hiatus or herniation of the proximal stomach 'through' the wrap. Diagnosis here requires both endoscopy and barium swallow and will almost certainly require revisional surgery.

References

1. Rantanen TK, Salo JA, Sipponen JT. Fatal and life threatening complications in anti-reflux surgery: analysis of 5502 operations. Br J Surg. 1999;86:1573–7.
2. Fitzgerald RC, di Pietro M, Ragunath K, Ang Y, Kang JY, Watson P, Trudgill N, Patel P, Kaye PV, Sanders S, O'Donovan M, Bird-Lieberman E, Bhandari P, Jankowski JA, Attwood S, Parsons SL, Loft D, Lagergren J, Moayyedi P, Lyratzopoulos G, de Caestecker J. British Society of Gastroenterology guidelines on the diagnosis and management of Barrett's oesophagus. Gut. 2014;63(1):7–42.
3. Kohn GP, Price RR, DeMeester SR, Zehetner J, Muensterer OJ, Awad Z, Mittal SK, Richardson WS, Stefanidis D, Fanelli RD, SAGES Guidelines Committee. Guidelines for the management of hiatal hernia. Surg Endosc. 2013;27(12):4409–28. https://doi.org/10.1007/s00464-013-3173-3. Epub 2013 Sep 10
4. Stylopoulos N, Gazelle GS, Rattner DW. Paraesophageal hernias: operation or observation. Ann Surg. 2002;236(4):492–501.
5. Joris A, Broeders JA, Roks DJ, Ali UA, Draaisma WA, Smout AJ, Hazebroek EJ. Laparoscopic anterior versus posterior fundoplication for gastroesophageal reflux disease systematic review and meta-analysis of randomized clinical trials. Ann Surg. 2011;254:39–47.
6. Broeders JA, Roks DJ, Ahmed Ali U, Watson DI, Baigrie RJ, Cao Z, Hartmann J, Maddern GJ. Laparoscopic anterior 180-degree versus Nissen fundoplication for gastroesophageal reflux disease: systematic review and meta-analysis of randomized clinical trials. Ann Surg. 2013;257(5):850–9. https://doi.org/10.1097/SLA.0b013e31828604dd.
7. Thompson AK, Watson DA. What is the best anti-reflux operation? All fundoplications are not created equal. World J Surg. 2015;39:997–9.
8. Lamb PJ, Myers JC, Jamieson GG, Thompson SK, Devitt PG, Watson DI. Long-term outcomes of revisional surgery following laparoscopic fundoplication. Br J Surg. 2009;96:391–7.
9. Lidor AO, Kawaji Q, Stem M, Fleming RM, Schweitzer MA, Steele KE, Marohn MR. Defining recurrence after paraesophageal hernia repair: correlating symptoms and radiographic findings. Surgery. 2013;154:171–8.

Part VIII

Diaphragm

Congenital Diaphragmatic Hernia

33

Ingo Jester

Abstract

Congenital diaphragmatic hernia (CDH) encountered in the neonates is generally diagnosed antenatally and tends to cause significant postnatal management challenges. In this context surgery is only one of the minor challenges. The procedure involves the gentle reposition of the herniated abdominal viscera back into abdomen and repairing the defect either by primary approximation of the defect or by using a patch to separate the abdomen and thoracic cavity. The morbidity in survivals is mainly related to persistence of pulmonary hypertension, gastro-oesophageal reflux with feeding intolerance and recurrence of hernia. The significant mortality associated with CDH is related to severity of pulmonary hypertension, associated cardiac and chromosomal anomalies. The chapter will deal with both open and minimally invasive method of the repair. The management of pulmonary hypertension is outside the scope of this chapter.

Keywords

Congenital diaphragmatic hernia · Bochdalek hernia · Morgagni hernia · Hiatus hernia · Thoracoscopy · Persistent pulmonary hypertension · Pulmonary hypoplasia

I. Jester, F.R.C.S. (Paeds), M.D.
Department of Pediatric Surgery, Birmingham Children's Hospital NHS FT, Birmingham, UK
e-mail: Ingo.Jester@bch.nhs.uk

D. Parikh, P.B. Rajesh (eds.), *Tips and Tricks in Thoracic Surgery*,
https://doi.org/10.1007/978-1-4471-7355-7_33

33.1 Introduction

Congenital diaphragmatic hernia (CDH) is classically a term used for a posterolateral defect and is associated with a variable degree of pulmonary hypoplasia. The diaphragmatic hernia can occur through various anatomical and developmental weak points: anterior defect (Morgagni hernia), posterolateral hernia (Bochdalek hernia) and hiatus hernia. Bochdalek hernias comprise about 80% of all diaphragmatic hernias and are most common on the left side (78%), about 20% on the right side and approximately 1% bilateral [1]. Morgagni hernias comprise about 2% of all diaphragmatic hernias and are typically asymptomatic in the neonatal period.

The exact causes and development of the defect within the diaphragm are not well understood. Pulmonary hypoplasia and associated abnormally thickened pulmonary arterial vasculature lead to the development of postnatal pulmonary hypertension. Significant challenges are in the postnatal management of pulmonary hypoplasia and persistent hypertension to maintain adequate oxygenation and circulation within vital organs [2].

CDH is identified in1:3000 live births accounting for 8% of all congenital malformations and in the majority of instances diagnosed antenatal on a routine prenatal ultrasound screen [3]. However, some infants can present postnatally with the respiratory distress and diagnosed to have a presence of a diaphragmatic hernia. Late diaphragmatic hernia presentations in infancy and childhood are rare and have variable clinical features of abdominal pain, recurrent intestinal obstruction or recurrent chest infections [4]. CDH cases are frequently associated with cardiovascular malformations and chromosomal abnormality and may contribute towards mortality. Improved survival in CDH is related to better understanding of the pathophysiology of persistent pulmonary hypertension and pulmonary hypoplasia and its postnatal management [5–7].

Mortality in CDH cases is high in the presence of:

- Cardiac and chromosomal abnormality [8].
- Size of the diaphragmatic defect [9].
- Degree of pulmonary hypoplasia.
- The liver above the diaphragm [10].
- Severity of pulmonary hypertension (perinatal or chronic).
- Right-sided hernias are associated with a greater mortality than left-sided defects [11].

Morbidity is considerably high in all survivors with CDH:

- Pulmonary symptoms with lifelong limited exercise tolerance and symptoms of airway obstruction requiring bronchodilators
- Gastrointestinal symptoms with failure to thrive (<3rd centile), oral food aversion and gastro-oesophageal reflux requiring medical treatment or fundoplication
- Developmental delay

- Chest deformity with pectus excavatum and scoliosis
- Sensorineural hearing defect

33.2 Tips and Tricks for the Surgical Repair of CDH

Mainstay of postnatal management of CDH is the preoperative stabilization of the pulmonary and cardiovascular status.

33.2.1 Open Approach

1. The diaphragmatic defect can be repaired either using abdominal subcostal or longitudinal midline incision. The herniated viscera are reduced gently into the abdomen and the defect closed with interrupted non-absorbable sutures without a chest drain.
2. Postoperative chest drain should not be used as it leads to overexpansion of the lung or persistent air leak from the hypoplastic lung. Occasionally postoperative effusion or chylothorax may cause respiratory distress. Difficulty in ventilation may require insertion of a chest drain [12].
3. In the presence of a large defect where primary approximation of a muscle defect is not feasible, a prosthetic material is used to patch the defect. The authors recommend polytetrafluoroethylene patch (PTFE or Gore-Tex®) repair which has been associated with better outcome and less recurrence than other synthetic and biological or absorbable patch materials [13, 14].
4. Higher recurrence rate of up to 10% is reported in literature in patients where a prosthetic patch CDH repair has been carried out [15].
5. Most recurrences occur within the first 2 years postoperatively and are often asymptomatic; hence, regular chest x-rays are recommended during this period to detect recurrence.

33.3 Technical Tips and Tricks in Open Hernia Repair of Large Diaphragmatic Defects (Bochdalek Hernia) with Gore-Tex® Patch

1. Intraoperative problem at the time of surgery is the lack of abdominal space following the reduction of viscera and patch repair of the hernia allowing a tension-free closure of the abdominal wall. This can be achieved by folding the flat Gore-Tex® patch into a cone shape (Fig. 33.1a–c). This creates an average additional space of at least 20 ml in the abdominal cavity. It also reduces the space in the chest cavity containing the hypoplastic lung that may reduce the risk over its over distention. It is our practice to fix the cone-shaped Gore-Tex® patch by an overlapping border of about 1 cm to the muscle rim and the edge separately to the diaphragmatic muscle to create a broad base fixation (Fig. 33.2). This has shown to reduce the risk of recurrence rate to about 3% [16].

17. Nam SH, Cho MJ, Kim DY, Kim SC. Shifting from laparotomy to thoracoscopic repair of congenital diaphragmatic hernia in neonates: early experience. World J Surg. 2013;37:2711–6.
18. Vijfhuize S, Deden AC, Costerus SA, Sloots CE, Wijnen RM. Minimal access surgery for repair of congenital diaphragmatic hernia: is it advantageous?--an open review. Eur J Pediatr Surg. 2012;22:364–73.
19. Bishay M, et al. Hypercapnia and acidosis during open and thoracoscopic repair of congenital diaphragmatic hernia and esophageal atresia: results of a pilot randomized controlled trial. Ann Surg. 2013;258:895–900.
20. Maier S, et al. Preventive antireflux surgery in neonates with congenital diaphragmatic hernia: a single-blinded prospective study. J Pediatr Surg. 2011;46:1510–5.

34 Diaphragmatic Eventration

Dakshesh Parikh

Abstract

Diaphragmatic eventration is referred to surgeons for plication not uncommonly by the intensivists as they are unable to wean the infants from the ventilator. The persistent elevation and paradoxical movements clinically, on fluoroscopy and on ultrasound, are diagnostic of paralysed diaphragm. The reduced thoracic capacity and paradoxical movement of the diaphragm, persistent collapse of the lower lobe or recurrent infection in the collapsed lung are indications for surgical intervention in children. Typically, these infants fail to thrive and are breathless on exertion and prone to recurrent chest infections in the collapsed lobe. Plication can be easily achieved thoracoscopically with minimal morbidity. Recurrence generally is rare but is seen in children with syndromes or associated with myopathy and/or poor muscle tone.

Keywords

Diaphragmatic eventration · Thoracoscopy · Plication · Diaphragmatic pacing · Diaphragmatic hernia with hernia sac

34.1 Introduction

Diaphragmatic eventration or abnormal elevation of diaphragm in the thoracic cavity can be either congenital or acquired as a result of phrenic nerve injury. Diaphragmatic eventration is not uncommonly seen in neonates after cardiac surgery and with birth injuries associated with brachial plexus trauma. On occasion it is idiopathic and

D. Parikh, MBBS, MS, FRCS (Ped.), MD
Department of Pediatric Surgery, Birmingham Women's and Children's Hospital NHS FT, Birmingham, UK
e-mail: dakshesh.parikh@nhs.net

D. Parikh, P.B. Rajesh (eds.), *Tips and Tricks in Thoracic Surgery*,
https://doi.org/10.1007/978-1-4471-7355-7_34

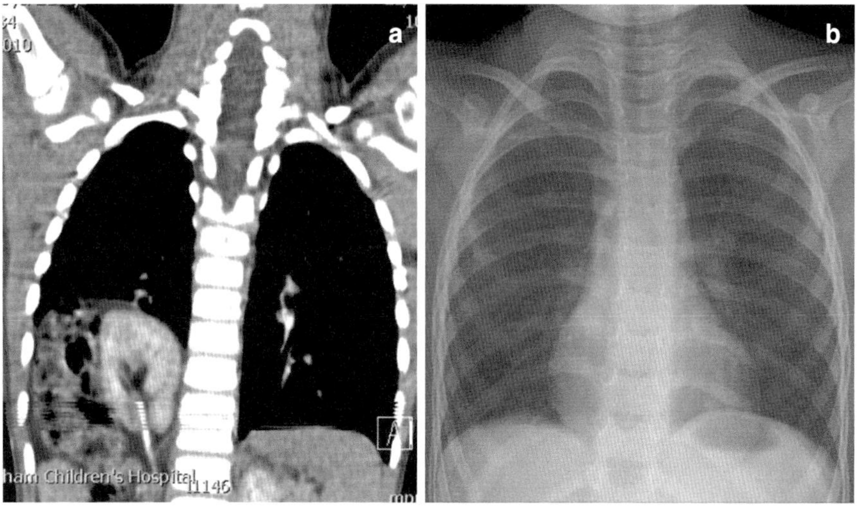

Fig. 34.2 Chest x-ray in a symptomatic child showed eventration. Ultrasound with M mode performed to document paradoxymal movement demonstrated the kidney above the diaphragm leading to CT scan (**a**) that confirmed the kidney rotated and above in the eventration. Postoperative chest x-ray is shown, repaired with thoracoscopic plication using three ports

Alternative method: Innovation by inserting a spinal needle from the intercostal space and taking diaphragmatic muscle interrupted creating pleats bringing the suture outside, and suturing on the ribs has been suggested to reduce a number of ports in the small chest cavity. This method is difficult to describe in words. Suture is introduced from outside brought in by the thoracoscopic needle holder, the spinal needle picks up interrupted muscle bites, and the end of suture is threaded into the needle and brought out. A second row is done in a similar fashion, and the other end of suture is threaded into the needle and brought out. These are then tightened outside the chest watching the diaphragm getting plicated. The sutures are then buried in the subcutaneous space. The disadvantage being the knots are palpable underneath the skin and can result in granuloma formation and a source of pain.

34.3 Postoperative Complications

- *Recurrence*: This is common in children with neuromuscular disorders or associated with syndrome that causes muscle weakness. It is also seen in cases where absorbable stiches or monofilament sutures are used. Recurrence can be managed either at open or with advanced minimally invasive techniques with redo plication using braided non-absorbable sutures. Adhesions should be gently separated avoiding damage to either intrathoracic or intra-abdominal viscera depending on the approach taken.

- *Damage to intra-abdominal viscera*: This can be avoided by lifting the diaphragm muscle rolling it between the jaws of the forceps and then taking the stich through the picked-up muscle [5]. Distended stomach should be emptied with a nasogastric tube. In cases where previous abdominal surgery is carried out, plication should be carried out with care as there could be adherent colon or small intestine. Many surgeons would prefer open intra-abdominal approach dissecting adhesions and then plicating the diaphragm. We had done redo thoracoscopic surgery after damage to phrenic nerve after resecting a large mediastinal teratoma.
- *Persistent respiratory failure despite plication*: Most times this is a result of failure to adequately manage chronic lung disease. In this cases an expert neonatal advice to manage chronic lung disease, allowing a degree of permissive hypercapnia, management of persistent pulmonary hypertension and gradual weaning of ventilation may be required. Weaning can be prolonged, and patience is necessary as pressure damage to already affected lung can affect the outcome. Recurrent pneumothorax is a problem in many instances. Localised pulmonary interstitial emphysema can be resected to improve the expansion of the collapsed lung. Nutrition should be given consideration as these chronically ventilated neonates can be malnourished and have atrophied respiratory muscles. Gastro-oesophageal reflux is also commonly associated in these infants and should be managed appropriately.

Conclusions

Plication can be performed either through chest or abdomen using either open or minimally invasive surgical approach. When performed in patients that are dependent on mechanical ventilation, it allows successful weaning and extubation. Long-term results after plication are very good and recurrences are rare in most instances.

References

1. Crabbe DCG. Diaphragmatic eventration. In: Parikh DH, DCG C, Rothenbergh S, Auldist A, editors. Pediatric thoracic surgery. New York: Springer; 2009. p. 501–9.
2. Bingham JAW. Two cases of unilateral paralysis of diaphragm in the newborn treated surgically. Thorax. 1954;9:248–52.
3. Bisgard J. Congenital eventration of diaphragm. J Thorac Surg. 1947;16:484–91.
4. Schwartz MZ, Filler RM. Plication of the diaphragm for symptomatic phrenic nerve paralysis. J Pediatr Surg. 1978;13:259–63.
5. Becmeur F, Talon I, Shaarschmidt K, et al. Thoracoscopic diaphragmatic eventration repair in children: about 10 cases. J Pediatr Surg. 2005;40:1412–5.

Part IX
Miscellaneous

Spontaneous Pneumothorax

35

Maninder Singh Kalkat

Abstract

Pneumothorax can be either primary with apparently normal lung parenchyma or secondary when associated with an underlying pathology. Primary spontaneous pneumothorax is idiopathic occurring in young healthy adults and adolescents; however, a causative aetiology should be suspected if encountered in younger children or recurring after surgical intervention. In older adults, it is invariably secondary to chronic obstructive pulmonary disease (COPD). Although, significant radiological investigations are considered unnecessary after its identification on chest X-ray in young healthy individuals, it may be necessary to investigate selected cases and children with CT scan of thorax. Surgical thoracoscopic intervention is both diagnostic and therapeutic and gives good outcomes if combined with parietal pleurectomy.

Keywords

Spontaneous pneumothorax · Sub-pleural blebs · Apical bullae · Tension pneumothorax · Marfan's syndrome · Emphysema · Pleurodesis · Pleurectomy Cystic fibrosis · Acquired immune deficiency syndrome

35.1 Introduction

The term pneumothorax—presence of free air in the pleural cavity—was first used by two French physicians Etard and Laennec in 1803 and 1826, respectively. However, Boerhaave described the presence of large amount of air in pleural cavity with collapsed lung in a patient with spontaneous rupture of oesophagus. The most

M.S. Kalkat, MBBS, MCh, FRCS(CTh)
Birmingham Heartlands Hospital, Birmingham, UK
e-mail: Maninder.kalkat@heartofengland.nhs.uk

D. Parikh, P.B. Rajesh (eds.), *Tips and Tricks in Thoracic Surgery*,
https://doi.org/10.1007/978-1-4471-7355-7_35

common cause of pneumothorax used to be tuberculosis for a long time, which still remains one in many parts of the world. There were few cases which occurred in apparently healthy individuals and were referred to as pneumothorax simple.

35.2 Pathophysiology

A pneumothorax can be spontaneous or secondary to trauma, diagnostic or therapeutic event. A spontaneous pneumothorax can be primary—occurring without evidence of underlying lung disease or secondary—in presence of disease process in the lung.

The intrapleural pressure is negative with respect to atmospheric pressure and varies between −3 and −8 cm of water. The intrabronchial pressure is higher than intrapleural pressure due to elastic recoil of the lung and ranges from −1 to +5. This difference of pressures holds the lung parenchyma closely applied to the chest wall, with parietal and visceral pleura opposed to each wither throughout the breathing cycle.

The disruption of either visceral or parietal pleura results in air entering the potential pleural space and loss of negative intrapleural pressure. This results in collapse of the lung parenchyma and pneumothorax ensues. The air leak into pleural space continues till there is either equalisation of pressure between communicating spaces or the leak gets sealed. The rupture of pleural bleb or bulla results in disruption of visceral pleura, and parietal pleura is involved secondary to injury to the chest wall, oesophagus and airways.

The pneumothorax decreases pulmonary volumes, compliance and diffusing capacity. The pathophysiological outcome is dependent on the size of the pneumothorax and condition of underlying lung parenchyma. With collapse of half or more normal lung, arterial hypoxemia occurs but often resolves as the perfusion to the collapsed lung diminishes. However, in patients with underlying lung disease and destroyed elastic recoil of the lung, the pneumothorax can be slow to develop and less extensive, but physiological effects and symptoms are more profound.

At times, a check valve effect can occur at the site of pleural disruption resulting in unilateral entry of air into the pleural cavity without any egress. This can result in progressive build-up of positive intrapleural pressure, compounded by deep laboured breathing, anxiety and coughing. This increasing positive pressure in the pleural cavity shifts the mediastinum and interferes with venous return and cardiac output, resulting in tension pneumothorax—a life-threatening emergency.

35.3 Clinical Presentation

The symptoms and signs depend on the cause of pneumothorax, the extent of lung collapse and underlying lung disease. The typical symptoms of chest pain and dyspnoea may be minor or absent, especially in patients with primary spontaneous pneumothorax. In patients with secondary pneumothorax, the symptoms are more

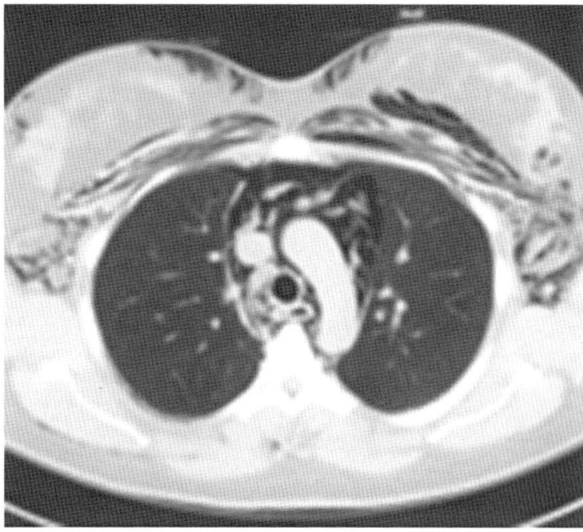

Fig. 35.1 CT scan demonstrating surgical emphysema and pneumomediastinum without pneumothorax

severe, and majority of patients have dyspnoea out of proportion to size of pneumothorax. The air can track into subcutaneous tissue and present as surgical emphysema. Occasionally, the air leaking from ruptured bleb can track along the peribronchial tissues into mediastinum, presenting as pneumomediastinum and surgical emphysema, without evidence of classical pneumothorax (Fig. 35.1). The tension pneumothorax is accompanied by severe dyspnoea and cardiovascular collapse.

The physical signs of pneumothorax can be subtle and include diminished motion of chest wall with respiration, hyper-resonance on percussion, reduced tactile fremitus and diminished breath sounds on the affected side. The presence of mediastinal emphysema is diagnosed by characteristic crunching sound on auscultation—Hamman's sign. In addition, cyanosis, sweating, tachycardia and hypotension may suggest presence of tension pneumothorax. The trachea and cardiac apex may be shifted to the uninvolved side in these patients.

Arterial blood gas measurements are frequently abnormal demonstrating arterial hypoxemia and degree of carbon dioxide retention, particularly in patients with secondary pneumothorax.

The diagnosis of pneumothorax is usually confirmed on a standard postero-anterior chest film taken in deep inspiration. The radiographic hallmark is displacement of visceral pleura from the parietal pleura by air in the pleural space. This appears as hyperlucent area with absence of pulmonary markings on the periphery of the hemithorax. The visceral pleura is seen as thin white line separating air in the pleural cavity and lung parenchyma (Fig. 35.2).

If no abnormality is seen on inspiratory film and suspicion of pneumothorax persists, chest film taken in expiration should be performed. The subtle pneumothorax becomes visible with reduction in the size of the lung volume and its increased radiographic density.

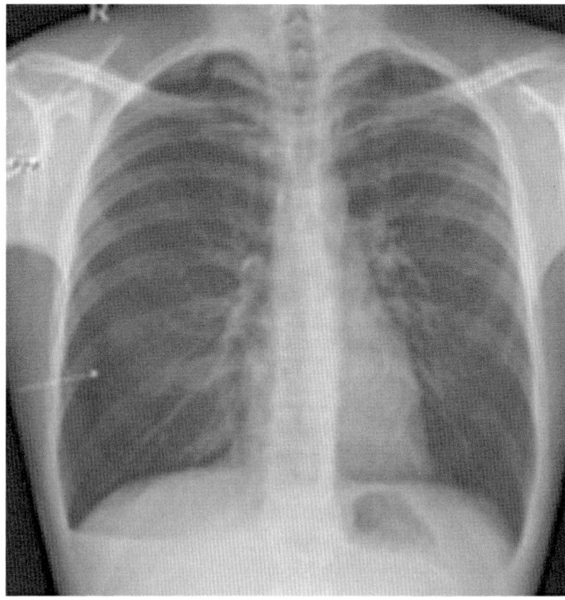

Fig. 35.2 Chest X-ray appearance of pneumothorax

The pneumothorax may be difficult to identify in patients with bullous emphysema, surgical emphysema or images taken in critically ill patients in supine or semirecumbent position. In particular, the differentiation from a large bulla is a common problem and has often resulted in an appropriate insertion of chest drain into the bulla.

The CT scan is recommended in such cases to identify septa of bullae traversing the hyperlucent area. It can also localise loculated pneumothorax and guide insertion of chest drains.

The CT scan can be regarded as the gold standard in detection of small pneumothoraces, size estimation and evaluating lung pathology. It is recommended that all patients with secondary pneumothorax should be investigated with CT scan of the chest.

The pneumothorax is not too often associated with haemothorax, due to tearing of vascular adhesion, bleeding from edges of parietal pleura or lung parenchyma.

Rapid accumulation of large amount of fluid, presence of pneumomediastinum and deteriorating clinical condition of patient should raise the suspicion of ruptured oesophagus (Fig. 35.3).

Pneumothorax present as a small rim at the periphery of the chest film may occupy 30% of the pleural cavity. The 2 cm pneumothorax approximates to a 50% pneumothorax by volume.

Portable chest X-ray performed supine position, particularly in sick patients, may not reveal pneumothorax, as the air will collect anteromedially or in the subpulmonic area.

The patient with pleural adhesions because of previous surgery, infection or trauma may have loculated pneumothorax which can be missed.

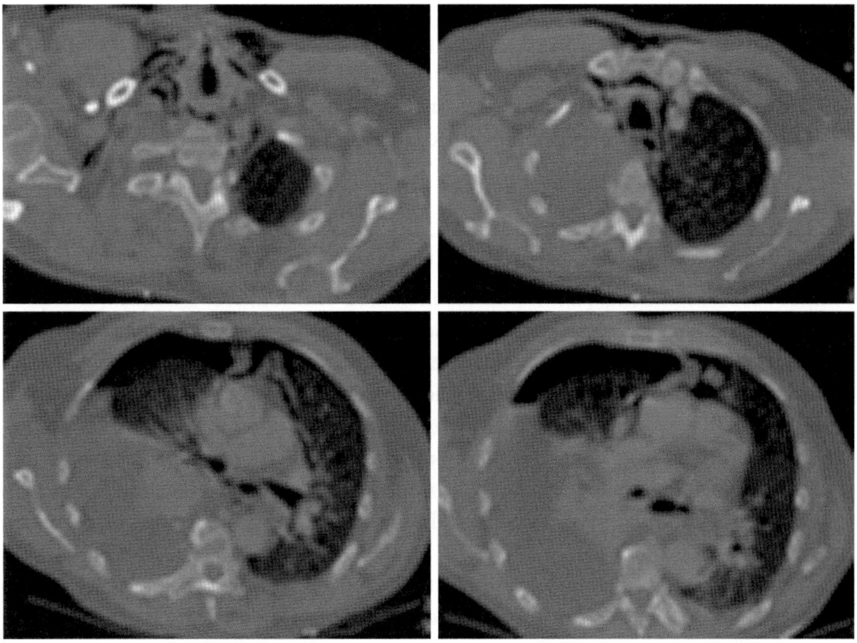

Fig. 35.3 CT scan appearance with ruptured oesophagus

Differentiation of pneumothorax from a large bulla is often a difficult and can lead to inadvertent insertion of the drain into the bulla.

CT scan of the thorax may be useful in identifying difficult to diagnose pneumothoraces and detect underlying lung condition. There may be presence of subpleural blebs, bullae, emphysema and interstitial lung disease accounting for pneumothorax. Presence of pleural adhesions and pleural fluid or haemorrhage can also be identified.

If the lung fails to expand after insertion of drain, bronchoscopic examination is warranted to rule endobronchial obstruction.

Patients with underlying lung disease may have smaller pneumothorax but can be sufficient to increase work of breathing and result in more severe symptoms.

35.4 Primary Spontaneous Pneumothorax

Primary spontaneous pneumothorax is disease of healthy young people, without underlying lung disease. More men are affected with incidence of 18–28/100,000 compared to 1.2–6/100,000 women [1]. There is increased incidence in smokers (12% vs. 0.1%) [2].

It usually results from rupture of sub-pleural blebs or bullae, which will be seen in 90% patients at surgery or 80% on the CT scan. It is more common in taller people, at the apex of the lung related to greater distending pressure in the apical alveoli.

Table 35.1 Indications for surgery in spontaneous pneumothorax

Significant air leak and failure of lung to expand fully
Persistent air leak for more than 5 days
Recurrent pneumothorax
Second ipsilateral pneumothorax
First contralateral pneumothorax
Synchronous bilateral pneumothorax
Complication of pneumothorax
Haemothorax
Empyema
Professions at risk
Airline pilots
Scuba divers
Underlying lung conditions resulting in pneumothorax
Pregnancy

35.7 Tips and Tricks for Thoracoscopic Bullectomy and Parietal Pleurectomy

The surgery involves resection of the lung parenchyma containing blebs or bullae, followed by pleurodesis. Blebs are found in about 85% of patients and well-defined bullae are seen in others. These are usually present at the apex of the lung and occasionally in relation to the apical segment of the lower lobe. Rarely, no obvious abnormality is seen in the lung parenchyma, and in such cases, adequate pleurodesis is relied on to prevent recurrence.

The procedure is usually carried using video-assisted thoracoscopic approach, using single or up to three ports. The large port to insert 12 mm stapler should be place more anteriorly as the intercostal spaces widen anteriorly reducing the risk of inadvertent intercostal nerve injury. Post-operative neuralgic pain is the most common complication following thoracoscopic resection of apical bullae. The apicectomy, removal of the apex of the upper lobe or bullectomy is carried out using staplers, ensuring healthy area of the lung is incorporated in the staple line. Lung parenchyma injury should be avoided by either using an optical port while inserting the first port or by an open method. The open method of port insertion is used in recurrences, after the use of an intercostal tube or previous thoracoscopic or open surgery.

The pleurodesis is carried out by stripping the parietal pleura off the chest wall – parietal pleurectomy. It is important to undertake a wide pleurectomy, particularly from the apex to prevent recurrence. The pleural abrasion has also been recommended to achieve pleural symphysis, but recurrence of pneumothorax is higher, 3% compared to 0.4% for pleurectomy. Intercostal nerve injury and injury to sympathetic system should be avoided while stripping the parietal pleura.

In patients with secondary pneumothorax, the thoracoscopic treatment can prove difficult and thoracotomy may be performed for assessing the pleural cavity. The lung in such cases is more friable and needs delicate handling. In diffuse lung disease, the site of leak may be difficult to discern with thoracoscopic approach.

Some patients with secondary pneumothorax may be unfit for an operative procedure on account of the lung disease or poor general condition. In such patients, conservative management is advised, including adequately placed, wide-bore chest drains, judicious suction and chemical pleurodesis, if the good lung expansion is achieved. Use of blood pleurodesis has also been recommended with satisfactory outcomes.

35.8 Tips and Tricks for Specific Aetiology

Acquired immune deficiency syndrome: Secondary pneumothorax may occur in AIDS related to secondary infection from pneumocystis carinii pneumonia (PCP) or infection related to cytomegalovirus and tuberculosis or atypical mycobacterial infection. Chronic interstitial inflammation may be responsible for formation of sub-pleural blebs and spontaneous pneumothorax in AIDS. Necrotising pneumonia may be responsible for pneumatocele formation in sub-pleural space. The surgical resection of sub-pleural blebs in association with parietal pleurectomy either thoracoscopic technique or open thoracotomy allows re-expansion of lung parenchyma. Associated infection should be actively managed with appropriate antibiotics.

Cystic fibrosis: The spontaneous pneumothorax secondary to cystic fibrosis reflects severe underlying parenchymal damage. Improvement in understanding of the disease, aggressive physiotherapy, postural drainage and timely management of secondary infections has reduced the risk of severity parenchymal damage. However, poor compliance with the regular prescribed management and self-neglect is associated with the end-stage respiratory failure. Lung transplantation in selected cases may be the only curative option in some cases. If the case has been selected for transplantation, it may be best managed conservatively and avoid using sclerosants for pleurodesis until transplantation. Management of secondary infection is vital in association with physiotherapy. In some localised cases, bullectomy and pleurectomy may result in success and reduce the risk of recurrence.

Malignancy: Secondary metastases especially from soft tissue sarcoma or osteogenic sarcoma or primary lung tumours have caused spontaneous pneumothorax. Management of these conditions by way of resection can diagnose the underlying pathology leading to investigations of occult primary. Survival depends on the pathology of the underlying tumour. Occasionally spontaneous pneumothorax is seen in patients with graft versus host disease in bone marrow transplants. Nonoperative management with chest tube drainage and appropriate management of infection and rejection have been associated with good success.

Pediatric and neonatal cases: Primary spontaneous pneumothorax normally encountered in thin, tall teenage boys. Rarely Marfan's syndrome and rib exostosis can also predispose pneumothorax in children. Spontaneously occurring pneumothorax in younger children should raise the possibility of a congenital pulmonary airway malformation (Fig. 35.4). A CT scan of the chest should be done in such instances [7].

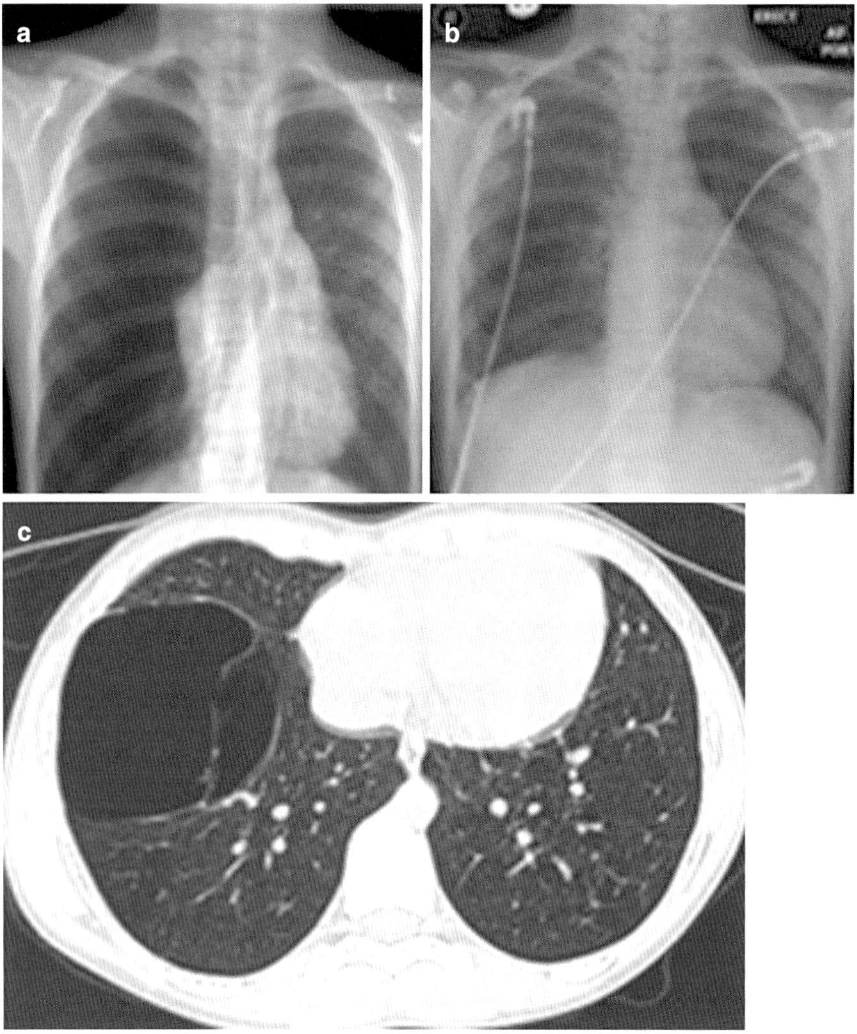

Fig. 35.4 (**a**) Chest X-ray showing a spontaneous pneumothorax in a 6-year-old child (**b**) managed initially with an intercostal chest drain. (**c**) CT scan showing a localised cystic lesion, which was resected thoracoscopically to confirm on histology as cystic adenomatoid malformation

In children primary spontaneous pneumothorax managed with chest tube alone has high chance of recurrence (up to 30%), while thoracoscopic bullectomy and pleurectomy has a reported recurrence rate of less than 5%.

Premature infants with surfactant deficiency and hypoplastic lungs (both primary and secondary lung hypoplasia) requiring prolonged mechanical ventilatory support are associated with pneumothorax. These are diagnosed on simple chest X-ray and managed with an insertion of intercostal chest drain by Seldinger technique. Recurrent pneumothoraces associated with prematurity are a challenge in neonatal intensive

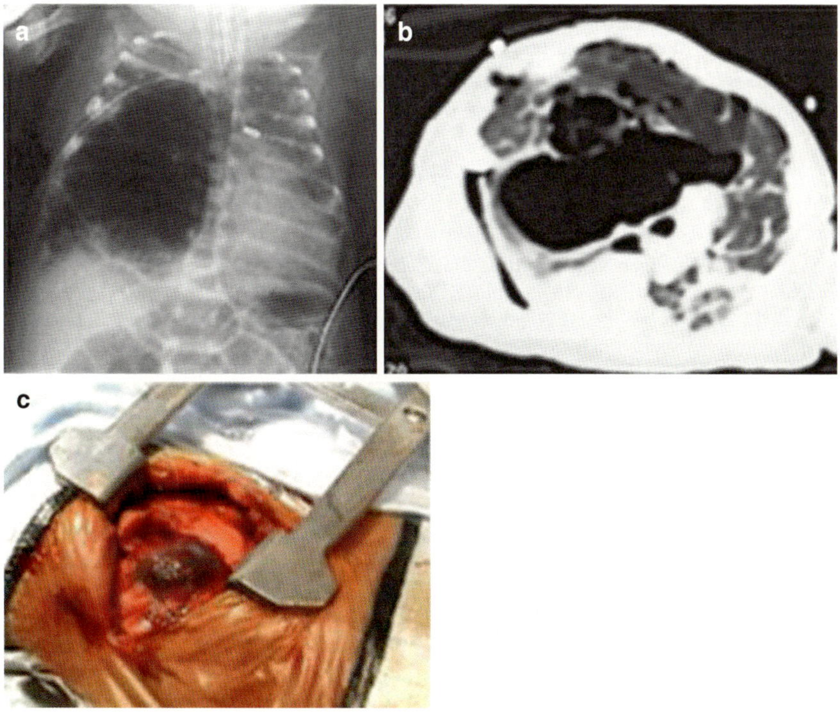

Fig. 35.5 (**a**) Chest X-ray showing emphysematous lesion responsible for recurrent unilateral pneumothoraxes in a premature infant, (**b**) CT scan confirming localised PIE, (**c**) operative picture of interstitial emphysema before resection

care management. Multiple conservative strategies are employed in order to improve lung expansion and tissue oxygenation. Managing infant on the side, high-frequency ventilation, management of consolidation, single-lung ventilation if possible and other manoeuvres are some of the options available depending on individual case scenarios. In spite of employing conservative strategies occasionally, recurrences and air leaks are significant and continuous and may require investigations such as CT scans. Pulmonary interstitial emphysema (PIE), a result of high-pressure ventilation, can be a cause of continuous air leaks and recurrent pneumothoraxes in premature infants. Localised PIE is amenable to surgery (Fig. 35.5) and improves the outcome, oxygenation after its resection. Generalised and bilateral PIE is not amenable to surgical intervention and is difficult to manage and can result in mortality if effective oxygenation cannot be achieved. Blood pleurodesis and povidone-iodine pleurodesis are used to contain air leaks in difficult cases.

Conclusion

Pneumothorax is uncommon in young children before adolescence and should be investigated for underlying case similar to older patients with associated parenchymal disease with CT chest. One recent study involving two Pediatric centres suggested primary surgery and investigation to include CT scans prior to surgery. Primary spontaneous pneumothorax managed with the guidelines of thoracoscopy and resection of bullae and parietal pleurectomy is associated with good outcome and low recurrence rate.

References

1. Melton LJ III, Hepper NG, Offord KP. Incidence of spontaneous pneumothorax in Olmsted County, Minnesota: 1950 to 1974. Am Rev Respir Dis. 1979;120:1379–82.
2. Bense L, Eklund G, Wiman LG. Smoking and the increased risk of contracting. Spontaneous pneumothorax. Chest. 1987;92:1009–12.
3. Gobbell WG, Rhea WG, Nelson IA, Daniel RA. Spontaneous pneumothorax. J Thorac Cardiovasc Surg. 1963;46:331.
4. Gupta D, Hansell A, Nichols T, et al. Epidemiology of pneumothorax in England. Thorax. 2000;55:666–71.
5. Davies HE, Davies RJ, Davies CW, BTS Pleural Disease Guideline Group. Management of pleural infection in adults: British Thoracic Society pleural disease guideline 2010. Thorax. 2010;65(Suppl 2):ii41–53.
6. Baldt MM, Bankier AA, Germann PS, et al. Complications after emergency tube thoracostomy: assessment with CT. Radiology. 1995;195:539–43.
7. Soccorso G, Anbarasan R, Singh M, Lindley RM, Marven SS, Parikh DH. Management of large primary spontaneous pneumothorax in children: radiological guidance, surgical intervention and proposed guideline. Pediatr Surg Int. 2015;31(12):1139–44.

Hyperhidrosis

36

Peter B. Licht

Abstract

Primary hyperhidrosis is a frequent disorder of unknown aetiology that most often affects the palm of the hands, the axillae, or the face to such an extent that it becomes a professional, psychological, and social burden to many patients. Non-surgical management by dermatologists is the first line of treatment, but if medical treatment fails, sympathectomy surgery is effective and offers the only permanent treatment option. Surgery basically blocks transmission of nerve impulse to the eccrine sweat glands by transecting, ablating, resecting, or clipping the sympathetic chain, and technically these are not difficult for the experienced VATS surgeon. The difficult part, and the most important key to success in sympathectomy surgery, is the critical and meticulous patient selection that includes thorough information about frequent side effects. Compensatory sweating is the most common, but gustatory sweating and bradycardia are also quite frequent. In some patients side effects are severe enough to regret surgery, which is considered irreversible by most. At present, application of a metal clip on the sympathetic chain is promising because of potential reversibility in theory, but the question of true reversibility remains controversial. Ideal patients, who are treated by sympathectomy, are among the most satisfied patients that thoracic surgeons will ever meet.

Keywords

Hyperhidrosis · Blushing · Surgery · Sympathectomy · Sympathicotomy Sympathetic Trunk · Side Effects · Compensatory Sweating · Anaesthesia Complications

P.B. Licht, M.D., Ph.D.
Department of Cardiothoracic Surgery, Odense University Hospital, Odense, Denmark
e-mail: peter.licht@rsyd.dk

D. Parikh, P.B. Rajesh (eds.), *Tips and Tricks in Thoracic Surgery*,
https://doi.org/10.1007/978-1-4471-7355-7_36

36.4 Anaesthesiological Considerations

Single-lumen intubated anaesthesia with brief periods of apnoea is considered adequate by most surgeons. To decrease the risk of parenchymal damage, the anaesthesiologist should disconnect the endotracheal tube from the ventilator during apnoea during introduction of the trocar(s). Less experienced surgeons may prefer single-lung ventilation by double-lumen intubation, but insufflation of CO_2 improves and is not necessary even though exposure is superior. Double-lumen intubation is particularly useful after previous thoracic surgery because apical adhesions, which are typically seen at reoperations, need careful dissection without damage to the stellate ganglion. Double-lumen intubation is also helpful in morbid obese patients where a high diaphragm can jeopardize adequate exposure during simple apnoea.

Most patients achieve sufficient pain relief after local infiltration analgesia combined with oral NSAIDs and paracetamol in the postoperative period, and all uncomplicated surgeries can be discharged on the same day of surgery. An epidural catheter for pain relief is obsolete, but intrapleural analgesia at end of the procedure, just prior to inflation of the lung, may significantly reduce pain postoperatively [8].

36.5 Surgical Technique

Over the last 30 years, hundreds of retrospective single-institution follow-up series have been published, and there is no clear consensus regarding which surgical technique is better. More than 30 different surgical approaches have been described that differ mainly in the use of resection, ablation, transection, or clipping at various levels of the sympathetic chain.

For many years resection of a segment of the sympathetic chain was preferred because it allowed histological proof, but it was never possible to prove that the correct segment or level(s) had been resected. Most surgeons now prefer simple transection, which is correctly named sympathicotomy, because it is easier and faster. Most surgeons consider outcome to be equivalent, but resection achieves a slightly better long-term result [9]. Some use cautery; others prefer ultrasonic energy devices, particularly when the sympathetic chain is targeted at the level of the second rib where it is feared that heat from cautery may dissipate and cause thermal injury to the stellate ganglion resulting in Horner's syndrome. Over the last decade, application of titanium clips that block nerve impulse transmission has become popular because of the theoretical possibility of a reversal operation if the patient develops intolerable side effects. The question of true reversibility, however, remains controversial as experimental studies found severe signs of nerve damage that were still present 6 weeks after the clip had been removed [10]. Recent data with longer observation periods demonstrated these signs of damage decreased suggesting that, in theory, application of metal clips may be a reversible procedure. It is not known whether such histological reversibility at cellular level translates into physiological reversibility, and there are only few reports on clinical outcomes following the reverse operation, but they are optimistic [11–15]. Clearly, all sympathetic surgeons should switch to the clipping method if the procedure is truly reversible. Conversely, they should abandon clipping completely if it is not, because some patients are likely to accept sympathetic surgery under false premises if they are told that the operation is reversible.

A staged procedure where just one side is operated at a time is still practiced by few, but the vast majority of surgeons safely perform the procedure bilaterally during the same anaesthesia. This is easily achieved with the patient in supine position, and slightly anti-Trendelenburg allows gravity to improve visualization of the apex when the lung collapses. Both arms are abducted to expose the axillae. Most surgeons use two ports but uniportal access is possible, and more than two ports are not necessary in uncomplicated cases. The first incision is typically made anteriorly in or above the axillary hairline because of better cosmetic results, but lower access can be used. The anaesthesiologist briefly disconnects the endotracheal tube to deflate the lung before the pleural cavity is entered to avoid damage to the lung parenchyma. A 5-mm (or even smaller depending on the diameter of the thoracoscope) blunt-tip trocar is introduced for the use of a 0° or 30° video-assisted thoracoscope, and an additional 5-mm incision is placed posteriorly in the hairline for the introduction of an ultrasonic instrument or a second trocar for cautery and/or a metal clip applier. The sympathetic chain is identified where it crosses the costal heads (Fig. 36.1). If a metal clip is applied, the parietal pleura is opened parallel to the desired level of the sympathetic chain by cautery (a hook is easier because it allows simultaneous traction and cautery). The sympathetic chain is freed completely on the backside before the metal clip is applied to ensure that the entire circumference is blocked. Others prefer to resect the sympathetic chain with ganglion(s) by cautery, ultrasound, or simple scissors, but the vast majority of surgeons just transect (sympathicotomy) where the sympathetic chain crosses the rib(s), which makes a fine solid background for transection, which can be difficult with soft intercostal tissue as a background. This also allows for better reporting of which level(s) the sympathetic chain was targeted as rib-oriented nomenclature is recommended by

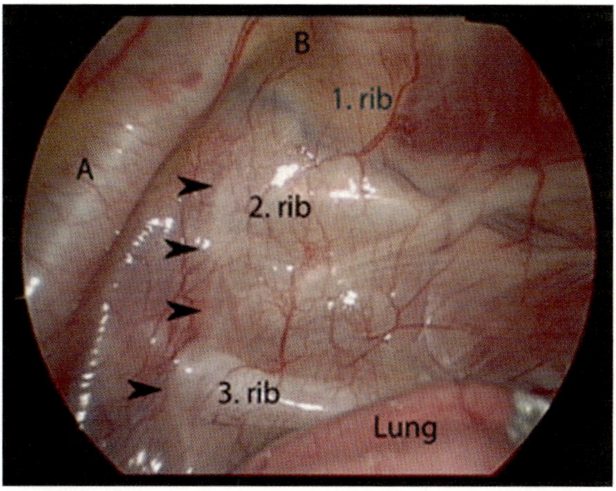

Fig. 36.1 Anatomical landmarks of the apex for sympathetic surgery (left side). A: subclavian artery, B: the fat pad that covers the stellate ganglion. Arrows: the sympathetic chain.

the Society of Thoracic Surgeons expert consensus for the surgical treatment of hyperhidrosis [16]. The pleural incision is typically extended laterally for approximately 2 cm on the second and third costa to include any accessory nerve fibres (the nerve of Kuntz). The procedure is performed bilaterally during the same anaesthesia, and recent data suggest fewer haemodynamic effects if surgery is started on the right side [17]. On either side, at the end of the procedure, the lung is reinflated under direct vision until it is fully expanded and reaches the parietal pleura. While the anaesthesiologist ventilates the patient manually, exerting continuous positive pressure for a few seconds to prevent pneumothorax, a small 4-mm chest tube may be left in the trocar to evacuate small air pockets before it is removed, but usually the trocar itself is sufficient as drainage when the surgeon's thumb is used as a one-way valve that is closed during expiration. The 5-mm surgical wounds can be sutured, but adhesive strips are usually sufficient for skin closure.

36.6 Level of Targeting the Sympathetic Chain

From hundreds of clinical reports on this topic, it is clear that for a long time there was no consensus regarding which level(s) of the sympathetic chain should be targeted for palmar, axillary, or facial hyperhidrosis, but the number of randomized clinical trials is slowly increasing. At present the most widely accepted recommendations by the "Society of Thoracic Surgeons expert consensus for the surgical treatment of hyperhidrosis" [16] recommend that the sympathetic chain should be targeted at the level of the third and/or fourth rib (R3 and/or R4) for isolated palmar hyperhidrosis. For combinations of palmar and axillary hyperhidrosis, they recommend targeting R4 and R5. For craniofacial hyperhidrosis, R3 is recommended although many still believe that R2 must be included in the patients and in those who are treated for facial blushing.

36.7 Tips and Tricks to Avoid and Deal with Intraoperative Anticipated and Unanticipated Complications

Bleeding is rarely seen in sympathetic surgery, but major catastrophic bleeding has happened following injury to the subclavian artery and intercostal vessels or even direct cardiac laceration. Most cases are handled by acute thoracotomy, but fatal outcome has occurred, and surgeons who do sympathetic surgery should be able to handle these complications. For the less experienced surgeon, particular care should be given during introduction of the cautery hook or the ultrasonic scalpel directly through the second 5-mm axillary skin incision where the direction and depth of the instrument tip is given careful attention because it can easily reach the mediastinum – particularly in small patients and/or when exposure is suboptimal if the lung does not deflate readily.

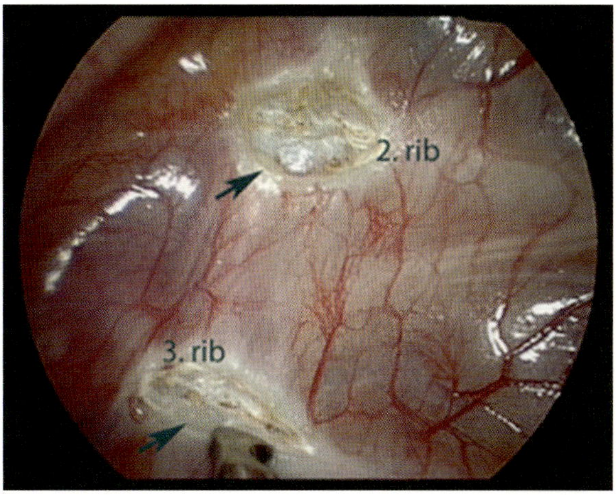

Fig. 36.2 Rib-oriented transection of the sympathetic chain (sympathicotomy) is the most frequent procedure. The ends (arrows) are typically pushed apart to ensure complete division of all sympathetic fibres.

Recurrences generally occur in a 5–8% of patients in the literature, but in facial blushing, mild recurrence has been reported in up to 30% after simple transection of the sympathetic chain [6]. Late recurrences are more common after simple transection [9]. Recurrences should be distinguished from primary "nonresponders" who never experienced any effect of surgery. If immediate lack of effect following sympathetic surgery is unilateral, it should be dealt with as a primary technical failure, which is more likely when the sympathetic chain is just transected or if a metal clip has been applied. In these case the patients should undergo a unilateral reoperation [18]. To avoid primary failure, it is important to see that the entire trunk is transected (Fig. 36.2) or included in the metal clip by careful observation. Sometimes pushing the cut ends in either direction reveals that some fibres remain intact.

36.8 Alternative Methods of Hyperhidrosis Management

Dermatologists should evaluate all patients who seek surgical assistance for disabling primary hyperhidrosis. Non-surgical treatment options are plenty and many patients satisfied although none provide any permanent relief. Non-surgical methods have been reviewed extensively [19] and consist of topical agents (antiperspirants that contain aluminium salts), repeated iontophoresis, or botulinum toxin injections and systemic medical therapy (anticholinergic agents).

As mentioned above, patients whose main complaint is axillary hyperhidrosis may be better off with local surgical treatment such as subcutaneous curettage or skin excision rather than sympathetic surgery because of significantly better local effect and fewer side effects.

36.9 Variations and Complex Presentations

Young and otherwise healthy patients rarely present with pleural adherences, but parenchymal tearing during introduction of the first 5-mm trocar does occur. It is readily identified during subsequent introduction of the camera and should not discourage from further thoracoscopic surgery. Re-intubation with a double-lumen tube may be necessary for severe cases allowing for single-lung ventilation, and with the addition of a third 5-mm port, even dense adherences can usually be cleared for full exposure of the apex.

Exposure of the sympathetic chain may be obscured by anatomical variations such as azygos lobe [20]. If so, the azygos lobe is retracted inferiorly and the pleural curtain that separated this lobe from the upper lobe is dissected for exposure of the sympathetic chain. It should not be necessary to divide the azygos vein. All dissection is facilitated if the patient is re-intubated with a double-lumen tube.

Large intercostal venous contributories to the azygos vein can sometimes cross or parallel the sympathetic chain, and if simple transection (sympathicotomy) is used, the vein is easily divided together with the sympathetic chain by ultrasonic energy at low amplitude without bleeding. If venous bleeding occurs, then 5 min of compression with the working instrument or an endoscopic sponge stick is usually enough to ensure complete haemostasis.

Subpleural fat may cover the entire sympathetic chain, so this is not readily visible even though the pleural space and the apex are free. In these situations the first rib is identified laterally as the uppermost rib where there is no intercostal musculature above but only the yellow fat pad, which covers the stellate ganglion. The direction of the subclavian artery may also be helpful as it passes over the first rib. The second and third ribs are identified below, and with the working instrument, the sympathetic chain can usually be palpated as a separate very slightly mobile structure over the medial part of the osseous rib. The parietal pleura may need to be opened to visualize the chain before it is divided because the longus colli muscle lies just medial and can be mistaken for the sympathetic chain by simple palpation.

References

1. Strutton DR, Kowalski JW, Glaser DA, Stang PE. US prevalence of hyperhidrosis and impact on individuals with axillary hyperhidrosis: results from a national survey. J Am Acad Dermatol. 2004;51(2):241–8.
2. Cina CS, Clase CM. The illness intrusiveness rating scale: a measure of severity in individuals with hyperhidrosis. Qual Life Res. 1999;8(8):693–8.
3. Vallieres E. Endoscopic upper thoracic sympathectomy. Neurosurg Clin N Am. 2001;12(2):321–7.
4. Smidfelt K, Drott C. Late results of endoscopic thoracic sympathectomy for hyperhidrosis and facial blushing. Br J Surg. 2011;98(12):1719–24.
5. Heidemann E, Licht PB. A comparative study of thoracoscopic sympathicotomy versus local surgical treatment for axillary hyperhidrosis. Ann Thorac Surg. 2013;95(1):264–8.
6. Licht PB, Pilegaard HK, Ladegaard L. Sympathicotomy for isolated facial blushing: a randomized clinical trial. Ann Thorac Surg. 2012;94(2):401–5.

7. Rex LO, Drott C, Claes G, Gothberg G, Dalman P. The boras experience of endoscopic thoracic sympathicotomy for palmar, axillary, facial hyperhidrosis and facial blushing. Eur J Surg Suppl. 1998;580:23–6.
8. Assalia A, Kopelman D, Markovits R, Hashmonai M. Intrapleural analgesia following thoracoscopic sympathectomy for palmar hyperhidrosis: a prospective, randomized trial. Surg Endosc. 2003;17(6):921–2.
9. Assalia A, Bahouth H, Ilivitzki A, Assi Z, Hashmonai M, Krausz MM. Thoracoscopic sympathectomy for primary palmar hyperhidrosis: resection versus transection -- a prospective trial. World J Surg. 2007;31(10):1976–9. discussion 80-1
10. Loscertales J, Congregado M, Jimenez-Merchan R, Gallardo G, Trivino A, Moreno S, et al. Sympathetic chain clipping for hyperhidrosis is not a reversible procedure. Surg Endosc. 2012;26(5):1258–63.
11. Chou SH, Kao EL, Lin CC, Chang YT, Huang MF. The importance of classification in sympathetic surgery and a proposed mechanism for compensatory hyperhidrosis: experience with 464 cases. Surg Endosc. 2006;20(11):1749–53.
12. Kang CW, Choi SY, Moon SW, Cho DG, Kwon JB, Sim SB, et al. Short-term and intermediate-term results after unclipping: what happened to primary hyperhidrosis and truncal reflex sweating after unclipping in patients who underwent endoscopic thoracic sympathetic clamping? Surg Laparosc Endosc Percutan Tech. 2008;18(5):469–73.
13. Lin CC, Mo LR, Lee LS, Ng SM, Hwang MH. Thoracoscopic T2-sympathetic block by clipping--a better and reversible operation for treatment of hyperhidrosis palmaris: experience with 326 cases. Eur J Surg Suppl. 1998;580:13–6.
14. Sugimura H, Spratt EH, Compeau CG, Kattail D, Shargall Y. Thoracoscopic sympathetic clipping for hyperhidrosis: long-term results and reversibility. J Thorac Cardiovasc Surg. 2009;137(6):1370–6. discussion 6–7
15. Whitson BA, Andrade RS, Dahlberg PS, Maddaus MA. Evolution of clipping for thoracoscopic sympathectomy in symptomatic hyperhidrosis. Surg Laparosc Endosc Percutan Tech. 2007;17(4):287–90.
16. Cerfolio RJ, De Campos JR, Bryant AS, Connery CP, Miller DL, DeCamp MM, et al. The Society of Thoracic Surgeons expert consensus for the surgical treatment of hyperhidrosis. Ann Thorac Surg. 2011;91(5):1642–8.
17. Kharbanda M, Prasad A, Malik A. Right or left first during bilateral thoracoscopy? Surg Endosc. 2013;27(8):2868–76.
18. Licht PB, Clausen A, Ladegaard L. Resympathicotomy. Ann Thorac Surg. 2010;89(4):1087–90.
19. Walling HW, Swick BL. Treatment options for hyperhidrosis. Am J Clin Dermatol. 2011;12(5):285–95.
20. Kauffman P, Wolosker N, de Campos JR, Yazbek G, Jatene FB. Azygos lobe: a difficulty in video-assisted thoracic sympathectomy. Ann Thorac Surg. 2010;89(6):e57–9.

Chylothorax

37

Dakshesh Parikh

Abstract

Congenital, idiopathic, pathological and iatrogenic chylothorax is encountered across all age groups. The aetiology and pathogenesis of the congenital chylothorax is unknown. Some congenital malformations and pathologies are known to be associated with chylothorax. Congenital diaphragmatic hernia after its correction can present with chylothorax as persisting and challenging problem. Thoracic chylous lymphatics can be accidentally injured during surgery or can leak after a blockage from an obstructing tumour or venous thrombosis of superior vena cava. Specific investigations to identify its causative aetiology are indicated in adult chylothorax. In infants and children, imaging is carried out after initial supportive measures have failed to resolve chylothorax. Respiratory compromise as a result of pleural collection of chyle may require drainage and ventilatory support. Chyle production can be reduced by withholding enteral nutrition and providing total parenteral nutrition. Surgical approach is considered in prolonged and intractable cases. Outcome can be variable depending on its aetiology, associated genetic and congenital malformations.

Keywords

Chylothorax · Thoracic duct · Congenital chylothorax · Iatrogenic chylothorax · Superior vena cava thrombosis · Congenital diaphragmatic hernia · Congenital lymphatic malformations · Antenatal pleural effusions

D. Parikh, MBBS, MS, FRCS (Ped.), MD
Department of Pediatric Surgery, Birmingham Women's and Children's Hospital NHS FT, Birmingham, UK
e-mail: dakshesh.parikh@nhs.net

D. Parikh, P.B. Rajesh (eds.), *Tips and Tricks in Thoracic Surgery*,
https://doi.org/10.1007/978-1-4471-7355-7_37

37.1 Introduction

Chylothorax is collection of chyle within the pleural cavity. Chyle is a milky lymphatic fluid containing chylomicrons composed of small fat globules and protein and lymphocytes. The intestinal chyle containing long-chain essential fatty acid and lower limb lymphatics drains into cisterna chyli situated on the second lumber vertebra and is then carried through thorax by mostly a single thoracic duct. Iatrogenic accidental thoracic duct injury may occur in cardiac, spinal and oesophageal surgery. Chylothorax is not uncommon after mediastinal tumour resection. Radiological investigations and sometimes tissue diagnosis are required to identify the pathological cause in spontaneous chylothorax. The pathogenesis and aetiology of the congenital chylothorax remains unclear while its management mostly conservative [1]. The management of congenital chylothorax can be challenging, as it is associated with prematurity, lung hypoplasia and pulmonary hypertension [1]. In addition, associated genetic and congenital malformation complicates multisystem management. The knowledge of the anatomical relationships of thoracic duct is essential for the surgeons wanting to ligate the duct for the management of chylothorax.

37.2 Typical Thoracic Duct Anatomy [2]

Thoracic duct originates from cisterna chyli at around 2nd lumber vertebral body in midline adjacent to the abdominal aorta. It then enters the thoracic cavity through the aortic crus of diaphragm between the aorta and vena azygous on the right. Typically the thoracic duct can be found on the right thoracic cavity lying on the vertebral bodies between the azygous vein laterally, aorta medially and behind the oesophagus. It then crosses the midline at the level of 4th thoracic vertebra. Thoracic duct then ascends towards the neck where it comes out from behind the internal jugular vein and drains into the left subclavian vein at its junction with left internal jugular vein. Thoracic duct carries lymph from the lower half of the body, left chest and the lymphatic system of the left arm and left side of head and neck. The right side of thoracic cavity along with right arm and head and neck drains either independently or by a right-sided thoracic duct into the right brachiocephalic vein. It is important to note that the anatomy of thoracic duct is variable and typical anatomical description of thoracic duct is seen in 65% of populations [3]. Between 9 and 12 different anatomical variations are described in literature [3, 4].

37.3 Technical Tips and Tricks

37.3.1 Establish the Diagnosis

The presence of milky fluid in a pleural aspirate raises the suspicion, and confirmation can be ascertained by its biochemistry and presence of chylomicrons in enterally fed patients. In antenatally diagnosed hydrothorax, a pleural aspirate sent for

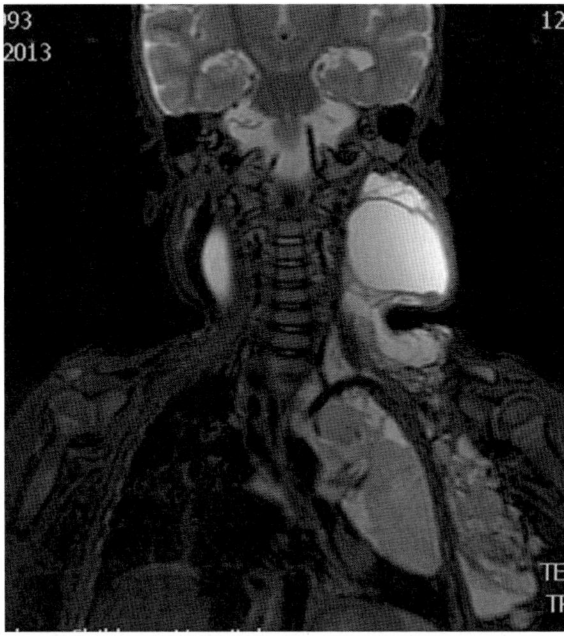

Fig. 37.1 MRI scan showing an extensive lymphatic malformation in the left axilla and neck and extending into mediastinum. He required tracheostomy as it caused significant respiratory compromise and required resection of neck cystic lymphatic malformation as injection of sclerosant caused significant respiratory distress.

biochemical analysis showing triglyceride content more than 1.2 mmol/L, protein levels greater than 2.5 g/dL, lactic-dehydrogenase above 110 IU/L and cell count predominantly of lymphocytes greater than 1000 cells/ml confirms the diagnosis of congenital chylothorax.

The radiological imaging is required to investigate its aetiology. Chest x-ray can only delineate the presence of pleural effusion and sometimes widened mediastinum, and indicates the presence of a pathological cause. In acquired spontaneous cases, in the absence of mediastinal or neck pathology and in resistant congenital cases, specific investigations are performed to identify and rule out any pathological cause before labelling as idiopathic chylothorax. Magnetic resonance imaging (MRI) is the investigation of choice for any soft tissue hamartomatous malformations (cystic hygroma, lymphangioma and lymphovenous malformation) (Fig. 37.1), lymph nodal disease (infective or malignant) and superior vena cava obstruction (primary or secondary). The lymphangiography with radionucleotide can demonstrate area of leak, lymphatic malformation. Lymphography is indicated in persistent leak that may require surgical intervention. Tissue diagnosis may become imperative in suspected malignant conditions.

37.3.2 Medical Management

- Prenatal intervention: Persistent hydrothorax detected antenatally may require either serial foetal thoracocentasis or pleuro-amniotic shunt. This prenatal intervention improves the pulmonary hypoplasia and pulmonary hypertension.

- Postnatal management: Initial diagnosis in newborn, which is not fed enterally is based on the biochemical analysis and cell content of pleural aspirate. Once the neonates are fed, the pleural fluid will contain chylomicrons and pleural fluid typically becomes milky. It is important to note that almost all congenital chylothorax cases are resolved with conservative measures. The associated mortality recorded in many series is generally related to associated congenital, genetic and cardiac defects, while some has been attributed to sepsis [5].
- Most antenatally diagnosed and postnatal early chylothoraxes generally have a degree of respiratory compromise, and many of them additionally have persistent pulmonary hypertension (PPH) that will require careful management along with the management of chylothorax. Most require insertion of intercostal tube drainage and ventilator support [5]. Supporting their nutrition initially with total parenteral nutrition and withholding the enteral nutrition have been found to be useful [5, 6]. Once there is stoppage of chyle production usually within 3–6 weeks, enteral nutrition with medium chain triglycerides can be commenced and continued up to approximately 3 months. Other supportive measures include administration of albumin, immunoglobulin, prophylactic antibiotics and fresh frozen plasma/blood products [5]. Some infants may benefit from administration of intravenous octreotide/somatostatin [5, 6]. Published regimens for administration of octreotide are variable, but the general agreement is to start with small dose and gradually increase the dose as necessary [7, 8].
- Monitoring: It is essential to monitor these infants regularly for blood counts, liver functions, serum albumin and immunoglobulins. They are prone to overwhelming sepsis, and therefore in addition to prophylactic antibiotics, regular blood inflammatory marker trends are helpful to detect sepsis in blood culture and intervene with appropriate antibiotics before fulminant sepsis.
- Most cases are successfully managed medically with supportive measures in congenital chylothorax and cases following the repair of congenital diaphragmatic hernia repair.

37.3.3 Operative Interventions

Pleuroperitoneal shunt: Some authors have claimed good success with diversion of chyle into peritoneal cavity in as high as 75% of cases along with dietary restriction of long-chain fatty acids on MCT diet [9]. This is a useful management option in intractable cases and can be palliative for incurable malignant conditions. In infants loss of chyle can cause overwhelming sepsis, and therefore its diversion into peritoneal cavity may be considered a viable option. Tube is passed both in pleural and peritoneal cavities with a pumping chamber containing one-way valve in the middle located on the thoracic wall in the subcutaneous space. The pumping chamber is pressed so as to divert the chyle into the abdominal cavity [10].

Ligation of thoracic duct: Continued significant drainage resistant to medical management despite total parenteral nutrition and bowel rest for a reasonable period would be an indication for thoracic duct ligation. Ligation of the duct should be undertaken as it emerges from diaphragm into the chest for it to be effective [6, 11, 12]. The reported success following thoracic duct ligation is equivocal which may be related to patient selection and the duct ligation performed as a last resort in sicker patients. Patients with poor outcome following surgery could have anatomical variations and anomalies of thoracic duct.

Thoracic duct ligation can be performed thoracoscopically by identifying the duct between azygous vein and aorta on the right side. This can be aided by giving the child or infant or adult a full fat milk or double cream approximately 6–8 h prior to surgery to make the duct more identifiable. The effectiveness of surgical thoracic duct ligation in management of congenital chylothorax is uncertain. Thoracoscopic duct ligation near its entrance through the right diaphragm is very effective in containing excessive chyle leakage after head neck surgery when it is difficult to identify and ligate the leak point in the neck.

Pleurodesis: We do not recommend this approach in infants and children. However many have attempted pleurodesis in the management of chylothorax with variable success. Various chemical agents have been used. The difficulty and disadvantage is that it is a blind procedure. Therefore continued chyle leakage results in loculated and medial collections that inevitably become inaccessible to percutaneous drainage. Recently some authors have used dilute Betadine for pleurodesis in persistent chylothorax through the intercostal tube.

Thoracic duct embolization: This minimally invasive interventional radiological technique has been recently employed successfully in adults to manage chylothorax. The technique involves lymphographic identification of cisterna chyli and percutaneous catheterization and embolization of thoracic duct [13, 14]. This technically demanding technique has also showed success in young infants [15].

37.4 Chylothorax Post Congenital Diaphragmatic Hernia (CDH) Repair

The occurrence of chylothorax is well recognized following repair of CDH in approximately 10–15% of cases. The postoperative chylothorax significantly increases the morbidity associated with CDH and inevitably increases the dependence of ventilation, need for oxygen, length of stay and the risk of infection [16]. The pathogenesis of its occurrence in CDH is unclear. It is believed to be associated with PPH as other cases in premature infants and cardiac surgical cases are also associated with PPH. The management of chylothorax in patients with CDH responds generally to conservative management, providing the infant with adequate respiratory support, draining the chylous pleural effusion and keeping the infant nil orally supported with parenteral nutrition. Some studies and our experience in intractable cases suggest a period of octreotide administration is useful in addition to other supportive and conservative measures.

Fig. 37.2 Thoracoscopic view of thoracic cavity containing chyle prior to resection of lymphatic mediastinal malformation.

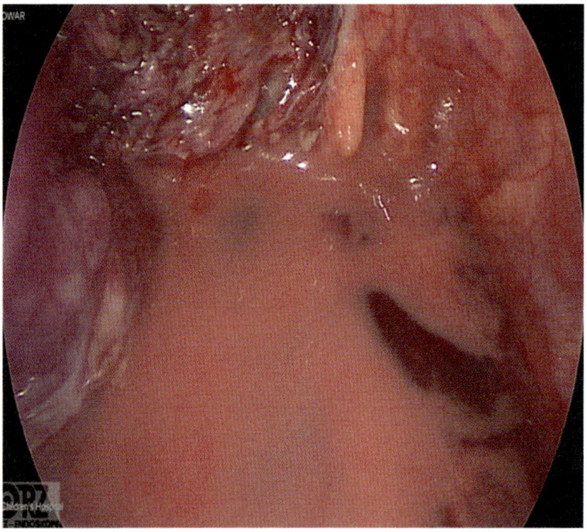

37.5 Chylothorax in Congenital Lymphatic Malformation and Mediastinal Cysts

Congenital lymphatic malformation with its anomalous and ectatic lymph channels results in leakage of lymphatic fluid and chyle into pleural or peritoneal cavity. The extensive cystic hygroma extending in the mediastinum obstructs the chyle drainage and may result in preoperative chylothorax even before surgery (Fig. 37.2). The leakage of chyle can happen after a resection surgery. The surgical accidental injury could be a result of the thoracic duct involvement in the lymphatic malformation or associated thoracic duct anomalies. Lymphangiectasia of the lung is a morbid condition and is not amenable to surgery. Chylothorax management in these cases has better chance of success with conservative approach. Surgery with thoracic duct ligation at its origin may be of value in selected cases.

Conclusions

Chylothorax can pause a management challenge. Most cases will require investigations for the diagnosis of its causative pathology. The management strategy can be tailored accordingly, both in adults and children. Conservative measures are mostly effective in infants and young children. The continuous loss of chyle results in loss of immunoglobulins and lymphocytes that may predispose infants and children to an overwhelming sepsis. Urgency to contain the chyle loss is indicated in cases that are intractable to conservative measures. Future in the management of refractory chylothorax lies in the advances in minimally invasive radiological embolization of thoracic duct techniques.

References

1. Guitierrez JCL, Tovar JA. Chylothorax and chylous ascites. Management and pitfalls. Semin Pediatr Surg. 2014;23(5):298–302. https://doi.org/10.1053/j.sempedsurg.2014.09.011
2. Parikh DH. Applied anatomy. In: Parikh D, DCG C, Auldist AW, Rothenberg SS, editors. Pediatric thoracic surgery. London: Spinger; 2009. p. 3–17.
3. Davies MK. A statistical study of the thoracic duct in man. Am J Anat. 1915;171:212.
4. Anson BJ. An atlas of anatomy. Philadelphia: WB Saunders; 1950. p. 336–7.
5. Bialkowski A, Poets CF, Franz AR. Congenital chylothorax: a prospective nationwide epidemiological study in Germany. Arch Dis Child Fetal Neonatal Ed. 2015;100(2):F169–72.
6. Lasko D, Langer JC. Chylothorax. In: Parikh D, DCG C, Auldist AW, Rothenberg SS, editors. Pediatric thoracic surgery. London: Springer; 2009. p. 573–88.
7. Das A, Shah PS. Octreotide for the treatment of chylothorax in neonates. Cochrane Database Syst Rev. 2007;9:CD006388.
8. Helin RD, Angeles ST, Bhat R. Octreotide therapy for chylothorax in infants and children. A brief review. Pediatr Crit Care Med. 2006;7:576–9.
9. Wolff AB, Silen ML, Kokodka ER, Rodgers BM. Treatment of refractory chylothorax with externalized pleuroperitoneal shunts in children. Ann Thorac Surg. 1999;68:1053–7.
10. Azizkhan RG, Canfield J, Alford BA, Rodgers BM. Pleuroperitoneal shunts in the management of neonatal chylothorax. J Pediatr Surg. 1989;18:842–50.
11. Lie CS, Tsai HL, Chin TW, Wei CF. Surgical treatment of chylothorax caused by cardiothoracic surgery in children. J Chin Med Assoc. 2005;68:234–6.
12. Milsom JW, Kron IL, Rheuban KS, Rodgers BM. Chylothorax: an assessment of current surgical management. J Thorac Cardiovasc Surg. 1985;89:221–7.
13. Itkin M, Kucharczuk JC, Kwak A, et al. Nonoperative thoracic duct embolization of traumatic thoracic duct leak: experience in 109 patients. J Thorac Cardiovasc Surg. 2010;139:584–9.
14. Nadolski GJ, Itkin M. Thoracic duct embolization for nontraumatic chlous effusion: experience in 34 patients. Chest. 2013;143:158–63.
15. Itkin M, Krishnamurthy G, Naim MY, et al. Percutaneous thoracic duct embolization as a treatment for intrathoracic chyle leaks in infants. Pediatrics. 2011;128:e237–41.
16. Mills J, Safavi A, Skarsgard ED. Chylothorax after congenital diaphragmatic hernia repair: a population-based study. J Pediatr Surg. 2012;47:842–6.

Index

D. Parikh, P.B. Rajesh (eds.), *Tips and Tricks in Thoracic Surgery*,
https://doi.org/10.1007/978-1-4471-7355-7

B

R